The Jossey-Bass Health Series brings together the most current information and ideas in health care from the leaders in the field. Titles from the Jossey-Bass Health Series include these essential health care resources:

Regulating Managed Care

Regulating Managed Care

Theory, Practice, and Future Options

Stuart H. Altman

Uwe E. Reinhardt

David Shactman

Editors

Foreword by Steven A. Schroeder

Developed under the auspices of the
Council on the Economic Impact
of Health System Change

A program supported by the
Robert Wood Johnson Foundation

Jossey-Bass Publishers • San Francisco

Jossey-Bass books and products are available through most bookstores. To contact Jossey-Bass directly, call (888) 378–2537, fax to (800) 605–2665, or visit our website at www.josseybass.com.

Substantial discounts on bulk quantities of Jossey-Bass books are available to corporations, professional associations, and other organizations. For details and discount information, contact the special sales department at Jossey-Bass.

 Manufactured in the United States of America on Lyons Falls Turin Book. This paper is acid-free and 100 percent totally chlorine-free.

Library of Congress Cataloging-in-Publication Data

Regulating managed care: theory, practice, and future options/
   Stuart H. Altman, Uwe E. Reinhardt, David Shactman, editors.
      p.   cm.
   Includes bibliographical references and index.
   ISBN 0-7879-4783-0 (alk. paper)
   1. Managed care plans (Medical care)—Law and legislation—United
States.   2. Insurance, Health—Law and legislation—United States.
3. Health care reform—United States.   I. Altman, Stuart H.
II. Reinhardt, Uwe E.   III. Shactman, David.
KF1183.R44   1999
344.73'032104258—dc21   99-24496
                                                                              CIP

FIRST EDITION
HB Printing   10 9 8 7 6 5 4 3 2 1

Contents

Foreword

In our pluralistic society, the trends in social policy often swing like a pendulum. They overcome inertia and gain momentum in one direction only to swing back the other way, ultimately settling somewhere near the gravitational center. In issues such as personal health, which touches the lives of all of us, interest in that center is likely to be strong. In 1994, the country rejected a large government role in health care and began to pursue a market-based system. But five years later, after sampling the benefits and detriments of market-based medicine, the pendulum has begun to swing the other way. Legislation to regulate managed care has proliferated at both the state and federal levels of government and is at the top of the congressional agenda as we advance through the last year of the millennium. Policymakers, clinicians, and consumers are struggling to find the right balance between competition and regulation that will result in a high-quality and compassionate health care system, accessible and affordable to all Americans. This volume, with contributions by many of the nation's leading experts in health care policy, provides a comprehensive examination of the issues from a broad range of political perspectives.

In the late 1980s and early 1990s, annual increases in health care inflation were in the double digits, and employers and consumers found health insurance increasingly unaffordable. In response, the Clinton administration attempted to legislate comprehensive health care reform. But the country rejected the government's large role in that plan, and instead pursued market-oriented reforms based on a system of competitive managed care.

Enrollment in managed care organizations grew rapidly during the 1980s, and many analysts have expounded on the potential virtues of managed care: to make the delivery of health care services more rational, to integrate service delivery, to reduce overtreatment and clinical variation, and to focus on disease prevention. In addition, managed care has achieved its primary objective of cost control, at least in the short run.

But some of the ways in which managed care achieves cost control, regardless of whether they are rational or beneficial, have drawn opposition from patients and providers. For example, managed care attempts to align the incentives of the physician and insurer by providing financial rewards for cost-efficient treatment (or penalties for high utilization). From one perspective, this results in a more rational use of resources and eliminates the tendency to overtreat that existed in fee-for-service medicine. From another perspective, however, it provides a perverse incentive to undertreat, and it could eventually undermine the quality of health care. Physicians and patients are concerned that the injection of money and profit into clinical decision making could destroy the sanctity and trust of the doctor-patient relationship.

Managed care also effects savings by channeling patients to physicians who are part of their system, who follow their clinical guidelines and protocols, and who work for discounted fees. However, patients resent having a limited choice of providers, and doctors resent the loss of autonomy, not to mention the discounting of their fees.

As a result of these kinds of conflicting trade-offs, managed care has been able to increase market penetration at the same time that dissatisfaction from patients and providers has continued to surface. This "managed care backlash" was prominently covered in the news media, which publicized both thoughtful concerns and alarming anecdotes. The degree of vilification of the managed care industry in such a short time period has been breathtaking. In a recent poll, only the tobacco industry was held in lower esteem. Thus, the pendulum began to swing back toward regulation, and both the industry and the government began to respond.

The industry's response can be seen partly in the proliferation of point-of-service plans and other options that grant patients a greater degree of choice. In addition, some important industry players have accepted many of the goals—as well as the apparent inevitability—of regulation and have put forth their own recommendations for a regulatory framework.

The response of government is evident in the number of regulatory measures proposed and enacted at the state and the federal levels. For example, the federal government has passed legislation guaranteeing a forty-eight-hour minimum hospital stay for normal births, banning "drive-through" mastectomies, and prohibiting so-called gag clauses in HMO contracts. A striking number of the proposed managed care regulatory initiatives focus on issues of women's health: in addition to delivery and mastectomy, coverage for in vitro fertilization, contraception, and screening for breast cancer, cervical cancer, and osteoporosis are frequently addressed in both federal and state legislatures. A wide variety of other consumer protection remedies also have been proposed, including mandatory benefits, access to emergency services, access to specialists, rights of grievance and appeal, legal liability of health plans, disclosure of financial incentives, and provision of information on quality of services.

In the future, if we expect managed care to control costs, it will have to do so by reducing utilization. This will inevitably lead to further conflict with patients and providers and to continued pressure to enact regulations. Regulating markets, however, is no easy task, and individuals—even those with similar objectives—differ on the major questions to be resolved. What is the proper role of governmental regulation in a market-oriented health care system? Who should regulate (for example, the states, the federal government, or a quasi-public authority)? What is the proper role of the courts, particularly in regard to issues involving liability? What existing models can we identify that might guide us in designing an effective regulatory structure?

In March 1998, the Robert Wood Johnson Foundation underwrote a conference to address these questions. The fifth Princeton conference, entitled The Role of Regulation in a Market-Oriented Health Care System, was conducted by the Council on the Economic Impact of Health System Change. With many leading national health policy experts in attendance, the conference participants presented original papers and discussed a variety of potential options for regulatory reform. The contributions for this volume came out of that conference.

Whether or not the 106th Congress and the fifty state legislatures enact regulatory legislation, the issues discussed in this collection are not ones that will soon go away. The miracles of modern medicine are producing technologies and treatments far beyond what we might have imagined a few decades ago. As our population ages, the cost of health care will consume an increasing proportion of our resources. It will become more and more difficult to ensure that either the market or the government provides our nation's citizens with affordable access to the life-enhancing drugs and technologies of medicine. That being the case, the issues discussed in this volume will be with us well into the next millennium.

April 1999

STEVEN A. SCHROEDER
President
Robert Wood Johnson Foundation
Princeton, New Jersey

Acknowledgments

The time and effort of many individuals made this publication possible. First and foremost, we were most fortunate to collaborate with such an extraordinary group of authors, who represent a wide range of expertise on the topic of this book and a broad diversity in politics and point of view. Their efforts were supported by many other individuals who brought this collection to fruition.

Particular thanks are due to the Robert Wood Johnson Foundation, not only for their generous funding but also for their active and substantive participation in planning the Princeton Conference, where many of these papers were presented. The foundation has supported the ongoing series of five Princeton Conferences, and this is the third book produced from that series. Steven Schroeder, M.D., the President of the Robert Wood Johnson Foundation, has taken a personal role in the planning of the conference series, and the final product has benefited from his wisdom and advice. Project officers who assisted in this effort include Nancy Barrand, David Colby, and Rush Russel. Robert Hughes, Paul Jellinek, James Knickman, and Lew Sandy also contributed to the planning process.

The Council on the Economic Impact of Health System Change conducts the series of Princeton Conferences. The Council is housed at the Institute for Health Policy in the Heller Graduate School at Brandeis University. Brian Rosman of the Council staff contributed substantially to this effort. Cindy Parks Thomas and David Keepnews also provided assistance. Administrative support was provided by Mary Flynn and Ann Cummings, who have successfully coordinated three of the conferences in this series.

The Woodrow Wilson School at Princeton University has generously hosted this series of conferences. Our thanks are extended to Dean Michael Rothschild, who has supported our efforts each year. Particular thanks are also due to Ruth Miller and Patricia Trinity, who have been instrumental in the meeting and conference planning as well as being the most gracious of hosts.

Our appreciation is also extended to the team at Jossey-Bass Publishers, who worked diligently to produce a high-quality product in a limited period of time. Andy Pasternack envisioned this collection even before we decided to publish it, and his ideas and enthusiasm played a major role in shaping and assembling the final product.

April 1999　　　　　　　　　　　　Stuart H. Altman
　　　　　　　　　　　　　　　　　Uwe E. Reinhardt
　　　　　　　　　　　　　　　　　David Shactman

The Editors

Stuart H. Altman, Ph.D., is Sol C. Chaikin Professor of National Health Policy, the Institute for Health Policy, Heller Graduate School, Brandeis University, Waltham, Massachusetts.

Uwe E. Reinhardt, Ph.D., is James Madison Professor of Political Economy, Woodrow Wilson School of Public and International Affairs, Princeton University, Princeton, New Jersey.

David Shactman, M.P.A., M.B.A., is senior research associate, the Institute for Health Policy, Heller Graduate School, Brandeis University, Waltham, Massachusetts.

The Contributors

Drew E. Altman, Ph.D., is president of the Henry J. Kaiser Family Foundation, Menlo Park, California.

John M. Benson, M.A., is deputy director of the Harvard Opinion Research Program, Harvard School of Public Health, Department of Health Policy and Management, Boston, Massachusetts.

William F. Benson is principal, The Benson Group, Washington, D.C.

Marc L. Berger, M.D., is executive director, Outcomes Research, Merck & Company, Inc., West Point, Pennsylvania.

Brian Biles, M.D., M.P.H., is senior vice president, the Commonwealth Fund, New York, New York.

Robert J. Blendon, Ph.D., is professor of health policy and political analysis, Harvard School of Public Health, Boston, Massachusetts.

Mollyann Brodie, Ph.D., is senior researcher, Henry J. Kaiser Family Foundation, Menlo Park, California.

Patricia A. Butler, Ph.D., is an independent health care analyst based in Boulder, Colorado.

Craig Copeland, Ph.D., is research assistant, Employee Benefit Research Institute, Washington, D.C.

Karen Davis, Ph.D., is president of the Commonwealth Fund, New York, New York.

Allen Dobson, Ph.D., is senior vice president, The Lewin Group, Fairfax, Virginia.

Alain C. Enthoven, Ph.D., is Marriner S. Eccles Professor of Public and Private Management, Stanford University, Graduate School of Business, Stanford, California.

Larry S. Gage, J.D., is president, National Association of Public Hospitals, Washington, D.C.

Bill Gradison is president, Health Insurance Association of America, Washington, D.C.

Tina Hoff is director of media relations and senior communications program officer, Henry J. Kaiser Family Foundation, Menlo Park, California.

Larry Hugick is director of media and political surveys, Princeton Survey Research Associates, Princeton, New Jersey.

Karen Ignagni, M.B.A., is president and CEO, American Association of Health Plans, Washington, D.C.

David M. Keepnews, R.N., M.P.H, J.D., is a senior researcher on the staff of the Institute for Health Policy, Heller Graduate School, Brandeis University, Waltham, Massachusetts.

Larry Levitt is director of California grants, Henry J. Kaiser Family Foundation, Menlo Park, California.

Phil Nudelman, Ph.D., is chairman and president, Kaiser-Group Health, Seattle, Washington.

Mark Pauly, Ph.D., is professor of health care systems, The Wharton School, University of Pennsylvania, Philadelphia.

William L. Pierron, J.D., is public affairs associate, Employee Benefit Research Institute, Washington, D.C.

Ronald F. Pollack, J.D, is executive director, Families USA Foundation, Washington, D.C.

Thomas Rice, Ph.D., is professor and chair, School of Public Health, University of California, Los Angeles, California.

William L. Roper, Ph.D., is dean, School of Public Health, University of North Carolina, Chapel Hill, North Carolina.

Brian Rosman, J.D., is research associate, the Institute for Health Policy, Heller Graduate School, Brandeis University, Waltham, Massachusetts.

David Sandman is program director of the Commonwealth Fund, New York, New York.

Steven A. Schroeder, M.D., is president, the Robert Wood Johnson Foundation, Princeton, New Jersey.

Sara J. Singer, M.B.A., is executive director, Center for Health Policy, Stanford University, Stanford, California.

Caroline Steinberg, M.B.A., is senior manager, The Lewin Group, Fairfax, Virginia.

Walter Zelman, Ph.D., is president and CEO, California Association of Health Plans, Sacramento, California.

Introduction: The Philosophy of Regulation

Stuart H. Altman and Brian Rosman

Policy analysts have reacted in a wide variety of ways to the sharp growth of managed health care and whether and in what form the actions of managed care organizations should be regulated by government. The chapters in this book demonstrate the wide spectrum of informed opinion. The diversity of responses, we believe, reflects more than differences over factual material or variations in interpretation. Rather, we postulate that fundamentally different premises are at the heart of many of the policy differences evident in their views.

Philosophical Foundations of Regulatory Policy

Policy analysts viewing issues like increased regulation of managed care often start from opposite points of view. Some start from the position that markets are ill-suited to the task of providing health care services. These analysts view health care as a public good to be provided to all citizens, as a matter of right, like education or our transportation infrastructure. They are particularly suspicious of managed care because it can be seen as altering financial incentives for providers toward providing less care. They also maintain that the private, for-profit delivery system siphons profits away from the health care system, potentially raising the costs of health care for society. Also, because consumers are not able to evaluate medical judgments, quality can suffer as market competition encourages providers to compete on the basis of cost by cutting corners.

These opponents of unregulated market forces thus start out with the position that the government should play the predominant role in organizing and regulating the health care system. To them, the burden of proof is on those who want to divest social control of health care from government or tightly controlled not-for-profit organizations and give it to the private sector. The key question from this point of view is, To what extent should the government allow market forces to play a role in structuring and operating health care?

One complicating factor for the interventionist view is determining which level of government—federal, state, or some other entity—should play the major role in regulating managed care. The federal Employee Retirement Income Security Act of 1974 (ERISA) constrains states from imposing regulations on health plans offered by employers who self-insure. (See Chapters Nine and Ten for more detailed discussion of ERISA and its impact on state regulation of employer-provided health care plans.) These plans encompass about 40 percent of individuals covered by employer-provided health insurance. Thus, to achieve maximal effect, federal regulation of all health insurance coverage is required. This is consistent with the general view of political liberals, who typically favor increased government intervention at the federal level. However, many strong interventionist policies have been enacted in recent years by state governments, whereas Congress has until now rejected comprehensive managed care reform. Thus, those supporting a strong government role oppose provisions in federal law that act to preempt stronger state laws. They prefer the federal government setting a common floor, with states permitted to establish more stringent regulations if they choose. Advocates of state regulation also point to the more potent ability of states to enforce their laws; the federal government's anemic response to its enforcement responsibilities under the Health Insurance Portability and Accountability Act of 1996 (HIPAA) exemplifies the difficulty with federal enforcement of traditionally state-based insurance regulations.[1]

On the other side from those who favor regulation are those who start from the premise that markets are the best way to allocate any resource, including health care. Such advocates believe that markets provide an efficient method of delivering care and are more capable of responding to patients' individual preferences for type of care. In their view, health care services generate real costs and cannot be provided in a vacuum that ignores economic considerations. As one adage puts it, "If you think health care is expensive now, you should see what it will cost when it is free!" The operating belief of those in this camp is that a market system will promote efficiency and quality as insurers vie to meet the demands of purchasers, usually employers. If employers are able to shop for the best plan for their firm, they will seek value by looking for the highest quality available at an affordable price. In time, the market will weed out providers or plans that offer poor quality care or care that does not effectively match benefits with costs.

Market-based systems also allow for the fact that individuals place different valuations and demands on the health care system; some might value the freedom to choose among any provider whereas others might value cost savings or access to alternative treatments. A free market allows customers and providers to maximize their individual preferences by seeking arrangements that best reflect their economic choices.

As can be seen, this point of view requires substantial justification for government intervention in the health care market. Still, proponents of this approach often support a limited government role in regulating health care, particularly to ensure adequate information about the different plans offered in a market. If evidence demonstrates deficiencies in a particular area, government may be required to step in to support goals such as helping consumers get fair value for purchases, preventing consumers from being harmed or assuming undue risks, improving consumer choice and education, encouraging products that promote consumer welfare, or promoting consumer autonomy and producer accountability. With regard to the federal-versus-state issue, often these advocates prefer to see any federal standards serve as a ceiling that preempts more potent state laws.

Models of Regulatory Policy

Of course, these philosophical foundations are only that: foundations for more sophisticated points of view. These starting points translate into a number of models of regulation along a continuum from least to most interventionist. We divide the models on the continuum into four basic archetypes, although the lines dividing them are not fixed and there are gray areas along the continuum. But these models, based on material originally developed by Stanley S. Wallack for analyzing long-term care regulation, do provide a framework for evaluating the policy options under discussion.[2]

Elective Model

The least interventionist point of view might be termed the elective model. In this approach, government only imposes regulations if required to correct market failures. There are several prerequisites for efficient market-based systems. For example, markets require a sufficient number of buyers and sellers to prevent domination by one party; buyers need good information on quality, price, and alternatives; and sellers and buyers must have an opportunity to enter or exit the market. If these or similar preconditions are definitively lacking, the elective approach favors modest government intervention to support the marketplace. Otherwise, the market should be allowed to function without governmental interference.

In general, proponents of the elective approach maintain that employers, who actually purchase most health insurance, have the resources to obtain sufficient information to make reasonable choices about health care insurance. The growth of employer purchasing groups indicates that even small firms can unite to get the information they find most valuable rather than depend on informational requirements that a government official might impose. By consolidating their members' bargaining power, these groups have also allowed small firms to negotiate discount prices as well as minimum quality standards. Also, private sources such as magazines (for example, *U.S. News and World Report, Consumer Reports*) regularly provide comparative quality information on health plans.[3] Consumers may seek out plans that are accredited by voluntary organizations, such as the National Committee for Quality Assurance (NCQA), a private nonprofit organization that assesses and reports on the quality of managed care plans. Consumers may also evaluate a plan's performance by checking the performance measures reported on the Health Plan Employer Data and Information Set (HEDIS), a set of standardized measures used to compare health plans that is managed by NCQA.

Proponents of the elective approach also emphasize the costs that increased regulation would impose on managed care. The growth of managed care in the late 1990s has substantially reduced the rate of growth of health care costs. The administrative costs of complying with bureaucratic dictates would invariably be reflected in premium rates. Adding to plans' costs would only exacerbate the problem for those who are uninsured because they cannot afford coverage. Thus, although the elective model accepts minimal governmental regulation of health plans, the fact that existing laws— already impose a substantial regulatory burden on managed care and the lack of substantial benefits relative to the costs of regulation—lead most of its supporters to reject any new regulation of managed care plans.

Directive Model

In the directive model, government acts as a voice for consumer interests by providing incentives for desired behavior. Rather than directly dictating what the market offers, government uses its influence as a regulator or purchaser to encourage the provision of a particular quality or type of good or service, thus lowering the cost to producers or consumers.

For managed care regulation, this may imply legislation to mandate valid comparative information on health plans. At a minimum, states or the federal government could establish standards for marketing materials and dictate the basic information that must be included (for example, formulary rules, specialist access rules, experimental treatment rules). Because most consumers are not experts on health services, they are unable to evaluate the quality of health plans. Hence, proponents of this model often support regulations requiring comparative "report cards," such as those produced in Maryland or Minnesota.[4] They may also support state "accreditation" of plans that meet minimum standards, but with no requirement that all plans be accredited. Some have proposed a state-run accreditation process; others have proposed piggybacking on industry standards such as NCQA.

Although the typical regulatory approach of this model is to provide information to consumers, some types of information mandates arguably belong in a more prescriptive model. For example, proposals requiring plans to make public how providers are paid are probably less of an attempt to get comparative information to consumers than to embarrass plans into making substantive changes in their policies. Thus, these proposals belong with a more aggressive model than the directive one.

Advocates of the directive model would also support the use of the government's purchasing power to set minimum standards for plans. In the past year, HCFA has imposed extensive standards on Medicare managed care plans. A recent report found that the experience of private purchasers who use quality data to evaluate and seek improvements in health plans could be of assistance to HCFA in its new obligations to monitor plan quality assurance programs.[5] States are also imposing a variety of standards in their Medicaid contracts with managed care organizations. These requirements are imposed not just to improve the quality of coverage to persons enrolled in the government plan but also to improve the quality of care offered to all purchasers, as plans may find it easier to use the same standards for all members.

Restrictive Model

The restrictive model is based on the supposition that, in particular situations, markets are incapable of producing a product that meets public goals. To remedy this, government steps in to dictate what may be offered on the market. This action is often taken to prevent a "race to the bottom," where firms compete on the basis of price leading to a decline in quality—the ValuJet syndrome. This approach is taken when policymakers believe that the social cost of a free market is greater than the social benefits of increased choice.

In regard to managed care regulation, advocates of this model support the bulk of proposals made by consumer groups, the Clinton administration, and congressional activists—such as bans on certain financial arrangements between plans and providers, requirements for managed care plans to use the "prudent layperson" standard for covering emergency room care, or regulations requiring plans to allow patients with chronic illness to have direct access to specialists. Also included in this category are various "mandated benefits" that states have imposed on plans, such as requiring infertility treatment or mandating minimum inpatient maternity stays. These policies are intended to set minimum requirements that plans may not undercut.

Supporters of this approach believe that under a free market system, managed care plans might not offer these benefits because of an asymmetry of interests between the insurer and the insured that results in *adverse selection*. Insurers benefit financially from enrolling relatively healthy members. The majority of their costs are due to a small percentage of ill patients. In the health insurance market, adverse selection refers to the tendency of people who know they are ill to gravitate to the plan with the best benefits for that illness. Hence, plans can profit by restricting benefits for expensive conditions and trying to attract the healthiest individuals. Consequently, supporters of regulation maintain that if plans were not required to offer a benefit, such as access to chronic disease specialists, no plan would do so, because they would not want to attract patients with chronic illnesses to their plan. This justifies government's intrusion into the market to require all plans to offer these and other legislated benefits.

Prescriptive Model

This most interventionist approach replaces consumer preferences with those of the government. In the health care field, this is often justified because of the possible disjunction between the interests of the health insurance purchaser (typically, an employer) and the ultimate consumer (the employee and the employee's family). In this model, government does more than set standards. It actively dictates on an ongoing basis the requirements for participation in the market.

Minnesota's prohibition on for-profit health maintenance organizations exemplifies this approach.[6] The policy represents a stark intrusion into the marketplace, based on a judgment that for-profit HMOs would per se be detrimental to the residents of that state. A less extreme policy is binding external reviews of managed care plan decisions. This allows consumers to appeal to a governmental body if they are dissatisfied with their health plan's decision on a treatment or service. The agency will hear both sides and, if it believes proper, issue an order directing the plan to provide the disputed treatment. Binding external review statutes allow government to dictate in an ongoing fashion what a private health plan should cover. For example, many health plans exclude experimental treatments. Binding external review statutes allow an official decision to move a particular treatment from the experimental category to the expected practices category. Because of both cost and adverse selection, absent this appeal provision, plans would have an incentive to treat expensive treatments as experimental for longer than might be dictated by medical practice alone. Proponents of this model may also support legislation to insure greater consumer choice in the market. Examples are requirements that employers offer more than one choice of plan or that plans include a point-of-service option that allows patients to see a provider outside the plan's network. Such policies would reflect the most activist government role in requiring that certain options always be made available to insureds.

Analyzing the Chapters in This Volume

Although more fluid and suggestive than fixed and deterministic, this typology will allow readers to analyze systematically many of the chapters in this book. Some of the chapters are descriptive and do not take a clear stand on the various policy options, but others can be evaluated using this framework.

We would place the views expressed by Ignagni and Gradison in their chapters into the *elective* category. For the most part, these representatives of the managed care industry oppose strong government intrusion into their operations and point out the benefits of self-regulation and market forces. Ignagni, president of the American Association of Health Plans, argues in Chapter Thirteen against further government mandates by pointing out the extensive regulation already imposed on health insurers as well as the voluntary code of conduct adopted by her organization's members. The code of conduct encompasses many of the demands being placed on managed care by the Clinton administration and congressional activists, although there is no external enforcement mechanism. Ignagni endorses a public-private partnership, with government's role augmented or partly superseded by voluntary standards accountable to consumers. In rejecting intensified regulation of managed care, she supports the elective model's focus on efficiency and consumer choice.

In Chapter Fifteen, Gradison, former president of the Health Insurance Association of America, emphasizes the strong role consumer demand plays in shaping the offerings of health plans. For example, the rapid growth of point-of-service coverage, which allows the policyholder to go outside the HMO network for an additional fee, demonstrates the managed care market's responsiveness to consumers. The flexible market-based system, Gradison argues, allows for coverage that accommodates consumer desires while still considering costs.

The directive approach is taken by Pauly and Berger, Reinhardt, Roper, and Nudelman. These authors, though fundamentally supporting a market approach, see a need for a modest degree of intervention to protect managed care consumers. Pauly and Berger's chapter (Chapter Three) starts from the premise that private markets are the best mechanism for delivering health care, if they can be made to function well. They identify a lack of sufficient information to justify government subsidization of valid comparative data. They also support some sort of minimum quality mandate, but only for workers who are offered a single plan by their employer.

In Chapter Five, Reinhardt, a Princeton economist, focuses on the need for adequate information and a choice of plans to allow consumers to make valid comparisons in the marketplace. Our system presupposes that consumers are able to make informed choices about which health plan will best suit their needs. Yet the lack of reliable comparative information about insurers' performance makes this an impossible task for most of them. Reinhardt calls for the government to finance the development of standardized performance measurement tools. The resulting data, he states, should be made available at government-sponsored "farmers markets" where all health plans in a market must provide complete, audited information on the cost and quality of their products.

Roper, dean of the School of Public Health at the University of North Carolina at Chapel Hill, focuses in Chapter Eight on regulating clinical quality of medical practice rather than on the consumer protection issues raised by most managed care reform advocates. He advocates a balance of government and private sector initiatives to encourage the establishment of clinical quality standards and to maintain systems for clinical quality improvement. He emphasizes that regulatory mechanisms must be flexible to allow for innovative new strategies. Nudelman (Chapter Seventeen) too emphasizes flexibility in regulatory strategies. The rapid growth of managed care systems has caused anxiety among consumers. Yet because of trade-offs implicit in various regulatory goals and methods, there is a need to vary the regulatory approach to different issues.

The more aggressive restrictive philosophy is illustrated by the contributions of Zelman, Rice, Davis and Sandman, and Singer and Enthoven. In Chapter One, Zelman recognizes that market forces alone are not sufficient in health insurance and that some combination of market forces and regulation is necessary. This applies particularly to managed care, which creates financial incentives to limit services. Zelman looks toward market-based regulation— such as controls on the conversion of nonprofit organizations to for-profit status and increased antitrust scrutiny of provider combinations—as well as ensuring consumer choice.

In Chapter Four, Rice, professor at the UCLA School of Public Health, explains that the preconditions necessary for markets to optimize social welfare do not exist in health care. Rice concludes that substantial *micro*regulation—regulation of specific services, rather than controls on prices or expenditures—is required to counteract the incentive to undertreat inherent in capitated provider arrangements.

Davis and Sandman, president and program officer, respectively, of the Commonwealth Fund, begin Chapter Twelve by presenting evidence of consumer and physician dissatisfaction with managed care. They endorse the Consumer Bill of Rights and Responsibilities formulated by the President's Advisory Commission on Consumer Protection and Quality in the Health Care Industry in March 1997. They warn, however, that regulatory reform must not ignore the impact rising costs will have on the number of uninsured.

In Chapter Eighteen, Singer and Enthoven reflect the views of other authors in this group when they start with the observation that "complete reliance on the free market for the distribution of health care is not appropriate." Although Enthoven is generally recognized for his support of market competition among health plans, the recommendations of the California Managed Health Care Improvement Task Force were quite restrictive. They include allowing women direct access to reproductive health care providers and disclosing provider compensation methods, with a prohibition on those deemed most risky to consumers. They warn against micro-management of medical care and reforms that benefit providers more than consumers.

Finally, Pollack's analysis in Chapter Fourteen represents the prescriptive point of view. Pollack, executive director of the health care consumer organization Families USA, supports strong federal regulation of managed care plans, including binding external appeals. He emphasizes the need to repeal ERISA's limitation on lawsuits against health plans for wrongful denial of care. Pollack also provides a counterpoint to Ignagni's chapter on the issue of the cost of increased regulation, by pointing out areas where proposed regulations would reduce costs.

Descriptive Chapters

The other chapters in this book describe the key issues and concerns surrounding managed care regulatory policy. In Chapter Two, Butler describes the existing federal and state regulatory framework governing managed care plans and enumerates proposals of recent years to regulate managed care further. Her chapter identifies trends in state regulation and summarizes proposals pending before Congress that call for intensified federal regulation of managed care.

Two chapters deal with issues of access to care. Biles and Sandman write about access concerns of members in HMOs, whereas Gage discusses the needs of those not in HMOs, that is, the uninsured. In Chapter Seven, Biles and Sandman, of the Commonwealth Fund, maintain that patients in managed care plans report greater difficulty with access than those in fee-for-service plans. They describe the various legislative proposals to address access problems and also comment on managed care's voluntary initiatives to improve access for members.

In Chapter Six, Benson describes an important component of most regulatory proposals: the ombudsman. Drawing on his experience evaluating ombudsman programs serving nursing home residents, Benson delineates the features of a successful program for managed care consumers.

Gage argues in Chapter Sixteen that the debate over managed care regulation ignores the more fundamental problem of the growing number of uninsured. Absent national universal coverage, Gage advocates strengthening safety net programs for the uninsured, such as Medicare and Medicaid's Disproportionate Share Hospital (DSH) programs for high-volume providers of care to the uninsured.

One of the greatest controversies in the managed care reform debate has been over how much cost the various regulatory provisions would add to health insurance. In Chapter Nineteen, Dobson and Steinberg of The Lewin Group, which produced one of the most widely cited estimates, analyze the substantial differences between the various cost projections. For example, the estimates produced by the consulting firm Milliman & Robertson and the accounting firm Coopers & Lybrand of the proposed federal Patient Access to Responsible Care Act (PARCA) varied by a factor of thirty. Dobson and Steinberg note that differences in key assumptions about how a particular legislative provision would be implemented significantly affected the cost estimates, as did the degree to which indirect effects were considered.

Two chapters consider aspects of the managed care debate related to the ERISA statute. Copeland and Pierron (Chapter Ten) explain ERISA's preemption of state laws governing group health plans. Keepnews (Chapter Nine) examines proposals to hold managed care plans legally liable for harm caused to patients. He analyzes the complex legal issues involved, and he describes both state and federal legislation to evade or amend ERISA's restrictions.

Notes

1. U.S. General Accounting Office. *Private Health Insurance: HCFA Cautious in Enforcing Federal HIPAA Standards in States Lacking Conforming Laws.* GAO/HEHS publication no. 98–217R. Washington, D.C.: Author, 1998.

2. Wallack, S., Cohen, M., Nanda Kumar, A., and Rodwin, M. *Consumer Protection and Long-Term Care Insurance: A Framework for Analysis and Policy Options.* Waltham, Mass.: LifePlans, 1991.

3. See, for example, *U.S. News and World Report*'s rankings on the Internet at www.usnews.com/usnews/nycu/health/hetophmo.htm.
4. Maryland's HMO report, produced by its Health Care Access & Cost Commission, can be viewed on the Internet at www.hcacc. state.md.us/hmo/98hmo/index.htm.
5. U.S. General Accounting Office. *Health Care Quality: Implications of Purchasers' Experiences for HCFA.* GAO/HEHS publication no. 98–69. Washington, D.C.: Author, 1998.
6. See Minnesota statutes, Chapter 62D, section 2(4)(a) (1997).

Regulating Managed Care

The Role of Regulation in a Market-Oriented Health Care System

The four chapters in the first section of this collection provide a broad perspective of the role of regulation in managed care health markets. In his overview, Walter Zelman urges a balance between a regulatory approach to protect individuals and one to encourage market efficiency. Zelman begins by explaining that the very nature of insurance has made it a heavily regulated industry, and the characteristics of managed care insurance, in particular, obviate the need for market intervention. Zelman classifies regulatory measures into five categories that differ from those of Altman and Rosman but clearly cover the range from elective to prescriptive. He examines the advantages and disadvantages of each category, and places them in the context of current industry trends. Zelman points out that many of the more direct or prescriptive regulations provide a quality floor for the few, whereas many of those regulations that are less intrusive and intended to improve market function are aimed at raising the quality ceiling for the many. Although the proregulation and promarket forces are often in political opposition, they ultimately share many similar goals. A balanced regulatory approach, he reasons, can offer both consumer protection and improved health care quality.

Whereas Zelman provides a theoretical overview, the purpose of Patricia Butler's chapter is to provide a practical landscape of the scope of state and federal regulatory legislation both existing and proposed. Butler begins by tracing the legal sources from which government derives its regulatory authority and the goals and objectives that state and federal authorities seek in promulgating regulatory legislation. She then provides a detailed survey of state regulatory initiatives and discusses recent trends. Moving to the federal arena, she covers similar ground, providing details on legislation that failed to pass in the 105th Congress. Butler concludes with a summary of the challenges lawmakers will confront in future attempts to enact regulatory measures.

Mark Pauly and Marc Berger provide economists' perspectives on why managed care should be regulated. While reassuring us of their preference for free markets, Pauly and Berger give "a resounding yes" to the question of whether health care markets need some regulation. They highlight the need for information in economically efficient markets and explain why markets by themselves may not provide sufficient amounts. Pauly and Berger recommend a governmental role in subsidizing the provision of such information, but they are opposed to governments providing it themselves or mandating specific rules for others to do so. They also claim that some product quality regulation is needed, because of the harmful effects of existing public policy. The chief public policy culprit they identify is the tax subsidy for employment-based health insurance. Pauly and Berger argue that the tax subsidy distorts consumer incentives, causing some individuals to settle for what they don't prefer and others to be trapped into choices they no longer want. They advocate that the current tax subsidy for employment-based insurance be replaced by a tax credit of predetermined value, available to all insurance buyers, regardless of the purchase method or the nature of the purchasing group. In the absence of such reform, they identify the need for some product quality regulation, particularly to protect those consumers with limited choice.

In contrast to Pauly and Berger, who single out the harmful effects of existing public policy as a major reason for regulation, Thomas Rice argues that the very nature of managed care brings about the need for prescriptive regulation by both the private and public sectors. Rice begins by asserting that economic theory cannot inform us about regulating health markets because the assumptions that economists require for efficient markets are not present in the health care industry. After listing fifteen such assumptions, he concludes that one must look to the individual case to see if markets, government regulation, or some mix of the two are most likely to maximize social welfare. Rice divides regulation into two categories, macro and micro—with macro being the most indirect, micro the most prescriptive. He contends that regulations such as global budgets are macro, or less prescriptive, because they set a target but allow a great deal of autonomy for firms attempting to reach the target. In contrast, capitation and competition necessitate microregulation. Insurance plans, for example, employ utilization review and other prescriptive techniques to control the quantity of services provided or they capitate providers to control prices. Providers, in turn, shouldering the risk of capitation, have a strong incentive to underprovide services, requiring prescriptive regulation by government to protect consumers. As long as health care is organized along the current managed care model, Rice asserts, both the private and public sectors will engage in expensive and intrusive regulation.

Chapter One

Regulating Managed Care: An Overview

Walter Zelman

Government regulation in insurance markets has always been considered necessary. The regulatory strategies available, some of which are as political as they are regulatory, reflect differing views of the role of government and the marketplace in protecting consumers. All of these strategies have their value as well as significant limitations and liabilities, and the search for regulatory solutions is complicated by continuing uncertainty and rapid change in the health care marketplace. A comprehensive consumer protection strategy will probably need to employ elements of several strategies, especially if it aims both to protect individuals from wrongdoing and to raise the quality of care delivered to all.

The Nature of Health Insurance: Circumstances Likely to Generate Intervention

Government-inspired consumer protection efforts are most likely to emerge when one or more of several conditions exist:[1]

- *Consumers have particular difficulty in assessing the value of products or services.* Value may be especially difficult to assess, even with the assistance of intermediaries, because a marketplace is undergoing rapid change and many products are new, or for a host of other reasons. (Economists might say that such circumstances lead to the inability to perceive or calculate hidden costs.)

- *The costs of a bad decision are very high.* This may happen either because the product is expensive or because the damage resulting from product failure or inadequate service may be considerable or even irreparable.
- *The product is such that the consumer is locked in or unable to switch easily to another brand.*
- *The marketplace lacks competition.* Thus the consumer may have limited choice, and some sellers or manufacturers may not care if the consumer is dissatisfied.

Based on such conditions it quickly becomes clear why health insurance probably will always be among the more heavily regulated industries.

A Sensitive and Risky Proposition

Insurance investments, in general, are almost always a source of critical concern to the public because insurance is a costly product and what is being insured is almost always highly valued. Indeed, the first consumer rule of insurance is, "Do not buy insurance for what you can afford to replace." (Although it could be said that preventive services in health care may pose an interesting exception to this rule.) Thus, insurance is almost always associated with things that are highly valued and perhaps not easily replaced.

The investment is even more sensitive and risky for consumers because they will spend sizable amounts to insure themselves against events that may not occur for years, if ever. The combination of the potential need for a very large payoff and a date in a possibly distant future renders the arrangement uneasy and uncertain. Concerns that the insurer may not be able to deliver at some distant future date generate a need for some entity (with government being the obvious choice) to guarantee that the insurer will, in fact, perform and pay as promised.

Prepayment and Conflict

Additional tension between consumer and insurer may flow from the prepayment mechanism inherent in all insurance. With prepaid premiums, insureds who need services or payouts may be more likely to demand as much service or payment as possible. In contrast, insurers will generally not want to pay out any more than may be necessary or appropriate—and in some cases perhaps less than that. Insurer-consumer conflict, then, may often be almost inevitable, and one result of this can be more government intervention.

A Lock-In Product

Insurance consumers may have many choices and be considered "sovereign" at the time of purchase, but once the accident, fire, theft, or illness has occurred, there is only one place they can turn for payment. In the case of health care, of course, the consumer's loss of sovereignty may be further compromised. Rules about preexisting conditions and other such requirements may make it particularly difficult or even impossible to switch insurers. And employer purchasing strategies may limit or eliminate the right to choose, let alone the right to switch. Today, close to half of those individuals with employer-provided insurance have *no* choice of insurer.[2] Indeed, the presence of employer-as-purchaser suggests another category of circumstances in which government regulation may be more likely: where the consumer end-user is not the purchaser, and as a result, the seller may be more interested in meeting the needs of someone other than the consumer.

Marketplace Imperatives of Risk

Risk-based pricing is common in the insurance marketplace. Some consumers, because of their place of residence, age, health status, or other factors, may find insurance costs prohibitive. Society may find this acceptable when considering high automobile insurance rates for accident-prone drivers or high homeowner insurance rates for those who choose to build houses in desert canyons piled high with dry brush. But what about the homeowners who learn ten years after their purchase that their houses sit on a fault? And what about the individual who does everything to maintain good health and still gets cancer? The moral imperatives here almost certainly compel some form of government-imposed equity. That the government, as society's agent, might feel compelled to step in and assume costs for those who are at high risk for illness and cannot afford insurance is yet another reason to anticipate government intervention.

Many states and the federal government have now addressed some of these issues: requiring insurers to "take all comers" (guaranteed issue) or renew policies and limiting the extent to which groups might be charged more or less because of health status or experience. But while these requirements certainly have value, they also can aggravate the selection problem, generating even more incentives for insurers—who can no longer charge higher risks much higher premiums—to avoid enrolling higher-risk groups.

The Customer Doesn't Always Come First

The need to husband "company goodwill" is generally one of those things that keeps sellers and manufacturers from becoming bad actors and abusing consumers. They *want* the customer to come back. But here, too, insurance can be different. The insurer is likely to profit less, not more, from its highest users, the ones who have the most claims. Especially if they are not allowed to charge more to high-risk groups, insurers will find themselves tempted to avoid enrolling high-risk, high-cost individuals or groups. And unlike most business organizations, insurers may have less interest in seeing their highest users renew their policies, a situation that can run counter to the construct of company goodwill.

Insurance, then—and health insurance in particular—may not always subscribe to the old adage that the customer is always right. A smart department store will quickly refund the price of the shirt that didn't work out; the supermarket will do the same with the meat that didn't taste right. Airlines will usually do their best to respond to a consumer's complaint, especially in the case of a frequent flyer. Above all, these businesses want their highest users to come back.

But because the insurer's highest users may be the biggest cause of lower profits, those are the ones the insurer is most prepared to lose to a competitor. With some elements of company goodwill not having quite the strength as in other industries, the biggest users of health insurance may get less protection in the marketplace and thus be more likely to seek protection elsewhere—for example, from the government. It should be emphasized that this is true in all health insurance arrangements, not just in managed care or capitated ones.

Government as Regulator and Purchaser

Finally, in health insurance, there is the merger of government roles as purchaser and regulator. Through the Medicare and Medicaid programs (serving about seventy-five million individuals), the purchase of insurance for public employees, and other public expenditures, government spends close to half of all health care dollars. Government purchases or provides insurance for the largest and most costly block of potential new managed care customers—Medicare beneficiaries, who constitute a considerable political force. Government also has assumed responsibility for delivering at least some care to the most vulnerable segments of the population—those eligible for Medicaid and the uninsured. Whether the government views itself as purchaser, guardian, fiduciary, or regulator, its multiple roles suggest that its involvement in health insurance oversight will be unique and substantial.

These hallmarks of the insurance marketplace explain the heavy presence of government regulation in health care—starting with megaissues of solvency and working down to one-on-one complaint-handling processes.

Managed Care as a Special Case

The rise of managed care, along with some associated marketplace developments, only increases the demand for consumer protection. To be sure, some demands (such as "any willing provider" laws) of the so-called managed care backlash have been generated by provider organizations seeking to serve interest group needs by linking them to concerns of consumers. But some consumer concerns about managed care are legitimate, and many are understandable (read politically actionable). As with conflict of interest in politics, both the perception and the reality of need must be addressed.

Risk Bearing and the Rise of Fear

Although consumers may have accepted that conflict with insurers is natural, their concern that managed care payment arrangements can move their *physicians* into the insurer's "do less" camp creates a fear of underservice. Under managed care, then, and especially when physician capitation strategies are deployed, the arm's length consumer-insurance conflict is shifted to the immediacy of the physician-patient relationship.

Shifting the risk to providers—the value of which is often not fully recognized by consumers—may also result in increased concerns about quality. Just as the fee-for-service system encouraged physicians to do too much, the new system may put pressure to do too little. Sooner or later the "low hanging fruit" will be picked and the imperative to reduce utilization could impact quality. This may be particularly true for the neediest and highest-risk consumers; not surprisingly, it is the advocates for the needy who are often at the forefront of those pressing for more consumer protection in managed care relationships.

In most marketplaces there is an answer if a consumer fears poor quality: go elsewhere, and usually pay more. But in the world of managed care, choices may be more restricted. First, many employers may not be willing to pay more, so that the insurer who tries to address consumer demands by offering more services, access, or benefits at a higher price may find itself with significantly fewer customers. Moreover, as part of efforts to reduce costs, health plans will almost certainly have to impose some limits on choice of and access to physicians, but in the absence of proven quality (still hard to define in the new industry) these may remain the surest indicators of quality for many consumers. Moreover, virtually all employers limit choice of plan. Indeed, as noted earlier, close to 50 percent of individuals with employer-based insurance have no choice of plan at all. In managed care, then, unlike in most lines of insurance where the consumer can at least choose their insurers, the consumer may seldom be sovereign.

Consolidation Heightens Worries

The dramatic trend toward consolidation among plans, hospitals, and physicians and toward conversion of nonprofit to for-profit systems may compound consumer worries. Consumers in general may not—as economists are more likely to do—see consolidation as a potential threat to competition or choice. Nor are they likely to attempt to weigh the balance—as will antitrust enforcers—of greater efficiency against reduced competition. Instead, they are more likely to see consolidation as the local community hospital growing less responsive to community needs and more responsive to outside pressures. Purchase of the institution by a distant for-profit entity, whatever the marketplace rationale, can cement negative perceptions of control by outside forces.

For many consumer advocates, especially those with more vulnerable constituencies, these trends are matters of real concern. Systems that once cared for the poor now find a more competitive marketplace punishing them for delivering charitable care. Conversion of some hospitals (certainly not all) further threatens care for the uninsured. And even if studies of quality in managed care reveal that it is as good or better than the fee-for-service system that preceded it, there will always be some exceptions.[3]

Perceptions of Who Benefits

Finally, because medical bills are paid by insurers and premiums are paid by employers, consumers don't see the full costs of health insurance or the savings that are being generated by managed care. (At least individual consumers pay their own automobile insurance premium.) Thus, health care consumers are less likely to see and understand the primary benefit of managed care—lower premiums—and less likely to accept some of the restrictions imposed as a means to those lower premiums. Accurately or not, many consumers may view managed care as providing lower premiums to employers and higher profits to insurers while they as consumers lose choice and access, which in turn they associate with lower quality. In fact, consumers today are paying higher percentages of premiums.[4] Thus, they see themselves as paying more and getting less, which may seem to provide evidence of a need for government intervention.

The rapid pace of change in the health care marketplace may heighten such consumer concerns. Managed care defenders and most economists maintain correctly that consumers are benefitting from the lower costs of managed care and will certainly do so in the long run. But for the consumer, that case is far from proven. All that is certain is change, much of which (pace and substance) can be disconcerting.

To sum up, insurance of all kinds has historically been subject to regulation, and managed care will no doubt experience regulation in the near future. The questions for policymakers are why, when, and how government should intervene or not intervene.

Five Strategies for Consumer Protection

Multiple regulatory strategies are employed to enhance consumer protection. Some aim directly at protecting the individual consumer. Others seek to make an impact on markets, with consumers as a class—not necessarily as individuals—the ultimate beneficiaries. For discussion purposes, we offer five strategy types, which, admittedly, may overlap.[5]

Direct Regulation and Marketing of Products

Most consumer protection efforts directly regulate products or services by imposing requirements that businesses must meet to get and retain the right to sell them. Health plans must meet solvency requirements, have adequate provider networks, disclose certain data, subject themselves to government oversight requirements, and so forth. Such regulations can run the gamut from outright bans of certain products to limited demands for disclosure of organizational processes.

Another category of regulatory activity focuses on the marketing of products, specifically on potentially deceptive and unfair marketing practices. Such regulations may impose limits or bans on door-to-door sales of certain products, require licensure of salespersons, put restrictions on misleading advertising, or require approval of marketing materials. Like regulation of products and services, restrictions related to marketing may be attached to the licensure process. They are most prevalent in the Medicaid and Medicare programs, where consumers are often viewed as more vulnerable to marketing abuses.

Underlying both of these approaches to consumer protection may be the assumption that the marketplace cannot always adequately protect consumers, and thus attention must be focused on what to do when markets fail.

Making the Marketplace Work

A third approach, while accepting some of the direct demands imposed by the first two (such as solvency requirements), focuses more on improving the functioning of the marketplace. The underlying assumption here is that the rights and opportunities of consumers as individuals would increase if the marketplace could better protect them as a whole—and as a result, direct demands on manufacturers and sellers might be less necessary. The goal of market-directed regulation, then, is not to protect individuals in the face of market failure but to reduce the probability of such failure in the first place.

Philosophically, this approach offers an interesting blend of liberal and conservative values. On the one hand, it aims at the big picture, trying to improve conditions for large blocks of consumers; on the other hand, it is often tied to more conservative theories and political forces whose main goal appears to be to minimize government regulation. For this reason, perhaps, its advocates are sometimes distrusted by more liberal consumer group leaders.

Examples of the market-directed approach include these:

- Insurance market reforms or requirements that employers provide a choice of plans. This may be offered as a means of protecting certain groups of purchasers and consumers, or of encouraging health plans to compete on quality, price, and service rather than on risk selection.
- Development and dissemination of data on plan performance, or investments in research aimed at improving consumers' capacity to compare plans. These may be offered as a means of encouraging competition.
- Reliance on incentives rather than requirements, as with proposals to link deductibility of premiums to enrollment in purchasing cooperatives or to collection and disclosure of specified data.
- Antitrust enforcement as a means of protecting consumers by maintaining a competitive marketplace.

Arguably, strategies involving accreditation could be included here because they may be seen as a means of improving market competition. But with the exception of circumstances in which government links accreditation to participation in a government program (as the Medicare program does today), accreditation is a private-sector strategy, not a government one.

Strengthening the Consumer Voice

Much less frequently invoked, or even debated today, a fourth strategy focuses on protecting consumers by enhancing their organizational or political leverage—some call it the "consumer voice."[6] This strategy can be viewed as expanding the concept of market intervention to include processes that give consumers more strength in the political-economic marketplace. Consumer protections might include creation of health plan–based or external ombudsman arrangements, direct public funding of consumer participation in regulatory proceedings, tax incentives for organizations that include consumers on health plan or hospital boards or advisory committees, and start-up funds for consumer-led or small-employer purchasing cooperatives.

Consumer voice strategies thrived in the 1960s and 1970s and even into the 1980s. They were a central part of the Johnson administration's War on Poverty. The HMO Act of 1973 required that federally qualified HMOs have at least one-third of their policymaking bodies drawn from their members, and many states provide financial support for consumer intervention in utility rate-setting proceedings. State attorney general offices may intervene for consumers and frequently include consumer protection units.[7] But consumer voice strategies fell on hard times during the Reagan years. Today they seem out of vogue and are rarely a part of public debate.

Interestingly, some consumer voice approaches, although generally controversial, should find at least theoretical support among those who prefer market-oriented interventions to direct regulation of managed care organizations. In fact, the most radical proposals might actually dovetail with the regulatory philosophy of those who generally espouse conservative viewpoints.

Court of Last Resort

The right to sue for malpractice and over denials of rights or benefits in managed care relationships is another consumer protection approach, although some may argue that government policy regarding right to sue is not a regulatory strategy. Today, this subject is fraught with uncertainty and controversy. Issues of who can sue whom, for what, and under what circumstances and laws (state law or the federal Employee Retirement Income Security Act [ERISA]) are very much on the front burner of policy and legal debate. Some consumer groups, trial attorneys, elements of the medical profession, and some Democrats usually are pitted against insurers, employers, and most Republicans.

The liability issue interacts in some interesting ways with other policy questions. Advocates of the right to sue, for example, view it as an essential—even the quintessential—element of consumer protection. Clearly, most such advocates argue that increasing health plan liability will make plans more accountable and more responsive. However, especially if plans are held liable for the actions of contracted professionals (as many advocates of greater liability would propose), the immediate results of increased plan liability could be very distasteful to consumers: networks would likely shrink in size as plans moved to reduce their exposure and insurers would grow more aggressive in questioning physicians' decision making, fearing that they would be charged with every error.

Of course, the various regulatory approaches do not have to conflict. Advocates of direct regulation of products or marketing often have few problems with market-oriented interventions, although the converse is much less frequently true. Common ground is often found in the area of disclosure, which can serve both as direct protection for individuals and as a means to enhance informed competition.

Advantages and Liabilities

All the strategies have their advantages and liabilities, some of which are described in the following paragraphs.

Direct Regulation

Given the lock-in nature of insurance and the new incentives of managed care, some enhanced level of direct consumer protection offers the advantage of firming up protection for individuals. Making direct demands about what insurers must provide offers a means of reducing the probability that some individuals will be mistreated or undertreated. When it comes to grievance procedures or guarantees that health insurers meet minimal quality assurance standards (such as providing adequate networks of physicians and hospitals), demands for certain government-imposed and monitored rules could be effective.

But many direct efforts aimed at enhancing consumer protection may actually reduce consumer choice, lock in the obsolete, or restrict innovation in a fast-changing industry. Or, despite the best intentions, these efforts may fail to achieve reform goals. For example, proposals to guarantee out-of-network access can unnecessarily restrict the options of those who will accept the trade-off of less choice for lower cost, and at the same time they reduce incentives for health plans to invest in integration.

Even strengthened grievance procedures, appropriate as they may be, can produce far less benefit than is commonly presumed. The procedures themselves may be so time consuming and expensive that many plan enrollees will be reluctant to invoke them, especially when they will have to remain in the same plan with the same physicians. Nor do such procedures necessarily solve the problem for the *next* individual. Without built-in means to turn legitimate grievances into policy change or aggressive follow-up by regulators, grievance proceedings tend to remain one-by-one solutions.

Moreover, some analysts who focus on quality issues point out other limitations of the direct regulation approach. Brennan and Berwick, for example, conclude that health plan quality improvement efforts have not generally been driven by demands of regulators but by the expectation of plans that those quality enhancements will prove valuable in the marketplace.[8] And they argue that regulators are often behind the innovation curve, unable to assess unique properties of new delivery systems. Further, regulators tend to be too focused on details and conformity to specified sets of rules, and are often punitive in their approach. Overall, Brennan and Berwick say, today's regulatory processes may be best able to regulate the *parts* of a system (such as physicians and hospitals) when increasingly it is the *whole* of the system that is more important.[9] This potential failing may be particularly obvious in regulators' focus on health plans when in many markets most of the functions (physician recruitment, utilization management, risk bearing, and so forth) are being performed by delivery systems that remain largely unregulated.

Most importantly, it can be argued that many of the current and proposed measures for directly regulating managed care plans will, at best, prevent wrongdoing. But they will not encourage or force plans to improve. Therefore, they are important but limited safety-net measures. Yet the most important goal of managed care today may be to *raise the quality of care for the many.*[10] To the extent that raising quality rather than securing a minimum standard of quality is the goal, many traditional, direct regulation approaches to consumer protection are of limited value.

Marketplace Strategies

By contrast, market-oriented approaches and some consumer-voice ones may hold more potential to produce behavioral changes on the part of managed care organizations, leading to widespread benefits for consumers and populations. Rather than offering a prescribed series of requirements, they aim at setting broader and more potent forces in motion, hoping the result will be enhanced value and quality. For example, a purchasing coalition strategy might envision skilled, professional purchasers or "sponsors" invoking sophisticated information about health plan performance and quality to assist consumers in choosing plans, thus driving competition on quality into the marketplace.

But many market-oriented strategies—such as tying tax deductibility of health plan premiums to various structural or performance goals—face formidable political obstacles. And even if politically viable, market-oriented approaches may fall short of producing adequate protections for consumers as individuals; they might need to be supplemented by more direct regulations on products, services, and processes. Even the best systemic efforts to reduce the probability of market failure, and thus the need for direct regulation, will not eliminate the necessity of protecting individuals. In health care, the stakes for individual consumers are simply too high.

Nor should we fail to point out the reality (often denied by advocates of market-based approaches) that such strategies often require sizable doses of direct regulation. Implementation of disclosure-based strategies, risk-adjustment mechanisms, rating-reform approaches, and managed competition types of purchasing arrangements may all require significant, even aggressive government intervention. Indeed, one flaw in the advocacy of managed competition has been the reluctance of some proponents to accept the level of government rule making or "management" that the strategy requires.

Health Plan Liability and Malpractice

Like the strategies of direct and market-oriented intervention, litigation approaches offer opportunities and liabilities. Some proponents of reform envision that increasing opportunities and rights to sue insurers would render the latter more accountable and reduce the likelihood of their inappropriately denying care or benefits. It is also argued that increasing their exposure to liability would encourage insurers to improve system integration and co-ordination, and to place greater emphasis on practicing evidence-based medicine. In short, the need to reduce the likelihood of lawsuits and increase the ability to defend against them might propel insurers to improve system processes, services, and quality.[11] In these ways the individual remedy of a lawsuit could benefit the larger population.

However, as discussed earlier, some results of increased plan liability—smaller networks and more insurer interference in physician decision making—would be very consumer-*un*friendly. In addition, expanding the right to sue raises the legitimate question of whether the gains would be worth the increases in premiums that could result as lawyers seek to exploit a new medical "deep pocket." Nor have malpractice rules generally performed as advocates might hope. Compensation has been provided unevenly, with some victims of malpractice receiving massive awards and many others getting little or nothing. It remains unproven that the system actually deters wrongdoing or increases quality. And without question, the current system is expensive and time consuming, with transaction costs, including attorney fees, devouring over half of jury awards.[12]

A Multiple-Strategy Approach

Clearly, then, although we may be able to distinguish categories of government intervention, a comprehensive consumer protection strategy that aims at both protecting individuals and encouraging managed care organizations to raise quality overall will likely require some blend of the several approaches.

Trends and Regulatory Needs

Ideally, policymakers would be able to adjust regulatory strategies (which, almost by definition, are less than perfectly flexible) to fit future marketplace and organizational configurations. Unfortunately, those predicting the future of the health care marketplace are much like stockbrokers: usually more confident than accurate. It remains difficult to distinguish isolated success from benchmark and benchmark from trend. In fact, the only way to depict a trend in health care markets accurately is to look backward—a point driven home by the awareness that some of the most obvious marketplace trends run counter to one another. Such uncertainty in the health care arena, as well as the difficulty of anticipating the effect of various regulatory strategies, complicates the regulatory task.

With such caveats in mind, however, we can attempt to define some trends and their potential impact. And we can begin to assess what regulatory or consumer protection strategies deserve the most attention.

Integration and Ever-Larger Networks

Health plans, physicians, and hospitals continue to seek new organizational arrangements. Integrated delivery systems are emerging in an almost unlimited variety of forms: real and virtual; more integrated or less; led by insurer, physician, hospital, and even physician management company. New legislation approved by Congress in 1997, facilitating the organization of provider-service organizations (PSOs), will accelerate this trend and expand its variety. As integrated systems grow in number we may expect that more will assume greater amounts of risk, many accepting full-risk capitation from insurers. But trends in risk bearing by physicians alone remain murky.

At the same time, consumer demand for choice of physician is generating ever-larger networks, leading to a preference for nonexclusive over exclusive physician contracting arrangements. The Washington-based consulting firm The Advisory Board is now informing its hospital clients that they no longer need fear being left out of networks, because networks will want them all.[13] "Welcome to the PPO network," writes one plan to new physician participants. "You are now part of a carefully selected panel of more than 300 hospitals and 21,000 physicians."[14] PPOs, once expected by many to serve only as a transition phase from fee-for-service to HMOs, continue to thrive. Indeed, in some respects at least, the most prominent trend in managed care is toward the old system of every physician in every plan. In this way, the trends toward integration and choice of physician appear to be on a collision course.

The tension between integration and choice makes it difficult to project the future of various managed care forms. In the short term, IPA-based systems—offering greater flexibility for organizers, more physician choice, lower start-up costs, some independence for physicians, and more capacity to take advantage of physician and bed surpluses—appear to have an advantage over traditional and more integrated staff and group models. But how this advantage will fare over time is unclear. IPAs that achieve substantial levels of integration—like some California systems—while still offering advantages such as those listed here, may be well-positioned. But others may be unable to compete with systems that have more name recognition, better information systems, fewer physicians, higher levels of physician integration and commitment, better capacity to improve and demonstrate quality, or other assets. The same realities may eventually catch up with the PPO.

Value-Based Purchasing and Other Purchasing Trends

Value-based purchasing dominates the headlines. But if you read carefully, you find that price rules, with choice of physician a close second, and quality improvement sometimes a stepchild. A variety of obstacles hinder those seriously interested in pursuing quality improvement: the high cost of quality-related investments, the difficulty of demonstrating higher quality, resistance from employers intent on obtaining lower prices, and avoidance of adverse selection that might accompany proven higher quality. Some large employers, public and private, are achieving gains here. But although they may constitute the majority of speakers at health care conferences, they remain the minority in the marketplace. Indeed, if the demand for lower price continues (and we can expect it will) and the demand for consumer choice of physician also remains high, quality may *remain* in third place. Moreover, with pressure for larger (and inevitably less integrated) networks reducing the capacity of plans to employ other cost-reduction tools of managed care, demands for low prices may eventually result in temptation to reduce quality.

Longer term, the prospects for quality may be brighter. Risk-adjustment methodologies will improve, as will the ability to assess and compare plan and provider quality. Still, these may be only necessary, not sufficient conditions for quality-based competition. That will require purchasers to reward quality and even be willing to pay more for it.

Consolidation and Conversion

Consolidation among plans, hospitals, and physicians is not likely to diminish, with consolidation among physicians beginning to catch up with that among plans and hospitals. Many markets soon may be distinguished by the prominence of a few plans, a few hospital systems, a few large medical groups, or even all three. The final verdict on consolidation is not yet in, although some analysts appear less concerned about consolidation among plans than among providers, largely because of the greater ease of market entry for plans. But balancing the values of consolidation (efficiency, lower cost, conceivably improved quality) against declines in competition remains a formidable task. However, many analysts offer the same warning: the majority of today's consolidation activity is aimed primarily at increasing market power, not at increasing levels of system integration or quality of care. Where integration is occurring, the clinical integration that may be most linked to quality lags behind.

Who will lead the new systems is an open question. Plans, hospital systems, and large physician groups all have the leadership assets and liabilities. Most probably, different configurations will emerge in different markets.

Conversion of nonprofit to for-profit organizations also continues, although not at the rate some imagine. Plan conversions will continue, but it is not clear—beyond ideological and image concerns—that the transition from nonprofit to for-profit status poses a substantial threat to consumers. Hospital conversions may be a different matter, because the loss of nonprofit capacity could affect the ability of the system as a whole to deliver uncompensated care to the poor and uninsured. The extent of that impact in any given community will depend largely on which hospitals in the community convert, those providing sizable amounts of charitable care or those that do not, and on conditions or demands placed by states on converting institutions. Even if conversions are few, the pressures of the new competitive managed care marketplace may reduce the willingness or ability of many hospitals, both for-profit and not-for-profit, to provide charitable care. This remains a source of serious concern for those attempting to represent or serve vulnerable populations.

Finally, it must be noted that, as a market driver, Medicare stands out. This is largely because of the dollars at stake as well as the reality that—as a result of its slow transition to managed care—Medicare is the richest source of new "covered lives." If nothing else, Medicare as market driver exemplifies the unique and multiple roles of government in the health care marketplace.

What to Do?

Based on the realities, uncertainties, and trends, what principles might guide policymakers in regulating managed care today and in the near future? What are the greatest needs and opportunities? What options offer more benefit than risk? We offer some broad themes and possible strategies.

Competing Regulatory Goals

In practice, comprehensive regulatory strategies are likely to include a mix of direct regulation of products, processes, and services; marketing restrictions; and efforts to affect the functioning of the marketplace. Which of these strategies leads may depend largely on the goals of the policymakers and those they are attempting to serve. If the goal remains (as is the case in most of the backlash agenda) increasing consumer protection against wrongdoing by plans or delivery systems, the focus will be on protecting the needs of individual consumers. This might include the right to visit the emergency room, grievance processes, restrictions on marketing materials, and so forth. In contrast, if the focus is more on the quest to raise quality for all then policy interventions will or at least should stress markets more than individuals, in order to increase competition based on quality and strengthen consumer power in the marketplace. The most likely meeting place between the two sets of strategies and goals may be disclosure.

We can see how, in practice, the two theoretical approaches to regulation often come together if we look at the current challenge of the Health Care Financing Administration (HCFA). It is possible that no greater regulatory burden has ever been handed to a government agency than the one bestowed by Congress in 1997. The list of regulatory tasks assigned—from structuring Medicare open enrollment, to devising risk-adjustment methodologies, to designing a regulatory framework for PSOs—suggests at least two equally unlikely and somewhat cynical explanations: first, that Congress has unparalleled faith in the agency, and second, that Congress was consciously setting up the agency for failure. More likely, Congress probably found that leaving the details—and much more—to the future was the most politically viable of several difficult options.

But where there is regulatory burden (not to mention unequaled purchasing power), there is also opportunity. The HCFA must find the right blend of explicit regulatory protection and market-based purchasing strategies. Its unique status might enable it to lead in both, if only its employees can find the time to think about it.

Protecting the Individual

Some additional, specific consumer protections will be required, at least in the short term, because of the following: legitimate public concerns about managed care arrangements and incentives;

uncertainty generated by the rapid pace of marketplace change; strong marketplace pressures to lower costs; and the high cost of undertreatment or error for the individual. Although many measures being proposed appear inappropriate, resulting from either exaggerated fears, provider-based agendas, or political motivations, some protections seem warranted and reasonable. Reports by a state task force in California and by a presidential commission in Washington, D.C., have sought to find a viable balance between adding protection and limiting burdens on managed care organizations and innovation.[15]

And although states will almost certainly remain the primary locus of insurance regulation, it will take federal action if consumer protection efforts are to be extended to self-insured plans governed by ERISA. Moreover, even as the Medicare reforms of 1997 increase choices and competition for beneficiaries (suggesting some success for market-oriented intervention advocates) there is little doubt that increased enrollment of these beneficiaries in managed care arrangements will require additional attention of managed care regulators. Stepped-up scrutiny will be inevitable, given the combination of political reality, the vulnerability of some elderly individuals, the anticipated turbulence of the Medicare marketplace, and the government and consumer dollars at stake.

Mature Versus Changing Industries

Finding the appropriate regulatory strategy is always more difficult when an industry is undergoing rapid change. There may be, simultaneously, more pressure to regulate *and* more reason to fear that regulation will stifle innovation and choice. Under such circumstances it may be wise to focus more restrictive regulatory efforts on areas where marketplace change is less likely to render regulation stifling and obsolete. The obvious candidate here may be grievance procedures, including rights to independent review of medical necessity decisions, which have some history and may not be very market-dependent. Moreover, they offer a means of easing consumers' worst fears. And if this could be accomplished, pressures for more intrusive and perhaps less appropriate interventions may lose momentum.

A focus on changing markets also leads to consideration of antitrust policy. If mergers are mainly about market power, antitrust enforcement agencies and courts may need to be particularly wary of organizational promises that proposed mergers and acquisitions will lead to heightened efficiency, integration, lower cost, or any other consumer benefit. Proof rather than promise may need to be the rule of the day.

Regulation of Organizations and New Actors

Some of the most suspect proposals in the backlash agenda include specific restrictions or demands to be imposed on managed care organizations: choice of physician or out-of-network access, limits on loss-ratios, and so forth. These emphasize process over performance or outcome, and they threaten to chill innovation and integration. It is somewhat surprising that consumers and those representing them have not stressed the market-based strategy of securing more choice of plan as a more potent means to attain these objectives.

Concerns about stifling new organizational relationships, however, should not obscure the reality that managed care regulation is focused almost exclusively on the health plan. As integrated systems of multiple forms emerge, accepting more risk and more functions traditionally performed by insurers, questions arise as to the most appropriate focal point for regulatory interventions. Keeping the focus on the insurer, and requiring it to secure guarantees that providers are meeting regulatory requirements, is one option. But as delivery systems pursue PSO avenues or direct contracting with self-insured employers, that option disappears. Determining what requirements PSOs should have to meet and how to measure their performance will be an additional challenge.

The Employer Role

The failure of the Clinton reform plan seems to have cemented in place the employer-based purchasing system. Notably, the public relations failure of the "alliance" construct may have led to a deemphasis on the issue of employee choice, a hallmark of the Clinton and managed competition approaches.

But a case can be made that, over time, employee choice may be the surest means to increasing competition based on quality and thus one of the more potent tools in the consumer protection arsenal. This value and the debate around it deserve to be resur-rected. The system may remain employer-based, with companies rather than individuals contracting for and paying for health in-surance. But as managed care evolves and the capacity to distin-guish between managed care organizations improves, leaving the choice of plan to the employer may become more problematic. As noted earlier, achieving quality goals—in addition to achieving goals on price, choice, service, product differentiation, and so on—may require far greater concern about quality on the part of pur-chasers—which suggests that consumers in particular may wish to focus more attention on the health care purchasing process.

The Burden of Malpractice

As managed care plans assume more responsibility over health care delivery, arguments for subjecting them to malpractice claims be-come more prevalent. But appearances may be deceiving. In fact, market trends may be leaning away from tightly knit, insurer-dominated systems. Networks are expanding, and as the pattern of almost-every-doctor-in-almost-every-plan grows more dominant, in-surers may have *less* rather than *more* control over participating physicians. Where integration is moving forward, it appears to be mostly on the delivery system side, with providers accepting more responsibility (including financial risk) for more decisions once con-trolled by insurers. This being the case, increasing the focus of the liability system on the insurer may not be the wisest course, even for those who believe that the right to sue is the key to accountability.

Organizing the Consumers

As Common Cause founder John Gardner has noted, "Everyone's organized but the consumer." Given their obvious stake in the sit-uation, and their limited health care purchasing power, consumers may need a more substantial role in the health care marketplace and even in the political process that affects it. Governments, foun-dations, and others might consider that very modest sums invested in consumer advocacy, organization, and education could have an enormous impact on consumer leverage in the marketplace, in policy discussions, and even with employers-purchasers. Guaranteeing genuine consumer participation in regulatory proceedings of insurance regulators may be another avenue to explore.

Indeed, such initiatives—often advocated by the most progressive forces—dovetail with the market-based strategies of those who prefer conservative approaches to regulation and policy in general.

Finding Common Ground

Advocates of direct and market-based intervention may wish to search for common ground. Demands imposed on health plans to protect consumers will have very limited capacity to secure and raise quality if the first priority of the marketplace is lower price. Thus marketplace forces and purchasing issues must be addressed. Still, even the boldest of market-oriented interventions will not likely address all of the concerns of individual patients in managed care plans.

The search for common ground might begin with a conscious focus on the ends rather than the means. Both those who tend to accept more government intervention and those who lean against it need to consider whether some of the strategies and means of the other might be necessary and appropriate to achieve the ends they hold dear. Government intervention is but a means. Traditional ideological inclinations to support or oppose it should remain secondary to the goals being sought.

Notes

1. Some of these circumstances are discussed in a 1979 law review article by Robert Reich. (Reich, R. B. "Toward a New Consumer Protection." *University of Pennsylvania Law Review,* 1979, *128*). They are listed here in a somewhat altered and less theoretical form.
2. Surveys vary depending largely on how the question is asked and how the choice is defined.
3. Miller, R. H., and Luft, H. S. "Does Managed Care Lead to Better or Worse Quality of Care?" *Health Affairs,* Sept.–Oct. 1997, pp. 7–25.
4. Gabel, J. R., Ginsburg, P. B., and Hunt, K. A. *Health Affairs,* Sept.–Oct. 1997, p. 107.
5. For a fuller discussion of these and related consumer protection options see Rodwin, M. A. "Consumer Protection and Managed Care," *Houston Law Review,* 1996, *32.*
6. Ibid.

7.   Rodwin, M. A. *Consumer Voice, Participation, and Representation in Managed Health Care.* Washington, D.C.: Consumer Federation of America, 1998.
8.   Brennan, T. A., and Berwick, D. M. *New Rules: Regulation, Markets, and the Quality of American Health Care.* San Francisco: Jossey-Bass, 1996.
9.   For further analysis of this line of argument, see Brennan and Berwick, *New Rules.*
10.   See Zelman, W., and Berenson, R. *The Managed Care Blues and How to Cure Them.* Washington, D.C.: Georgetown University Press, 1998.
11.   Professor Craig Havighurst of Duke University School of Law is perhaps the foremost exponent of this point of view.
12.   Sage, W. M. "Enterprise Liability and the Emerging Managed Health Care System." *Law and Contemporary Problems,* Winter–Spring 1997, pp. 161–162.
13.   Health Care Advisory Board. *Resurgence of Choice.* Washington, D.C.: The Advisory Board Company, 1996.
14.   Zelman, W., and Berenson, R. *The Managed Care Blues . . . and How to Cure Them.* Washington, D.C.: Georgetown University Press, 1998.
15.   See reports from President Clinton's Advisory Commission on Consumer Protection and Quality in the Health Care Industry, Nov. 1997, and from the California Managed Health Care Improvement Task Force, Jan. 1998.

Chapter Two

The Current Status of State and Federal Regulation

Patricia A. Butler

Although government regulation of health care is no longer as active as it was in the 1970s and early 1980s, states continue their traditional roles in licensing providers (practitioners and institutions) and insurers. As health insurance has moved from an indemnity model to managed care, insurance regulation has evolved to oversee not only plan solvency but also the availability and accessibility of promised care. And as managed care organizations have moved from traditional health maintenance organizations (HMOs) to a variety of integrated provider arrangements, many of which bear insurance risk, states have had to develop policy to define and oversee these new types of health plans.

The federal government has traditionally played a limited role in regulating health care providers and insurers. But through its function as a purchaser of Medicare services, it has set provider standards (for example, for hospitals and laboratories) that have influenced the broader health care environment. And this influence will continue with Medicare's emphasis on enrolling its beneficiaries in managed care organizations. Recently, Congress also developed standards for insurance market practices—the customary province of states—in enacting the Health Insurance Portability and Accessibility Act of 1996 (HIPAA).

Legal and Historical Role of State and Federal Regulation

Following is a brief description of the legal and historical roles of the state and federal governments in regulating health care providers and insurers.

Sources of Authority

The United States Constitution delegates specific "enumerated" powers to the federal government and reserves other types of governmental authority to the states. Among these reserved powers is the so-called police power to legislate for the public's health, safety, and welfare (*Jacobsen v. Massachusetts*, 1905). Police power is the source of authority for states to regulate health care providers, such as physicians and hospitals, and insurance entities operating solely within state boundaries. The U.S. Supreme Court held in 1944 that states cannot regulate insurers operating across state lines (*U.S. v. South-Eastern Underwriters Association*). But in the 1946 McCarran-Ferguson Act—and again in ERISA, the Employee Retirement Income Security Act of 1974—Congress delegated to the states the power to regulate such insurers, unless Congress specifically chooses to do so. Consequently, all states regulate at least some practices and policies of health insurers, including HMOs, operating within their borders. Furthermore, states have direct responsibility to set contract standards for health plans that serve Medicaid beneficiaries and state employees.

The federal government's authority is limited to powers enumerated in the Constitution. There is no general federal police power (*U.S. v. Lopez*, 1995). Of relevance to health care delivery system regulation are the taxing and interstate commerce powers. Constitution article I, section 8, authorizes Congress to tax, which has been held to imply a power to spend and to condition spending on meeting standards. For example, highway funds are conditioned on states' enacting certain safety laws. And funds under Medicaid and the recently enacted Child Health Plan are conditioned on states complying with federal standards.

The same constitutional provision (article I, section 8) gives the federal government exclusive authorization to regulate interstate commerce. The definition of what commerce flows across state lines has been broadened considerably in the last sixty years. The provision has been held to include, for example, authorization to regulate any businesses that purchase goods that are sold among states and the power to prohibit racial discrimination in public accommodations. But the power still has some limits. For instance, the Court recently invalidated a federal law prohibiting possessing a gun in school zones on the ground that such activities are not "substantially related" to interstate commerce (*U.S. v. Lopez*). Consequently, it is not clear that the federal government could directly regulate purely local activities such as physician practice. But the federal government can regulate insurance operating in interstate commerce (as it recently did in enacting HIPAA) as well as other health care activities that substantially affect interstate commerce.

In the federal Health Maintenance Organization Act of 1973 (P.L. 93–222), Congress relied on both sources of constitutional power. Under the taxing-spending authority, it provided grants to develop and expand HMOs meeting certain qualifications. And under the interstate commerce power, it required businesses with more than twenty-five employees and subject to the federal minimum wage law (previously upheld as regulation of interstate commerce) to offer their employees an HMO option if one existed in the service area. For purposes of grants and the "dual choice" provisions, federal law preempted state laws that would inhibit HMO operations. No grants have been available for many years, but this law served to promote the creation of HMOs.

Consumer Protection as Rationale

States currently regulate insurers to protect consumers from the consequences of insurer fraud and insolvency. Because managed care plans add a promise to arrange for or provide care to the risk-spreading function of indemnity insurers, government has two additional justifications for overseeing managed care plans: to assure that promised services are available and accessible, and to overcome managed care's financial incentives to underserve (in contrast to the overservice incentive of fee-for-service payment).

The protection of consumers under managed care derives from several concerns. First, consumers generally have limited information about such complex subjects as the delivery of medical care or the contents of an insurance policy. Furthermore, even given more information, consumers are usually unsophisticated health care buyers relative to providers or health plans. Finally, individual consumers have little bargaining leverage in dealing with large organizations such as health plans, and their ability to "vote with their feet" by changing plans may be constrained by lack of choice offered by employers.

Although state-level regulation is usually proposed to address consumer concerns, some of these laws appear designed more to protect providers against managed care plan practices than to protect consumers directly. For example, although so-called any willing provider laws are justified as expanding consumer access to providers, most have been promoted by pharmacists who fear losing business from plans that use mail-order pharmacies or otherwise limit their contracts.

Tension Between Market Forces and Consumer Protection

The national movement toward a more market-oriented health care system raises questions about the government's regulatory role. Why is government regulation needed if consumers can choose health plans or providers, much like other commodities? One response is that health care falls short of the ideal of a perfectly competitive market for several reasons: barriers to entry for providers and insurers; lack of homogeneous "products" for which consumers can shop; consumer insulation from most health care costs because of the presence of insurance; limited role employed consumers play in choosing among health plans and making treatment decisions; limited information about quality and price; and limited bargaining power (between consumers and plans or providers, and between plans and providers).

Nevertheless, through various public and private-sector interventions, the U.S. health care environment has moved closer to a competitive model in recent years. Among the examples are cost sharing (for premiums and at point of service) to increase price sensitivity of consumer choices; standardized health plan products that facilitate comparison shopping; integrated delivery systems that eliminate the need to shop for individual services; gradual improvement in information on health plan quality; purchasing cooperatives that allow consumer choice among plans; and risk-sharing payment arrangements that align provider financial incentives with those of plans. Nevertheless, the health care market will fall short of the perfectly competitive ideal as long as health insurance remains the primary means of financing health care, employers continue to play a major role in choosing and subsidizing insurance, measurement of quality is imperfect, and health care remains technically complex.

State and federal policymakers seek to balance the current preference for market forces over regulation with a concern that as long as health care remains different from other commodities, government needs to protect consumers. The policy dilemma is how to assure that consumers receive what they are promised without limiting managed care plan flexibility, inhibiting managed care's ability to control costs, encouraging employers to self-fund or drop coverage, and stifling care delivery innovation.

Potential Roles for Public Oversight

There are several potential roles for government oversight of managed care under a more market-oriented system. Public agencies can prescribe standards to increase the likelihood that the market can function most efficiently and fairly. They also can oversee specific health plan activities to protect consumers who are vulnerable because they have limited information, lack of technical expertise, or unequal bargaining power.

Facilitating Market Function

State and federal governments can use several tools to enhance the functioning of a market in health care, including enforcing antitrust laws, fostering alternative delivery arrangements (including provider-sponsored networks), and supporting technology assessment and development of quality measures. Regulatory standards that improve the chance that a health care market will evolve and function fairly to allocate insurance products based on prices and benefit levels include these:

- Mandating useful consumer information to help people choose among managed care plans based on price and quality
- Mandating standardized health plans to facilitate price comparisons
- Establishing fair insurance market practices to prohibit plans from avoiding risk by refusing to sell to or renew products for people in poor health
- Facilitating purchasing cooperatives to extend bargaining power to small firms and individual insurance purchasers and to provide choice of plans to employee groups

Protecting Consumers

There remains a role for public regulation to protect consumers when a market does not function effectively. Such a responsibility may be particularly appropriate when consumers are disadvantaged because they have unequal bargaining power with suppliers such as health plans and providers, when consumers have limited choice among health plans (and cannot "vote with their feet") or limited choice of providers within a plan, or when the product is a technically complex service whose quality can affect consumers' lives and well-being. For these reasons, state governments have traditionally regulated:

- Solvency standards for health plan financial capacity, such as minimum capital and surplus requirements, limitations on investments, reserve and deposit requirements, financial reporting and examination requirements, and state guarantee funds
- Consumer "hold harmless" provisions that forbid providers from seeking payment from enrollees if a plan becomes insolvent
- Marketing rules to prohibit unfair, false, or misleading advertising and marketing techniques
- Grievance resolution procedures for enrollees and authority for government to investigate consumer complaints
- Medical care quality oversight by government agencies or outside contractors
- Care availability and accessibility standards to assure plans can meet their promise to provide or arrange (not just pay for) care

- Rate regulation, at least requiring that insurance rates be neither inadequate nor excessive

In addition to their roles as regulators and purchasers, state and federal governments also establish contract terms to address particular needs. For example, state Medicaid managed care contracts often require culturally sensitive services, transportation, and other means to facilitate use of care among low-income populations.

ERISA poses a challenge to some types of state insurance regulation because it preempts state laws that "relate to" employee health plans while "saving" from preemption state laws regulating the business of insurance (Butler, 1998). Consequently, ERISA prohibits states from regulating self-insured employee plans. Although ERISA authorizes states to regulate the business of insurance, some courts have interpreted this "savings clause" narrowly to hold that certain insurance standards, such as any willing provider laws, are not insurance regulation and cannot be applied to either insured or self-insured employee health plans. Although few state managed-care regulations have been challenged in court, until the Supreme Court clarifies the meaning of ERISA's savings clause, more litigation is likely. (The ERISA preemption is discussed in some detail in Chapters Nine and Ten.)

State Regulation

States began to regulate health insurers more actively over twenty years ago with definitions of minimum benefits that all health carriers must offer (Laudicina, Yerby, and Pardo, 1998). All states currently mandate some health coverage benefits (such as alcoholism treatment or home health care) as well as types of providers (such as chiropractors and optometrists) and persons who must be covered in a family policy (such as dependent students or disabled children). Since the mid-1980s when the first any willing provider law was enacted to permit all pharmacies to participate in health plan networks, states have increasingly regulated various aspects of managed care.

A managed health care plan usually is defined as one that agrees to provide or arrange for health services (in addition to its insurance function) and that generally imposes some limits on the providers that enrollees may use (including primary care gate-keeper requirements, network limits, and cost-sharing differentials for in-network and out-of-network use) and mechanisms to influence provider cost-consciousness (such as financial risk-sharing arrangements or administrative review of proposed treatments).

In most states, an insurance department or insurance commissioner (to regulate insurance carriers) is primarily responsible for overseeing managed care organizations such as HMOs, often in collaboration with public health agencies. In a few states, like New York and Minnesota, the state public health department has primary jurisdiction to license HMOs (Horvath and Snow, 1996). Regardless of which agency takes the lead, insurance regulators generally enforce financial and marketing standards, and public health agencies generally monitor compliance with quality and access requirements.

National Association of Insurance Commissioners Model Laws

The National Association of Insurance Commissioners (NAIC) has developed a set of model laws to regulate managed care. Called the CLEAR initiative (Consolidated Licensure of Entities Assuming Risk), the objective of this series of five acts is to bring all health-insuring organizations under a single set of standards rather than separate licensure categories such as HMOs, PPOs, indemnity carriers, and health care service (Blue Cross–Blue Shield) plans. To the extent that these organizations include managed care features, they would be regulated similarly. Because some plans bear different levels of insurance risk (for example, when a plan shares risk with its providers), the NAIC has also developed a model act (risk-based capital model act) for establishing different levels of reserves depending on the type and amount of risk assumed. The five model acts are these:

Health Care Professional Credentialing Verification Model Act (NAIC Model Regulation Service, July 1996)

This model requires managed care plans to establish a program to assure that participating professionals meet minimum standards of clinical competency. The model act prescribes minimum information that health plans must obtain and gives providers a right to review credentialing information and correct errors.

Quality Assessment and Improvement Model Act
(NAIC Model Regulation Service, July 1996)

This model sets forth standards for programs of quality assessment (QA)—to measure and evaluate medical care quality—for all managed care plans, and quality improvement (QI)—to enhance health plans' processes and outcomes—for closed-network plans. Quality improvement plans are required to identify practices that ameliorate health outcomes as well as problematic use patterns and to foster an environment of continuous quality improvement (including integration of public health goals and coordination with public health agencies). Plans must include a description of their QA and QI plans in marketing and enrollee materials and provide an annual summary of QA activities to enrollees, providers, and (on request) the public.

Managed Care Plan Network Adequacy Model Act
(NAIC Model Regulation Service, October 1996)

This model requires that health plan networks are adequate to assure that all services to covered persons will be accessible without unreasonable delay. If a network is not sufficient, the plan must allow enrollees to obtain out-of-network benefits at no extra cost. Managed care plans must file with the state an "access plan" that includes descriptions of the network; referral policies; monitoring to assure network adequacy; prohibition of clauses limiting providers' discussion of treatment options; means to address needs of enrollees with physical and mental disabilities and different languages and cultures; a mechanism to assess enrollee health care needs; information to enrollees on the grievance system and emergency and specialty care approval processes; and a system to ensure coordination and continuity of care (including when a provider leaves the plan). The model act also prohibits inducements to provide less than "medically necessary" services to enrollees.

Grievance Procedures Model Act (NAIC Model
Regulation Service, October 1996)

This model prescribes procedures for a system to allow managed care enrollees to resolve grievances about availability, delivery, and quality of care, claims payment and handling, and other enrollee-plan contract disputes. Plans must maintain records of grievances accessible to state agency officials and file annual summaries of grievances with the state. The model act proposes procedures and time frames for two levels of standard review as well as expedited review if the standard review time frames would seriously jeopardize life, health, or the ability to regain maximum function. This model act is designed as a companion to the Utilization Review Model Act.

Utilization Review Model Act (NAIC Model
Regulation Service, October 1996)

This model provides standards for the structure and operation of utilization review (UR) processes (whose purpose is to evaluate the necessity, appropriateness, efficacy, and efficiency of the plan's health care). Information on a managed care plan's UR procedures must be included in marketing and enrollee information. The act prescribes time frames for providing a decision on prospective, concurrent, and retrospective review, an informal reconsideration of an adverse decision, an appeal within the UR process, and an appeal to the second grievance procedure appeal level. (This act is designed to mesh with the Grievance Procedures Model Act.) It includes an expedited appeal process for urgent cases, and prohibits a plan from requiring prior authorization for emergency services, defined from the viewpoint of the "prudent layperson."

Regulation to Promote Market Function

Most states that have regulated HMOs for many years have standards similar to those in the NAIC's 1995 model HMO act covering requirements for consumer information, grievance procedures, hold harmless provisions, quality assurance system, premium setting, and insolvency protections (Dallek, Jimenez, and Schwartz, 1995). In addition to these long-standing licensure standards, over the past ten years states have begun to consider other regulations of managed care practices. Since the mid-1980s, for example, many states have enacted any willing provider laws requiring managed care plans to permit certain providers (usually pharmacies) that agree to the plan's payment, administrative, and other terms, to participate in its network. Within the last few years, states have considered many other proposals to regulate managed care plans, usually through insurance and HMO licensure laws, the most common of which are summarized in the following section.

Consumer Information

All state HMO laws require plans to provide information to enrollees on benefits, exclusions, choice of providers, and how to obtain services (Dallek, Jimenez, and Schwartz, 1995). Several states have adopted broader disclosure standards. Although consumers may need different types of information to choose among plans or to use a plan effectively, few states seem to distinguish among these categories of disclosure.

• *Information on how to use a plan.* Most states require HMOs to provide information to enrollees about premiums, benefits and exclusions, cost-sharing, participating providers, and grievance mechanisms; and some states require disclosure of the plan's referral and authorization processes, quality assurance plans, or utilization data (Dallek, Jimenez, and Schwartz, 1995). A few states also require plans to disclose information on how to use the plan, such as procedures for obtaining referrals or prior authorization. Many states require HMOs to notify affected enrollees when their primary care provider is no longer participating in the plan. Several states require plans to notify enrollees about how to obtain emergency care, renewal terms, conversion or continuation options, and the right to complain to state agencies. (California and Minnesota require plans to include the state licensing agency's phone number on enrollee materials.)

• *Information to help choose among plans.* A few states mandate information for applicants. Colorado, for example, requires uniform plan descriptions that are compiled into a single form to permit comparisons between plans. Responding to consumer concerns that plan incentive payments may discourage appropriate treatment, several states have enacted laws requiring plans to disclose how they compensate providers ("Consumers and Providers Lobby for State Oversight," 1996). Texas requires that all information provided to enrollees also be made available to prospective enrollees.

• *"Gag clause" limitations.* Although the General Accounting Office reported no explicit so-called gag clauses in the contracts of 529 HMOs it reviewed (U.S. General Accounting Office, 1997), media reports that managed care plans were discouraging contracting providers from discussing treatment options with patients led forty-one states to ban these types of contract terms as of April 1998 (Families USA Foundation, 1998).

• *Standardized quality information.* Most states collect data on health care costs and use (Health Policy Tracking Service, 1998). Many have discussed collecting and publishing standardized information on selected elements of health plan quality, by using the HEDIS instrument or the CAHPS (Consumer Assessment of Health Plan Survey) instrument, for example, to create "report cards" by which consumers can compare plans. Among the few states that have done this, Nevada compiles selected indicators of health plan quality and Maryland and New Jersey published health plan "report cards" in late 1997 (New Jersey Department of Health and Senior Services, 1997; State of Maryland Health Care Access and Cost Commission, 1997).

Insurance Market Practices

By 1996 almost all states had enacted laws to restore stability to the small-group insurance market, requiring issue and renewal of products without regard to health status, crediting satisfaction of preexisting exclusion periods when an insured person changed plans, and narrowing the range of premiums. At least fifteen states provided similar protections in the individual insurance market (Mitchell, Pernice, and Riley, 1997).

Building on these state reforms of the small group and individual insurance markets, in 1996 Congress enacted the Health Insurance Portability and Accessibility Act (HIPAA), which created similar standards for preexisting condition exclusions and guaranteed issue and renewal and, in firms with fewer than fifty workers, coverage of persons in poor health. Although HIPAA also requires access to insurance products for individuals leaving a workplace group plan and gives states several individual coverage access options, the law does not assure these products will be affordable. These standards apply to insured plans and self-insured plans (which ERISA exempts from state regulation). States are authorized to enforce HIPAA insurance requirements and can set higher standards. Because legislatures in California, Missouri, and Rhode Island failed to enact HIPAA-enabling legislation in 1997, the federal Health Care Financing Administration is implementing HIPAA in those states.

Standardized Plan Requirements

As part of small-group market reform, about half the states required health plans in the small group market to offer at least one or two standardized plans (usually with more or less generous benefits or cost-sharing features) regardless of enrollee health status (guaranteed issue) (Laudicina, Yerby, and Pardo, 1998). A useful consequence of these laws was the opportunity to shop for price among plans with the same benefits. The federal HIPAA requires that all plans in the small group market must be issued regardless of health status. Although HIPAA does not invalidate state standardization requirements, neither does it require them, making it unclear whether such provisions will remain or whether other states will adopt them.

Plan Choice

In 1996, 80 percent of firms with fewer than two hundred employees and 47 percent of larger firms offered only one health plan (Gabel, Ginsburg, and Hunt, 1997). ERISA limits states from mandating that all employers offer workers a choice among insurance products. But some large employers offer such choice. And states can facilitate this type of choice by authorizing small employers to participate in purchasing cooperatives, as twenty states have done (Laudicina, Yerby, and Pardo, 1998). However, these cooperatives have been particularly successful in only a few states, including California and Florida.

Direct Consumer Protection Regulations

Regulations that seek to protect consumers directly include solvency standards, prohibition of false advertising, dispute resolution, availability and accessibility of services, and quality assurance.

Solvency Protections

Because consumers cannot easily evaluate the financial security of insurers, all states impose capital, reserve, and other financial standards on HMOs and other health insurers. Several states, such as Missouri, Ohio, and Texas, have established different financial standards for provider-sponsored health plans. State HMO laws also protect consumers in case of plan insolvency by requiring plans to prohibit providers from seeking payment from plan enrollees if the plan defaults on its payment (consumer hold harmless clauses).

Prohibition of False Advertising

Another traditional area of state insurance regulation is standards for accurate advertising and marketing activities.

Dispute Resolution

State insurance and HMO licensure laws all require that plans have a process whereby enrollees can file complaints about their coverage. Indemnity plan disputes usually are about who will pay a claim for a service already rendered. But because managed care plans provide or arrange for care, a dispute may involve whether the plan will authorize coverage for the service and a plan's coverage denial may result in an enrollee's practical inability to obtain care. In the case of expensive services and life-threatening conditions, coverage disputes may involve urgent situations that must be resolved quickly. Therefore, the provisions discussed in the following paragraphs have been applied in some states.

To enhance the fairness of the enrollee grievance process, laws and regulations in many states prescribe criteria for appeals, such as an independent decision maker to hear appeals and multiple levels of appeal (Dallek, Jimenez, and Schwartz, 1995). Twenty-eight states specify time frames for appeals to be resolved (Families USA Foundation, 1998). About half the states require expedited appeals of coverage denials for urgent or experimental care (Families USA Foundation, 1998), and several states also require HMOs to establish procedures for providers to file grievances regarding patient coverage.

Although about half the states set out in law the right of HMO enrollees to file complaints with the state, it is likely that all states investigate HMO enrollee complaints. Most states will accept enrollee complaints at any time, but some require enrollees to complete the HMO's grievance process before engaging the state agency review.

Several states authorize an appeal to an organization independent of the health plan. Florida authorizes an appeal to its Statewide Provider and Subscriber Assistance Panel. In 1997, Missouri, New Jersey, and Texas authorized the creation of independent review organizations to hear appeals of health plan coverage denials. As of November 1998, eighteen states provided a mechanism for enrollees to appeal to some type of independent decision maker (Pollitz, Dallek, and Tàpày, 1998).

Finally, in response to criticisms of managed care plan coverage denials, in 1997 Texas adopted the first statute explicitly authorizing enrollees to sue plans for damages resulting from inappropriate decisions to deny or delay coverage (Butler, 1997). And in 1998 New Mexico enacted a law allowing enrollees to sue to enforce their health plan contract rights.

Availability and Accessibility of Services

Many states have adopted standards designed to enhance availability of and access to services for managed care plan enrollees in order to assure that consumers receive promised services. Some of these laws prescribe specific clinical practice standards, such as hospital lengths of stay for certain conditions. Other examples follow:

- *Network adequacy.* Fifteen state HMO laws or regulations require that plan networks be "adequate to meet enrollee needs" (Families USA Foundation, 1998). Several states set forth maximum distance or travel times between enrollees and providers to assure reasonable geographic accessibility or physician-patient ratios. A few states also require that appointments be available within a reasonable period of time (Dallek, Jimenez, and Schwartz, 1995). States are increasingly requiring that if an enrollee needs a provider—such as a specialist—not in a plan's network, the plan must pay for an out-of-network provider.
- *Consumer choice of providers.* Responding to consumer opposition to restrictive plan networks or primary care gatekeeper requirements, many states have enacted laws expanding consumer choice of providers. For example, thirty-three states allow enrollees

to visit an ob/gyn without obtaining a referral from a primary care physician (some plans consider ob/gyns to be primary care physicians, but others do not). Nine states require plans to allow enrollees to use specialists as primary care providers in certain cases (Families USA Foundation, 1998). Eleven states require plans to offer a point-of-service option—generally with a higher premium—or allow enrollees to seek care from nonnetwork providers, although in some cases enrollees pay a greater share of the bill. Twenty states require plans to allow consumers to go outside networks, most often for pharmacy services (Health Policy Tracking Service, 1998). And ten states require plans to provide for a "standing referral" to a specialist for enrollees who have chronic or other conditions requiring routine specialist care (Families USA Foundation, 1998).

• *Any willing provider laws.* Between 1985 and 1996, half the states enacted laws requiring plans to permit any provider willing to comply with contract terms to participate in the network. Three-quarters of these laws apply only to pharmacies. Increasingly, states are enacting provider "due process" laws permitting them to apply to plans, receive notice of standards used to select or terminate providers, and appeal a denial of plan participation (Laudicina, Yerby, and Pardo,. 1998).

• *Continuity of care.* To address concerns of enrollees whose providers leave a network during the course of treatment, thirteen states require plans to pay for care by these providers for a specified time after the provider leaves the plan (Families USA Foundation, 1998). In some cases the requirement is limited to a continuing course of medically necessary care or terminal illness. Other states require plans to assist enrollees in finding a new provider.

• *Emergency services.* Almost half the states (twenty-three of them) have recently established standards for emergency care—for example, prohibiting prior approval for emergency care and requiring a plan to determine whether a visit is an emergency based on the viewpoint of a prudent layperson rather than a post facto clinical judgment (Families USA Foundation, 1998).

• *Experimental procedures.* Many plans exclude coverage for experimental services. In addition to requiring consumer information about such exclusions and expediting appeals regarding them, laws in California and Ohio require plans to use external reviewers to determine if a service is experimental.

• *Hospital length of stay.* Most (forty-one) states, and Congress, have enacted laws regulating the length of hospital stay after childbirth. In 1996 and 1997, thirteen states enacted hospital length-of-stay legislation for mastectomy and seventeen states enacted hospital length-of-stay laws for reconstructive breast surgery (Health Policy Tracking Service, 1998).

• *Off-label prescription drug mandates.* Through 1997, twenty-nine states have required health plans covering prescription drugs to include uses for which they are not approved by the FDA (primarily to treat cancer) (Health Policy Tracking Service, 1998).

• *Physician incentive payment limits.* Responding to concerns that some forms of managed care risk-sharing might discourage appropriate care, fifteen states have enacted laws attempting to curb incentive payments (Families USA Foundation, 1998). For example, Maryland prohibits withholds, and Georgia, Rhode Island, and Texas ban incentives that limit provision of medically necessary or appropriate care ("Consumers and Providers Lobby for State Oversight," 1996).

• *Utilization review standards.* Many state HMO licensing standards regulate the utilization review activities of managed care plans and about half the states license independent UR firms. To protect consumers and assist providers, these standards prescribe reviewer qualifications, time limits, appeals procedures, and information-sharing requirements.

Quality Assurance

Managed care plans can promote quality of care through an orientation to preventive care, service integration and coordination, medical practice protocols, unified medical records, and internal peer review. But because these plans provide or arrange for services, rather than merely pay claims, and because risk-sharing reimbursement creates incentives for underservice, protecting managed care consumers can involve mechanisms for assuring quality. The following are examples:

• *QA programs.* Most states require HMOs to develop and implement a quality assurance plan, and about half specify the minimum QA plan elements. These may include a written plan with goals and objectives, standards for assessing quality and taking corrective action for problems, regularly scheduled meetings, review of enrollee utilization and complaints, and reports to the governing board. Minnesota's regulations require plan QA programs to review activities in referrals, case management, discharge planning, appointment scheduling, second opinions, prior authorization, and provider reimbursement. In addition, states are beginning to require HMOs to conduct enrollee satisfaction surveys (Dallek, Jimenez, and Schwartz, 1995).

• *External review of plan quality.* In addition to the plan's internal QA process, most states require that quality be assessed by an outside organization, such as the state agency or an approved independent organization (like a PRO or accrediting body), usually every two to three years. Some of these state laws, such as those in California and Colorado, outline the areas for the external audit, including the peer review system, grievance procedures, staff and facilities, record systems, and cost and use control systems (Dallek, Jimenez, and Schwartz, 1995).

• *Physician credentialing.* Many states require HMOs to develop minimum standards for contracting physicians, such as hospital licensure or board certification or eligibility, and a process to review credentials. Maryland has established more detailed standards, requiring HMOs to review information not only on training but also on physical and mental status, adverse hospital actions and malpractice claims, and reports from the National Practitioner Data Bank (Dallek, Jimenez, and Schwartz, 1995).

Trends in State Managed Care Regulation

Several trends are evident in state regulation of managed care plans, including movement toward comprehensive standards. Although all states have adopted a variety of insurance reforms and managed care standards over the last ten to twelve years, since 1994 the NCSL Health Policy Tracking Service reports that thirty states enacted managed care laws drawn from the American Medical Association's Patient Protection Act or the Managed Care Consumers' Bill of Rights (developed by a New York consumer advocacy group)

(Health Policy Tracking Service, 1998). The NAIC model managed care laws also are a source of recent state initiatives. In 1996 and 1997, for example, Missouri, New York, Ohio, and Texas enacted comprehensive managed care standards, and a few states—Maine, New Jersey, New Mexico, and Vermont—adopted comprehensive regulations based on general legislative authority. It seems likely that other states will adopt some or all of the NAIC models regarding quality credentialing, network adequacy, grievance resolution, and UR, and may use this opportunity to revise and update their overall managed care standards.

Some individual managed care initiatives remain popular, as the following suggest:

- The number of states with emergency department standards (such as the prudent layperson definition of emergency) quadrupled to twenty-three in 1997 (Families USA Foundation, 1998).
- The number of laws requiring plans to pay providers leaving the plan so that they continue to treat patients under a course of treatment more than doubled to thirteen in 1997 (Families USA Foundation, 1998).
- The number of states requiring HMOs to offer point-of-service (POS) plans doubled to eleven in 1997 (Health Policy Tracking Service, 1998).
- The number of states prohibiting gag clauses doubled to forty-three in 1997 (Families USA Foundation 1998).
- The number of hospital maternity length-of-stay laws increased by 40 percent (to forty-one) in 1997, even though Congress had already enacted a national law on the subject in 1996 (Health Policy Tracking Service, 1998).
- The number of laws requiring direct access to ob/gyns increased by one-third to thirty-three in 1997 (Health Policy Tracking Service, 1998).
- Thirteen states regulated hospitalization for mastectomy patients and seventeen for breast reconstructive surgery patients in 1997 (Health Policy Tracking Service, 1998).
- The number of states enacting limited versions of mental health "parity" (with physical health coverage) doubled to ten in 1997 (National Conference of State Legislatures, 1997).

Some prospects for the immediate future are as follows:

- Several states have considered HMO liability laws like the one passed in Texas (Health Policy Tracking Service, 1998), although as of this writing none had yet been enacted.
- States are also likely to consider whether to treat provider-sponsored network plans differently than other managed care plans, particularly with respect to financial requirements.
- Several of the most popular laws of 1997, such as those providing mastectomy standards, are likely to be considered by other states.
- More ERISA challenges to state managed care laws are likely, even as applied to insured plans.

Federal Activities

The federal government has little experience in actively regulating insurers in general or managed care plans in particular. The HMO Act of 1973 was less a regulatory program than a means to encourage HMO development through grants and contracts. In almost forty years of operation, the Federal Employees Health Benefits Program (FEHBP) has offered multiple health plans, including managed care plans, to federal employees, but the Office of Personnel Management (OPM), which administers the program, has not been selective in contracting with plans (Polzer, 1998). The federal government has increased its role in overseeing both general insurance and managed care plans. Under HIPAA, the federal Health Care Financing Administration (HCFA) oversees implementation of insurance market reforms in three states (California, Missouri, and Rhode Island) whose legislatures failed to enact conforming legislation in 1997. No additional appropriations were made for this purpose in fiscal year 1997. HCFA also is charged with expanding opportunities for Medicare beneficiaries to enroll in managed care plans under the Medicare+Choice program.

The U.S. Department of Labor (DoL) administers ERISA and is responsible for overseeing the provisions of HIPAA that relate to self-insured employee plans. Considering its history and resources, it is unclear how actively DoL will enforce these provisions. Because of both resource limits and its interpretation of ERISA, DoL does not pursue remedies on behalf of individual health plan participants but only on behalf of aggregate plan members (Butler and Polzer, 1996). Nor does DoL routinely review health plan documents for compliance with, for example, disclosure requirements. (Partly in recognition of this fact, in 1997 Congress repealed the requirement that employee plans submit health plan descriptions to DoL.)

Insurance Mandates

A rare example of federal health insurance benefits mandates were the requirements in the 1997 appropriations act for the Departments of Veterans' Affairs and HUD that employee health plans (both insured and self-insured) offer limited parity in coverage of mental and physical conditions and postdelivery hospitalization. The mental health provisions apply to firms with more than fifty employees and require that if the group plan imposes a lifetime or annual limit on medical benefits, mental health benefits must have no lower cap (except if the provisions would increase premiums by 1 percent or more). The maternity care amendments require all group health plans that cover childbirth to pay for at least forty-eight hours of inpatient care after normal childbirth and ninety-six hours after a cesarean section (unless the patient and attending physician agree on an earlier discharge).

Managed Care Regulation Proposals

Several proposals made in the 105th Congress would have regulated other aspects of managed care. The most comprehensive and prominent was S. 644, sponsored by Senator D'Amato, and its companion, H.R. 1415, sponsored by Congressman Norwood. The Patient Access to Responsible Care Act of 1997 (PARCA) would have amended HIPAA, setting federal standards for insured plans under the Public Health Service Act and for self-insured plans under ERISA, and preempting state laws providing less stringent standards.

PARCA would have covered a number of areas. It would have outlined standards for enrollee access to primary and specialty care; mandated emergency care coverage under the "prudent layperson" standard; prohibited provider incentive payments designed to limit medically necessary care; limited provider risk-sharing arrangements (like limits recently adopted for Medicare); mandated a POS option (for a "fair" additional premium); required direct access to specialists; prohibited gag clauses (regarding patient treatment options, utilization review requirements, and provider financial incentives); prohibited discrimination against enrollees or health professionals; established UR standards (for review decisions, reviewer qualifications, and appeals); required provider due process standards (permitting providers to apply for participation, be reviewed under objective standards, and appeal participation denials and nonrenewals); and outlined information that plans must supply to enrollees and prospective enrollees. State solvency standards would have applied.

Finally, PARCA would have amended ERISA to eliminate from preemption state suits to recover damages for personal injury caused by a health plan or its administrators. Such a law is needed to overcome a 1987 Supreme Court case (*Pilot Life Ins. Co. v. Dedeaux*) that has been held to prohibit damages claims against both insured and self-insured employee health plans (Butler, 1997). Another bill (H.R. 1960) by Congressman Norwood would have addressed only this ERISA preemption issue.

Difficult Challenges Ahead

State and federal policymakers face several difficult policy issues in the current health care delivery environment. The challenges, discussed more fully by other authors in this volume, include these:

Balancing Market Forces and Regulation

The preference of policymakers for market forces to control cost and quality must be balanced against the need for regulation to facilitate market function and calls from consumers and providers for other direct protections. The trade-offs between the conflicting desires for market forces and consumer protection have not generally been discussed in public debates about managed care regulation.

Defining Risk-Bearing Entities Subject to Regulation

Decisions need to be made about what types of organizations should be regulated, the extent to which risk-bearing providers should be regulated, whether different standards should apply, and whether provider systems that do not bear risk should be regulated (NAIC, 1997).

Considering the Role of Private Organizations

Policymakers must consider the role of private organizations that monitor and accredit health plans. For example, should health plans be required to be accredited by these organizations? Should accreditation be permitted to satisfy various government standards? Or should accreditation remain entirely separate from government oversight activities?

Determining Which Level of Government Fits the Task

Finally, policymakers need to determine the level of government most capable of establishing and enforcing standards for health plans and providers. Even aside from ERISA (which imposes substantial limits on state authority to regulate consistently across health plans because it allows states to regulate insurance but not self-insured employee plans), an important policy question is whether nationally uniform standards, if they could be developed and consistently enforced, are preferable to variations that permit response to local conditions. HIPAA offers one approach to this question, creating national standards to which states can add but not subtract and leaving primary enforcement responsibility at the state level. But other models also are possible.

References

Butler, P. *Managed Care Plan Liability: An Analysis of Texas and Missouri Legislation*. Menlo Park, Calif.: Henry J. Kaiser Family Foundation, 1997.

Butler, P. *State Managed Care Oversight: Policy Implications of Recent ERISA Court Decisions*. Washington, D.C.: Health Policy Studies Division Center for Best Practices, National Governors' Association, 1998.

Butler, P., and Polzer, K. *Private Sector Health Coverage: Variation in Consumer Protections under ERISA and State Law*. Washington, D.C.: Health Policy Forum, George Washington University, 1996.

"Consumers and Providers Lobby for State Oversight of Managed Care's Compensation Plans, Incentives." *State Health Watch*, Dec. 1996, pp. 1, 4.

Dallek, G., Jimenez, C., and Schwartz, M. *Consumer Protection in State HMO Laws*. Vol. 1: *Analysis and Recommendations*. Vol. 2: *State-by-State Summary*. Los Angeles: Center for Health Care Rights, 1995.

Families USA Foundation. *Hit and Miss: State Managed Care Laws*. Washington, D.C.: Author, 1998.

Gabel, J. R., Ginsburg, P. B., and Hunt, K. A. "Small Employers and Their Benefits: An Awkward Adolescence." *Health Affairs*, 1997, *16*, 103–110.

Health Policy Tracking Service. *Major State Health Care Policies: Fifty State Profiles, 1997*. Washington, D.C.: National Conference of State Legislatures, 1998.

Horvath, J., and Snow, K. I. *Emerging Challenges in State Regulation of Managed Care: Report on a Survey of Agency Regulation of Prepaid Managed Care Entities*. Portland, Maine: National Academy for State Health Policy, 1996.

Laudicina, S., Yerby, J., and Pardo, K. *State Legislature Health Care and Insurance Issues*. Washington, D.C.: Blue Cross–Blue Shield Association, 1998.

Mitchell, E., Pernice, C., and Riley, T. *The Health Insurance Portability and Accountability Act of 1996: A Guide for State Action*. Portland, Maine: National Academy for State Health Policy, 1997.

National Association of Insurance Commissioners. *The Regulation of Health Risk-Bearing Entities*. Washington, D.C.: Author, 1997.

National Conference of State Legislatures. "Tracking Trends: State Action on Parity Laws." *State Health Notes*, 1997, *18*(260), 7.

New Jersey Department of Health and Senior Services. *New Jersey HMOs: Performance Report*. Trenton, N.J.: Office of Managed Care, 1997.

Pollitz, K., Dallek, G., and Tàpày, N. *External Review of Health Plan Decisions: An Overview of Key Program Features in the States and Medicare*. Menlo Park, Calif.: Henry J. Kaiser Family Foundation, 1998.

Polzer, K. *The Federal Employees Health Benefits Program: What Lessons Can It Offer Policymakers?* Washington, D.C.: Health Policy Forum, George Washington University, 1998.

State of Maryland Health Care Access and Cost Commission. *Health Maintenance Organizations: A Comprehensive Performance Report*. Baltimore: Author, 1997.

U.S. General Accounting Office. *Managed Care: Explicit Gag Clauses Not Found in HMO Contracts, But Physician Concerns Remain*. HEHS publication no. 97–175. Washington, D.C.: Author, 1997.

Chapter Three

Why Should Managed Care Be Regulated?

Mark Pauly and Marc L. Berger

The economic metamorphosis of private health insurance in a little more than a decade has been accompanied by an equally amazing political transformation. Managed care went from bipartisan embrace to near-universal scorn, attacked in both state and federal capitals by populist politicians, targeted by physician associations of the left and the right, and subject to critical exposés nightly on national TV.

We share the general predisposition of most Americans toward reliance on private markets rather than government to allocate resources for the production of goods and services. Health care, of course, is fundamentally different from other goods and services, but we postulate that markets ought to drive allocation of medical care services if they function well or can be *made* to function well (assuming government makes transfers to help those unable to afford as much care as society deems appropriate).

Because state and federal governments thus far have not provided as large a transfer as needed to achieve universal health insurance coverage, the sociopolitical problem of the uninsured regrettably has not been much affected one way or another by the managed care revolution.

The users of privately financed managed care so far have been overwhelmingly the middle-class (upper and lower) nonelderly, and so it is to their welfare that we should look in evaluating the effects of managed care and possible regulatory interventions. We will not address the potential consequences of government becoming a dominant purchaser of managed care for Medicare and Medicaid beneficiaries.

Kinds of Regulation

Have markets functioned well—or are they likely to—in providing insurance and medical services to working and nonelderly Americans under the current regulatory structure? In the following discussion we consider both regulation of managed care plans and regulation of the care they manage. But first, we make a crucial distinction between two kinds of regulation: that intended to improve the flow of information to consumers, and that intended to mandate the quality of specific types of care.

Does managed care need some regulation? Our answer is a resounding yes. Regulation aimed at improving the flow of information to insurance consumers is unequivocally desirable, based either on equity or efficiency grounds. There are many things associated with buying managed care insurance that make this choice a complex one, easy to get wrong; satisfaction may be problematic even when one does make the right choice. Old-style indemnity insurance was difficult enough for consumers to choose correctly and feel good about later, because selecting insurance requires buyers to estimate how frequently illness will strike, and what their needs or preferences will be when they do get sick.

Managed care insurance is even more complex, because buyers must in addition estimate how much care they will be allowed to have in the event of each illness. The unease associated with managed care insurance is fundamental because of a perceived gap of fiduciary trust; consumers must pay up front before they know for sure what they are going to get. For this reason, information to assist and reassure choosers, and then to enforce the decisions that have been made, is *more* needed under a managed care arrangement than an indemnity one.

We would not give a blanket endorsement to regulation intended to prohibit or discourage the sales of goods or services with perceived undesirable characteristics under what might be called product quality (really, product characteristics) legislation. Such regulation, beyond standard requirements for licensure and certification, is largely unneeded when buyers are well-informed and when the market is functioning well.

Unintended Consequences of Existing Policy

However, *some* product quality regulation may be called for to offset the harmful effects of existing public policy. Some of these effects are well-known. For example, regulations requiring community rating of insurance create incentives to insurers to tailor their benefit packages to attract lower risks. This, in turn, leads to demand for regulation to prevent such "cream-skimming" provisions.

A less well-known but perhaps more important existing public policy is the tax subsidy for employment-related health insurance. This encourages the majority of citizens to obtain their health insurance in connection with their jobs, rather than purchase it directly themselves as they do other products or insurances. By distorting consumers' expectations and choices, this public policy adds to the perception of need for product quality regulation. If the distortion is not removed, more regulation of managed care may be needed.

Indeed, an important reason for the need for government intervention often is the need to offset the harmful effects of prior government policy. Rather than accept this kind of "demand inducement" for regulation—which is, of course, not unknown in the political arena—it would be better to remove the root cause of the problem instead of calling for more government to patch up its own mistakes. However, in the case of health insurance, a preferred policy by far would be the removal of this distortion due to government policy, which would diminish the need for product quality regulation in the first place.

In fact, the presence of that tax subsidization of employer-related health insurance may well be partially responsible for the strong upsurge in consumer dissatisfaction with managed care and the demand for laws and regulations intended to alleviate it. (Provider dissatisfaction is a foregone conclusion.) Thus, government policy can be harmful not only because it leads some consumers to make choices that need regulation to correct (imperfectly) but also because it leads many more consumers to believe that their situations are not the best and that regulation could improve matters, even if in reality it could not.

Misperceptions of Employees and Employers

The current policy also fosters misperceptions among employees and employers alike: workers believe the employer is giving them insurance for free so they need not care what it costs, and employers think the premiums they pay are like any other cost of production—to be ruthlessly minimized in order to maximize profits. This bad situation is compounded by the fact that consumers-employees feel they do not have truly free choice because employers make prior decisions about which insurance plan or plans to make available. It is perhaps natural to be less satisfied with a given insurance chosen for you than with the exact same insurance chosen by yourself. In another instance, people are known to be much more concerned about risk when it is imposed on them (such as when a toxic waste dump moves into the neighborhood) than when they choose dangerous activities themselves (skydiving, for example).

Differing Preferences for Coverage

However, the harm of current policy extends beyond misperceptions among employees and employers. In many circumstances, the set of workers grouped together to obtain insurance do not have identical demands and desires for insurance. In particular, they may have differing preferences for their ideal mix between low premiums and managed care restrictions. Although workers in competitive labor markets do initially make choices among jobs based on both money wages and benefits, several factors can lead to workers with different insurance demands to be grouped together. This may happen, in particular, in smaller labor markets with a limited number of groups; when worker demands and circumstances change over time; and where production requires a mix of workers with different skills that may be associated with worker characteristics that imply different demands for or valuation of insurance.

How then do employers decide which of their workers to please? The profit-maximizing, nonunionized employer chooses the level and types of benefits based on their appeal to the typical worker, who is indifferent between the job at his firm and other potential jobs and who might be called the *average marginal worker*. If all workers have equally attractive options, the employer will at least take their preferences into account. The crucial problem, however, is that some workers may be *inframarginal*, that is, they will not jump to another job even if the value of their compensation changes by a relatively large amount. Because these employees' desires will be rationally ignored by profit-maximizing employers (Pauly and Goldstein, 1976), they are likely to be the most frustrated workers, and legitimately so even if their desires were consistent and correct. In many firms, such inframarginal workers are likely to be older workers with seniority and few employment opportunities, or they may be employees of any age who have developed a chronic condition that they would like their insurance coverage to emphasize. (Interestingly, some inframarginal workers may want less insurance than the group chooses; generally, these are younger or lower-income individuals.)

Three Ingredients for Dissatisfaction

Thus, the price employees pay for lower administrative costs of group health insurance and the favorable tax treatment provided to such insurance they receive include both limits on choice and disregard for the preferences of inframarginal workers. Some groups may be willing to pay this price. However, current tax policy causes more people to get their insurance in employment-related groups than would be the case in the absence of this policy, because compensation in the form of employer payments of health insurance premiums is not taxable income for the employer and is a tax-deductible business expense for the employer.

This artificial stimulus for imposed uniformity has three important consequences, all active ingredients for dissatisfaction. First, it causes more people to choose employment-related groups that do not provide them with exactly what they want but instead cater to a sort of average of all preferences. Second, more people are in groups in which their preferences are ignored entirely because they are inframarginal. And third, more people choose employment-related groups to obtain their insurance than other types of groups that might fit them better.

These consequences create an environment in which dissatisfaction with the quality of health insurance is to be expected. However, history also plays a significant role in the mounting public frustration and disappointment with managed care. The history of health care spending and quality in the United States until around 1994 was quite simple: for privately insured individuals, quality increased each year along with expenditures. Consumers (and their employers) both praised the increasing quality and decried the "inflation," but did nothing.

In the early 1990s, things began to change. An accelerated shift to managed care of various types was accompanied by a substantial slowing in the growth rate of health insurance premiums. This slowdown in premium inflation was also accompanied, after a lag, by higher growth rates in real money wages. However, public criticism—aided by the myopia of human nature—did not disappear. Instead, it shifted from complaints about low wage growth (which politicians threatened to do something about) to complaints about the deficiencies of managed care health insurance (with the same set of office-seekers eager to help).

We believe that this "time series" change in the focus of public outrage, which contributes to the current demand for regulation, has not been fully appreciated by analysts or by workers.

Regulation for Consumer Welfare

Do these problems of mismatched preferences and bad feelings require regulatory solutions? Some managed care regulation would improve consumer welfare even in an otherwise perfect world with no tax subsidy, so we begin by describing this benchmark case and the type of regulation it would entail.

First, it must be noted that whether we are talking about health insurance or lawn mowers, consumers cannot be expected to be endowed before purchase with full knowledge about positive and negative aspects of product quality. As one of us observed some time ago (Pauly, 1978), when information is costly for consumers, the strongest case for quality regulation is for regulation that forbids products of quality (or with qualities) that no well-informed consumer would ever prefer, given a plausible range of prices. In other words, no harm is done by outlawing products the buyer would be a fool to select.

If, as is likely, buyers have different preferences, this rule tells us to forbid products of quality so low that consumers who have the lowest valid or true tastes for quality would reject them. Such regulations, if they are feasible, are beneficial, both because they prevent choices that would always be mistaken and because they eliminate the need for consumers to spend effort avoiding those choices.

This policy may still leave many other consumers sorting out products of lower quality than they (but not all consumers) would prefer. Under politics as usual, there is a possibility here for a kind of tyranny of the average, in which voters with average preferences try to legislate away the existence of all products except the ones they like—so that shopping can be less stressful for them. If this means forbidding a lower-quality but lower-cost product a minority would have preferred, too bad for the losers. However, there is no obvious endorsement for this kind of heavy-handedness, though it might sometimes be justified on aggregate cost-benefit grounds, especially if there is a small minority of consumers with tastes for very low quality. When it comes to health insurance, however, there is no evidence that this is true.

It is ultimately an empirical matter. It is not necessarily foolish to buy insurance that sends mothers home after one night's stay following an uncomplicated delivery if the premium is thereby reduced enough and if some follow-up at home is provided with the savings. The average buyer, and even the majority of all buyers, might not choose this policy, but no one can refute the hypothesis that many buyers would properly be willing to make this sacrifice in return for a lower premium.

To work perfectly, this minimum quality regulatory process requires that buyers be well informed about the quality levels above the minimum, and know (for example) that their plan does not provide certain benefits or qualities. At least some buyers have been surprised at the existence of some of the managed care restrictions that have been proposed to be regulated. Information to prevent unpleasantly surprised buyers is unequivocally desirable.

Information About Quality

The strongest argument for government regulation *and* subsidization refers, therefore, not to product quality per se but to information about product quality. Markets will never have a chance of working well unless at least some buyers are well-informed. However, this level of information may not be achieved without regulation or subsidization if information is costly. There is in theory a role for government in subsidizing information, especially the kind of information that cannot be sold at a profit.

The main problem with this proposition is not the theory but rather its application. How is the government to know what information it is efficient to subsidize? And will actual governments always choose to do the right thing? There is room for substantial improvement in efficiency here but also strong possibilities for wasting time and resources. Research to discover the information that both improves the choices people make and that would otherwise not be provided privately is key, but so far not available.

Subsidizing Versus Providing Information

It should be noted that the strongest argument gives government the role of *subsidizing* information the market would not otherwise supply but gives it no necessary role in *providing* that information. Vouchers or credits that could be used to support private entities furnishing information might be sufficient. The alternative and politically more popular approach—requiring insurance firms themselves to bear the cost of providing information—is not ideally efficient, because such requirements artificially increase the price of insurance. Furthermore, it is not necessarily desirable to have a single or monopoly source or program for information.

There is a trade-off here: whereas comparison requires consistent data, the multiple dimensions of buyers' needs and the absence of a single scientifically valid method for measuring quality argue for the variety and the discipline of market competition in the supply of information, at least for a while.

Nevertheless, we view the development and promulgation of minimum data sets as critical to providing good information to consumers and purchasers. The creation of Health Employer Data

Information Set (HEDIS) measures, and its competitors, is an important first step. Significant obstacles to the development of comprehensive health plan performance measures make this a longer-term goal, one that includes the construction of an adequate infrastructure and its significant investment costs. Government activities supporting the development and implementation of quality and performance measures may be useful, and subsidization of the market to support the investment required may solve the "spillover benefits" problem of developing information that benefits all providers.

Critical Mass of Informed Buyers

Even here there is a potential shortcut to market efficiency without complete regulation or subsidization. Efficient markets do not require every buyer to be well-informed, they just need to have a critical mass of informed buyers. For instance, if a product will be supplied only at a single quality level, all one needs is this critical mass, because the informed buyers will make sure that the only product profitable to supply on the market is of high quality.

The solution is not so easy if there ought to be several quality levels; then not all products will be of equal quality. Buyers with a high cost or a low taste for information would be well advised to acquire the products preferred by informed buyers. Picking the HMO that large firms with well-financed benefits departments choose is the wise strategy for the individual or small group; the best strategy is to say, "I'll have whatever they are having."

Specificity in Advance

The other possibility is to require plans to specify up front the conditions under which they will provide services. Consider, for example, one of the most controversial issues in medical services quality: What new or experimental products and procedures should a plan be required to provide? Rather than endorse the concept of medical necessity, a notion that is medically subjective and economically nonsensical, plans could specify or be required to specify which procedures they will follow to determine whether or not to pay for new procedures.

A plan could choose to be more skeptical, or (in its view) more prudent than others, in adopting new technology—and in return offer lower premiums. Buyers could then choose whatever options they preferred, and disputes would become matters of contract enforcement, a task for which the public sector is more suited than for legislative determination of the cost-benefit trade-off for specific medical procedures.

To sum up, the conventional theory of product quality argues most strongly for government intervention in the financing of information provision but not for rules prohibiting some types of plans. Regulations that set limits to quality levels harmful to all consumers' utility (not just their health, because lower premiums may offset discomfort) are acceptable. Even then, a requirement that limits be publicized might be preferable when it is hard to establish for certain that no one would like some limitation. Warning statements, such as "This HMO will send you home the day after a normal uncomplicated delivery" or "This HMO does not provide services where the additional cost per quality-adjusted life year added exceeds $80,000" would help. The political process under majority rule is likely to lead to overprovision of some regulations that, although good for some, are not necessary for all.

Product Quality Regulation

The simple model of the political process just described helps to explain why there might be political demand for regulations that are ultimately harmful. But the current pressure for regulation of managed care plans seems so strong and so near-universal that one suspects there is more at work than just buyer confusion and special interests. For purposes of discussion, we assume that buyers have access to good information about HMO policies and procedures (whether or not they use it) and would not impose rules on others just to benefit themselves. Instead we ask: Are there reasons why a set of buyers might choose to constrain managed care firms from offering types of plans that they themselves might in some circumstances freely and knowledgeably choose? It turns out that, for a number of reasons, the answer is yes.

Misperceptions About Trade-Offs

One reason for dissatisfaction, even among knowledgeable insurance buyers, arises because employees may not be so well-informed about other aspects of compensation, especially about wages and their relationship to benefits. A worker faced with compensation cuts, who had for many years been offered fully paid fee-for-service (FFS) insurance, may well choose substantially lower raises in money wages while retaining FFS coverage rather than accept a somewhat larger raise along with HMO coverage. But newer workers, used to less lucrative alternatives, may be willing to accept more restrictive health coverage in return for higher wages.

Dissatisfaction arises because some individuals, formerly better off, feel that they have been forced to sacrifice a benefit that they knew was worth much more to them than the managed care substitute and for which they do not feel they have been adequately compensated. Their desires may lag their reduced circumstances.

Contrast this case with one in which accurate, before-the-fact knowledge about insurance is not assumed. A high likelihood of dissatisfaction remains, but now its basis is a mirror image of the previous one. The reason for imperfect choice may not be that knowledge is available, but rather that employees do not choose to use it. It has been estimated that most employees spend less than thirty minutes deciding which health benefit option to select from among those offered by their employers. If nothing else, this indicates that most employees, as consumers of health care coverage, do not perceive that the marginal value of investing time in making a more careful choice about their health benefits is worth it.

To some extent this reflects the discounted value of potential future benefits versus that of more immediate demands on people's time. It also reflects their lack of understanding of the marginal value of different benefit packages, or their perception—perhaps based on past experience when all insurance options were very similar except for the deductible—that such differences really aren't meaningful. Consumers may retain the expectation from their Blue Cross days that whatever medical problems they might encounter will generally be covered and that the real differences between plans involve cost sharing and perhaps process issues (such as choice of physician, access to specialists, and choice of hospital).

Even when employed individuals have access to reasonably clear information comparing benefit packages, it appears that the majority make their selection largely based on their out-of-pocket costs (employee contribution to premiums, deductibles, copays), rather than differences in the quantity or quality of medical service coverage, especially because a fixed-dollar employer contribution is the exception.

Adverse Selection

Some individuals may engage in adverse selection, choosing a medical benefit package because they know that specific treatments or benefits they plan to use are provided (such as in vitro fertilization); they are clearly upset when such coverage is proposed to be rescinded. However, these individuals represent the minority of health care purchasers. Moreover, insurers often make the judgment that reductions in coverage will not negatively affect their bottom lines, indeed rescinding coverage for costly treatment targeted to a small segment of their covered population will likely improve it for a while.

Even if individuals have access to better information on the marginal value of different benefit packages, other factors mitigate against their giving such differences full consideration. Before becoming ill with any given disease, people's valuation of "higher-quality" medical care to affect outcomes positively is lower than if they become ill.

What the Experts Perceive as Quality

The dimensions of health care delivery that individuals perceive as markers of quality generally differ from those of experts. Although experts will focus on (and offer measures of) the efficiency and effectiveness of medical care (outcomes), individuals are generally more concerned with issues of access (choice of doctor, geographic location, waiting times, for example), amenities (such as facilities and parking), and customer service (staff friendliness, responsiveness to phone queries). Indeed, these issues, along with premium costs, are the most common causes for changes in HMO affiliation in employed individuals, after changes in coverage due to changing employment.

Hidden Wage Trade-Offs

Finally and most importantly, even workers well-informed about different insurance options may not see that there is a connection between the cost of this fringe benefit and their wages. They notice the new HMO, whose restrictions they mildly dislike, but they do not see that this new insurance is linked to the more generous raise they have just received. Even in the best of circumstances, the "American way" of choosing your health insurance by choosing your job is likely to lead to disconnection and dissatisfaction.

Marketplace Factors

Confusion about the value and true cost of health benefits by consumers has been reinforced by recent events in the marketplace. Intense competition among managed care providers has resulted in price competition. Insurer premium increases were deferred or were smaller than increases in costs, as insurers attempted to buy significant shares of covered lives in local markets. This was reflected in substantial declines in the average revenue per member per month, with more than half of the HMOs in the country posting financial losses in 1997.

But benefit packages remained largely unchanged during this period, making real the disconnect between premium costs and coverage. So consumers were unconcerned or unaware of the financial losses sustained by insurers. And because they have been generally aware of the real and inflationary cost increases in the overall economy, consumers have viewed the stability of health premiums and apparent benefits as one less thing to worry about. Now, however, we are seeing the eventual premium increases, and consumers are becoming more unhappy.

Two Sets of Angry Consumers

So which is it? Is the average consumer unhappy with managed care (if indeed she really is) because: (1) she thought she could save a few dollars a month without giving anything up? or (2) she knew from the start that, even with savings, the sacrifice in quality or access associated with giving up the old fee-for-service system would never be worth it?

If the former situation, the remedy is not quality regulation but improved provision of information: the message that trade-offs are (ultimately) inevitable. Also, consumers need a better choice mechanism, one that allows them to spend more on insurance if they wish and to see the connection between the insurance they get and the amount of money they have to spend on other things. If the latter is the case, then we are left with the puzzle of why there should appear to be a "missing market" in high-quality, high-convenience, high-cost plans.

Both sets of angry consumers have converged on hapless HMOs. The most important role for regulation, in our view, is to address the cause of the missing markets—the most important of which is the tax treatment of employer payments for health insurance—rather than the symptoms of outrage and dissatisfaction.

Mismatching Informed Consumers

We now consider these arguments in somewhat more detail. First, even if every consumer is both rational and well-informed, there may still exist a subset of this group with a legitimate gripe against HMOs.

Such a result would seem implausible. In well-functioning markets, with many sellers and many buyers, the market should supply consumers what they want. People often choose lower-quality products because they are cheaper, and they do not usually complain when they get what they expect. So if people prefer more restrictive but less costly HMOs to less restrictive but more costly plans, should they not complain about the restrictions or expect a sympathetic response if they do complain? But this story of unimpeded individual choice does not match the situation of many American workers when it comes to health insurance. They do not buy it directly but instead receive payment for at least part of the premium as a portion of their compensation. Once they have chosen to work for a particular firm, they have a strong incentive to take the insurance plan or plans the firm offers.

We do not want to exaggerate here: if my employer pays part of my compensation as the premium for an HMO I hate, I could refuse to join (or use) that HMO and instead take my after-tax wages and enroll in the plan I like. Although this dropout option in principle sets a boundary to how bad off I can be under my current benefit offering, there is virtually no evidence of people rejecting group health plans and buying individual plans when the employer pays the full premium. So HMOs must not be *that* bad. Indeed, this view is consistent with the results of the Kaiser Family Foundation–Harvard University National Survey of Americans' Views on Consumer Protections in Managed Care (1998). According to this study, although many Americans have experienced problems with their managed care plans, only a minority would support a consumer bill of rights if it either resulted in increased insurance premiums or caused some employers to drop health coverage for their workers.

There is accumulating evidence that when people pay part of the premium themselves (an amount they can retain in cash if they refuse to join), more employees choose not to have any employer-paid insurance. Whether they then select another plan or remain uninsured is not known, but one suspects that the latter is more common.

Why Not Offer What Employees Want?

But suppose most employees decide the HMO (paid for by the employer) is better than nothing; it is easy to see why they still could be vocal about wanting something different. But this presents a problem: Why wouldn't the employer then offer them the plan they like rather than one they like less? Except in Hawaii, the employer is under no obligation to offer any benefit at all; if the employer does voluntarily go to the trouble of arranging benefits, why not select something employees like?

There are two answers to this rhetorical question, one common but nonsensical, the other rational but subtle. The answer the employer commonly gives: "I am trying to hold down my benefits costs, and what the employees want is too expensive." This is an illogical answer for two reasons: First, if employees all prefer a more expensive plan to the one currently offered, it makes sense for the employer to spend the same contribution on the plan the employees really like and let *them* pay any additional premium. If they refuse, they must not like it that much. Second, as economists argue, the money paid by the employer is not ultimately a cost to the employer; instead, it is paid by the employee in the form of lower cash wage (Pauly, 1997). So a solution would be to offer the more costly plan, take the extra premiums out of future raises, and even keep the employee premium share (and the tax breaks) the same. The conclusion is that if all employees actually value (in the sense of willingness to sacrifice wages) a more costly plan, sensible employers ought to be delighted to supply it. This theoretical conclusion may be frustrated by thickheaded or paternalistic benefits managers, by misinformed employees, or by silo thinking within the firm—but it shouldn't be.

There is another more serious problem, however. Employees are different. Some probably do like the current restrictive HMO, because they like the lower employee premium or the higher cash wages it allows them to have. However, others prefer a less restrictive plan, where "prefer" means they would choose a wage level reduced by the higher premium of the less restrictive plan to higher wages and a more restrictive offering. An essential aspect of group insurance is that not all participants can get what they want. The argument implies they should, nevertheless, not complain because they really prefer the lower administrative costs and higher wages associated with one-size-fits-all insurance to the more costly custom-tailored solution.

Tax Subsidy Undermines the Arrangement

The foregoing would be the case if two conditions were also true: workers understood the deal they had made and the deal was actually in their interest. The tax subsidy undermines each. Take the last argument first. The preferences of workers at a firm may be said to have been considered in the deal if they had many good alternatives to working at this firm. Give them a package they do not like, and they will walk. The key insight, however, is that some workers may not have this alternative, or (more precisely) may have an alternative that is less attractive at the margin.

The Ignored Worker

Consider the following example. Suppose a firm is going to offer only one insurance plan that it will fully pay for and that plans that are more restrictive in variety of providers and coverage of less-than-essential services (in vitro fertilization, long-term psychotherapy, long hospital stays) are less costly. Call this dimension *quality*. At some high initial level of quality, the firm could lower the premium cost by cutting quality, but doing so would reduce the value of the compensation package to its employees. For some employees, the marginal value of this reduction will be low, whereas for others it will be high. If the firm nevertheless reduces quality, it will have to increase money wages to retain its workforce. Thus, the firm faces a trade-off between benefits quality (and premiums) and money wages. What level of quality will it choose?

Employers always have problems reconciling different desires or values among their employees, especially when other employers are also making changes. There will be difficulties as long as employees with different preferences are grouped together, even if all preferences are taken into account. Some will be more pleased than others. An especially serious difficulty occurs if all workers are not equally responsive to changes in the value of the compensation package. If there are some who are less responsive than average *and* if the valuation of insurance is correlated with the degree of responsiveness, some workers' preferences will not be properly taken into account.

For instance, if workers with seniority, workers with strong attachment to their neighborhoods and their jobs, or high-risk workers subject to job-lock place higher-than-average value on quality but will quit in proportionately fewer numbers than others if quality is reduced, their desires will carry less weight than their presence in the firm's workforce implies. It is important to note that their desires will be ignored even if they dominate the workforce; if younger, healthier, risk-loving workers have more and better employment options, it will be *their* preferences, not those of the trapped or inframarginal workers, that the profit-maximizing employer will respond to.

It is then only a small step to imagine that these ignored workers, frustrated by the failure of their benefits department to pay attention to them, become sympathetic to or even lobby for regulation to inhibit low quality. Indeed, from a longer time perspective, all of us—even if we are young and putatively immortal now—should favor such rules, because becoming inframarginal could happen to anyone.

The problem is not group insurance per se; the problem is linking the insurance choice decision with employment choices, with the result of discrimination against workers unlucky enough to end up with few employment choices. Had these workers bought their insurance in some other way—either individually or as members of some other kind of group, such as professional associations or fraternal organizations—at least their preferences would be taken into account under majority rule. They still might not get exactly what they want, but at least they would not be ignored.

But if employment-based insurance leads to this kind of inefficiency, why do people participate in it in the first place? The answer is simple: it is a cheaper way to buy insurance, and the key point here is that it is made *artificially* cheaper by the tax subsidy. Tax breaks bribe workers into getting their insurance in this fashion, insurance that is very likely to leave them frustrated and angry. Remove the tax subsidy, cut tax rates so people get the money back, and they will be better off because they will be more likely to get the insurance they want.

A Guarantee of Conflict

Now consider the first assumption stated earlier: that workers understand the deal they made. The employee notes the nice wages and the less attractive benefits at his firm, but he may not see the connection between them. By encouraging the erroneous belief that the employer chooses and pays for health insurance, the tax subsidy virtually guarantees conflict. Moreover, the fact that this subsidy only applies to employment-based group insurance—not to all group insurance—promotes a grouping mechanism that is probably not the one that minimizes conflict. It thus guarantees that there will be some households willing to offer a negative opinion of their insurance (even while acknowledging it was the best deal they could find) than with other methods of grouping.

There is another distortion associated with the tax subsidy. Managed care controls cost by means of supply-side limits and incentives. Indemnity insurance controls cost by increasing patient cost sharing. Some consumers prefer one method to the other. However, the tax system does not treat these two methods equally.

In particular, if total spending is limited similarly by a managed care plan and by a catastrophic indemnity plan, the latter will receive a lesser subsidy than the former. Here again, the tax system subsidizes the kind of insurance most likely to generate complaints.

Managed care operates to limit what the patient and doctor can agree on, either directly through guidelines and protocols or indirectly through incentives to the doctor to limit overall services to a covered population. This allows the patient to avoid much of the dreaded patient cost sharing that was the primary way old-style insurance tried to keep the lid on costs, but it also provides a recipe for conflict. The amount of care (or the quality) the consumer as patient will want when it is free will be greater than the amount the consumer as insurance-premium-payer will want to see provided. Before the fact, people want their managed care plan to charge them low premiums, and they may be willing to accept prospective limits on the care they receive as an evil necessary to produce those low premiums. After the fact, when they get sick, they will protest if the plan tries to hold back.

As we have seen, current tax incentives cause workers to choose insurance that is more restrictive and less well-matched to their preference than ought to occur. However, the people who make these distorted choices are not, with the exception of the infra-marginal workers, forced into them; they are rewarded with lower taxes. The choices are, nevertheless, inefficient because those persons would have preferred the same tax break (which leaves the rest of us no worse off) *and* different insurance. It is not job-based insurance per se that ought to go, but rather tax-induced *excessive* job-basing of the health insurance choice.

Even going beyond economic arguments, we can see that employees who were bribed into making the wrong choice will be more likely to complain about it. After all, they can see what they would really like better—the same low taxes but the health plan they want. Because they are hardly likely to give back their tax break, they may complain that their plan is not the choice they would make. The same is true to an even greater extent for the trapped inframarginal workers. These people may have recognized, years earlier when they chose a career with a company that pays on the basis of seniority, that they might eventually become trapped. But that is an easy lesson to forget when your managed care plan refuses to allow an MRI for your sore shoulder or knee, and instead tries to talk you into exercising first.

What Should Be Done?

Would the best way out of this sorry mess be to abolish employment-based insurance entirely? Such an extreme measure is both inappropriate and unnecessary. There are benefits to many in using the employment group as a way of obtaining insurance, both in the form of lower administrative costs and in terms of implicit protection of the insured worker against unexpected surges in nongroup premiums that might accompany the random onset of chronic conditions. (Whether alternatives might also provide such protection remains an open question.)

Although not recommending a specific solution, we believe three general kinds of changes are needed.

Better Information

Information should include measures of the performance and "quality" of services provided by a managed care plan, as well as information about how providers are incentivized. Consumers should have sufficient information on the health plans' actual practice patterns to permit analysis of the relationship between incentives and what care is delivered. Developing uniform sets of performance measures to provide benchmarks and promote the development of standards for both quality and incentives would help, although it would be undesirable to prohibit other arrangements some buyers might like. Instead, we should ensure that the deviation from the standard is flagged for the buyer in big bold print. Government should play a productive role in subsidizing the development of these standards and measures, but maybe a less productive role in regulating them. As it becomes a significant purchaser of managed care services for Medicare, government may wish to pursue this role in its narrow self-interest.

In addition to providing information about the specific product, government could help even more by offering wise counsel about managed care in general, alerting managed care consumers to the inconvenient but important fact that, compared with the traditional Blue Cross insurance, they will be sometimes giving something up to get this bargain. Managed care has suffered as much from being oversold by its advocates as it has from being overcriticized by its opponents. A welcome relief would be a true consumer report that tells consumers to expect to give up something in exchange for lower premiums.

Further, workers need information about consequences. Telling them they are getting employer payments for health benefits in lieu of wages or other benefits, and requiring employers to quantify what this cost is, would be a major step to better understanding. Of course, what a plan costs the employer can be either greater or less than its value to the worker, so some quantification of each plan's monetary value (as well as its cost) to various types of consumers would be valuable.

Tax Credit

We also need to do something about the government-created source of the problem. The current policy could be replaced with a tax credit of predetermined value, made available to all who obtain insurance regardless of the method (Pauly and Goodman, 1995). This step should not lead to the demise of any group insurance that is worth what it costs but would prevent excessive "grouping" of insurance purchasers. It would probably lead some small firms with heterogeneous workforces—who can only offer administratively costly group insurance because of the tax break—to change. They would drop coverage and pay employees cash instead. It might well also lead to the emergence of group insurance provided by other types of organizations (such as the AARP or TIAA-CREF), the same types of organizations that now quite effectively provide portable group life and pension insurance.

Groups That Need Protection

Finally, no matter whether the tax treatment is modified anytime soon, our analysis shows which groups need regulation of product quality and which do not. People in HMOs chosen from a wide range of options (federal government employees, as a prime example) and with state-of-the-art information, do not need to be subject to product quality regulation or "consumer protection" laws. In contrast, those who work in small firms that only offer one tax-subsidized HMO to deliver a tax break might need help. The implication here—that product quality regulation, if it is to be present at all, should be strong in nonchoice settings but can be minimal when choices are present—is very important.

References

"Henry J. Kaiser Family Foundation–Harvard University National Survey of Americans' Views on Consumer Protections in Managed Care." Menlo Park, Calif.: Kaiser Family Foundation, January 1998.

Pauly, M. V. "Is Medical Care Different?" In W. Greenberg (ed.), *Competition in the Health Care Sector: Past Present and Future.* Germantown, Md.: Aspen Systems Corp., 1978.

Pauly, M. V. *Health Benefits at Work: An Economic and Political Analysis of Employment-Related Health Insurance.* Ann Arbor: University of Michigan Press, 1997.

Pauly, M. V., and Goldstein, G. S. "Group Health Insurance as a Local Public Good." In R. Rosett (ed.), *The Role of Health Insurance in the Health Services Sector.* New York: National Bureau of Economic Research, 1976.

Pauly, M. V., and Goodman, J. "Tax Credits for Health Insurance and Medical Savings Accounts." *Health Affairs,* 1995, *14*(1), 125–139.

Chapter Four

Macro- Versus Microregulation

Thomas Rice

Economic theory holds that if certain assumptions are met, then allowing markets to operate free of government interference will result in a state called *pareto optimality*. This is a state in which it is impossible to make someone better off without making someone else worse off. This is generally thought of as an "efficient" state of the world. *Efficiency* so defined, however, is only one measure of overall social welfare. The other is the public's satisfaction with the distribution of resources that results from reliance on markets, which is often referred to as *equity*. What assumptions must be met to ensure that a competitive market will lead to the highest possible levels of social welfare, which includes both efficiency and equity considerations?

Of fifteen assumptions (listed in Exhibit 4.1), fourteen are related to economic efficiency and one is related to equity. None of them is met in health care markets (Rice, 1998). So theory does not provide a justification for reliance on markets to improve efficiency in health care or to assure equity. Rather, such questions must be answered by examining each policy choice, compiling information on its expected effects, and drawing conclusions about the policy measures that will result in the highest gain in social welfare.

What has been missing in much past analysis is consideration of the range of assumptions necessary. It is well known, for example, that markets may fail to be efficient in the presence of a monopoly, or when consumers do not have good information. But

Exhibit 4.1. Assumptions Necessary for a Competitive Market to Optimize Social Welfare.

1. There are no negative externalities of consumption.
2. There are no positive externalities of consumption.
3. Consumer tastes are predetermined.
4. A person is the best judge of his or her own welfare.
5. Consumers have sufficient information to make good choices.
6. Consumers know, with certainty, the results of their consumption decisions.
7. Individuals are rational.
8. Individuals reveal their preferences through their actions.
9. Social welfare is based solely on individual utilities, which in turn are based solely on the goods and services consumed.
10. Supply and demand are independently determined.
11. Firms do not have any monopoly power.
12. Firms maximize profits.
13. There are not increasing returns to scale.
14. Production is independent of the distribution of wealth.
15. The distribution of wealth is approved of by society.

Source: Rice, 1998.

many other assumptions have been ignored. Just four are noted here:

• If people care not only about what goods and services they consume but also how this consumption compares with that of other people (Assumption 1), then markets, which often lead to the production of more goods but not their equitable distribution, can lead to lower social welfare if those not receiving the fruits of higher productivity object to their worsened relative status (Robbins, 1984; Bator, 1963). In health markets, this can occur if new technologies are developed that can save lives but are affordable only to well-to-do patients (Reinhardt, 1992).

• If people's tastes are determined by their environment and experiences rather than being fully endemic to them (Assumption 3), then markets may produce products that are not what people really want (Pollak, 1978). Instead, markets may produce what people are used to (the status quo), what they are addicted to, or what advertisers wish them to purchase. In the health care area, preventive services might be underproduced compared with medical technologies, for example.

• If people do not act rationally (Assumption 7), then the choices they make in the marketplace may not be the ones that will benefit them most. Much research has shown that people tend to engage in "cognitive dissonance"—that is, they make choices not rationally but rather for self-justification. This may, for example, lead them to underestimate the risk of (or overemphasize the pleasure derived from) cigarette smoking (Aronson, 1972) or to save too little money for old age because they do not wish to contemplate their diminished capacity to earn or function independently (Akerlof and Dickens, 1992).

• If people do not reveal their preferences through their actions (Assumption 8), then we do not know whether the things they choose are the ones they prefer (Sen, 1982, 1992). For example, a person's decision not to contribute to a charity aimed at improving the health of poor people might not be the result of a preference to spend the money on himself. Rather, it might be because he believes others might "free-ride" on his donation (Nath, 1969).

Thus, the overwhelming degree to which health services deviate from the assumptions of a competitive market makes it impossible to support the position that free market policies will necessarily be superior to regulated markets. In some instances free market policies may be better than government intervention, but such a belief can only come from examining particular experiences, not from economic theory.

Opinions about the proper role of government change with the times. During the 1960s and 1970s much of the U.S. public believed government should play a large role in the operation of markets. However, since the Reagan administration in the 1980s there has been an increasing belief that markets are good and government involvement is not; in the health arena and more broadly, markets are viewed as "efficient" and government "inefficient." Although no one is eschewing government involvement altogether, as Robert Kuttner (1997) has written, "America . . . is in one of its cyclical romances with a utopian view of laissez-faire" (p. 4). There is concern that economic theory is being used inappropriately to support further market-based policies in health care.

Micro- and Macroregulation

Regulation may be classified in different ways. One way is to demonstrate how regulatory strategies have changed over time. In such a schema, the first regulatory policies were primarily antitrust. These were followed by "old-style" regulations, such as controlling the prices charged in particular industries (natural gas, for example), which gave way in turn to "new wave" regulations, focusing on such things as consumer information and safety that cut across industries (Gordon, 1994). Another way to categorize regulation is to focus on its intent. For example, one recent text divides regulations into three categories: supply altering, demand altering, and price-output altering (Goff, 1996).

In this discussion, we take a somewhat different tack, first defining the term *regulate*. Four alternative definitions are given in *The American Heritage College Dictionary* (1997): (1) to control or direct according to rule, principle, or law; (2) to adjust to a particular specification or requirement; (3) to adjust for accurate and proper functioning; (4) to put or maintain in order.

The first definition—which implies government exerting control over a market through direct control of individual decisions—is the one most commonly used in the field of regulatory policy in general and health policy in particular. The other three definitions imply something different: making adjustments to improve performance. In health care, these definitions suggest a more indirect role for government—setting certain ground rules to meet societal goals, which, although influencing individual decisions, are less intrusive. In this discussion, the first kind of regulation—more direct—is referred to as *micro* and the second—less direct kind of regulation—as *macro*.

It must be stressed that regulation can come out of both government and markets. Consider a situation in which an individual practice association (IPA) attempts to control costs by such processes as requiring preadmission certification of hospital stays, requiring second opinions for surgery, using a formulary for pharmaceuticals, and profiling its physicians' practices and letting them know that exceedingly high costs will result in their expulsion from the plan. This seems to fit with the micro definition of regulation—"to control or direct according to rule, principle, or law."

Which types of regulation would be considered macro and which micro? Although there is some danger in generalizing, policies aimed at putting controls on prices or expenditures tend to be more macro in nature, whereas those targeting specific services provided are more micro. Consider the equation $E = P \times Q$, where E is expenditures, P is price, and Q is quantity. If controls are put on prices—by setting a maximum amount that physicians can charge Medicare, for example—the effect on providers is indirect. They are not told what services to provide; rather, they make their own decisions, based in part on the regulated prices. This is also true of most regulations on expenditures. For example, Part B of Medicare has expenditure controls based on volume performance standards; these standards do not tell physicians what services they can provide but control how much money is spent in the aggregate. In both cases the regulation is less intrusive because it is indirect.

Quantity Controls

Contrast the foregoing with the many controls put on quantity, which, interestingly, are more common in the private than the public sector. Among the standard quantity controls are utilization management tools, such as preadmission certification for hospital stays. Most insurers require that patients obtain permission from the insurer before they can be covered for a hospital stay. This is an example of microregulation because permission must be granted in each instance. It involves, at a minimum, having a provider contact the insurer and talk with a representative about whether the stay will be allowed. If there is disagreement, appeals can be initiated, which in turn can result in a very large administrative effort.

Similarly, most managed care companies now require that a patient must be referred by a primary care physician to receive coverage for specialist services. To determine whether this has occurred, an insurer must examine every case. And the patient may very well appeal a denial, which results in another cycle of administrative costs. Both are instances of more intrusive and administratively intense microregulation. Although these examples of microregulation are from the private sector, government can and does also engage in such activities.

Global Budgets

Most of the regulations used in other countries fall into the macro category. The most prominent example is the use of global budgets, which has been defined as follows: "prospectively set caps on spending for some portion of the health care industry" (Wolfe and Moran, 1993, p. 55). The exact meaning, however, varies from country to country. In Canada, for example, hospitals are paid a global budget by their provincial governments to cover their annual variable costs. Once this budget is established, hospitals are free to practice as they wish; there is little oversight of the appropriateness of each admission.

Similarly, most European countries employ global budgets, not necessarily for hospital care but for health expenditures in general. A survey of nine European nations revealed that all used some form of global budgeting. Most studies have found them to be helpful in controlling health care spending (Wolfe and Moran, 1993; U.S. General Accounting Office, 1991; Abel-Smith, 1992). Global budgets tend to be implemented on a regional level and are used in conjunction with other macroregulations, such as rationing the diffusion of medical technologies (Jonsson, 1989).

Increase in Microregulation

It is ironic that as the U.S. health care system has become more reliant on the market the amount of regulation has increased dramatically, mostly from the private sector itself. Studies have documented the high cost of administering the system (Evans, 1990). In fact, since 1980, when competitive strategies were starting to be introduced, the cost of administering the U.S. health care system (both private and public) has risen considerably faster than overall health care expenditures (Levit et al., 1998).

Two related forces have driven this increase in microregulation carried out by the private sector. The first is capitation. Health plans that receive a capitation payment from employers need to find ways to control expenditures by providers. Although some of the strategies might be viewed as more macro (physician payment incentives, for example), others are micro (such as utilization management techniques). This alone, however, cannot explain the increase in private microregulation.

Historically, health plans have received a fixed payment per year from employers and thus have had an incentive to control their costs. Something else must also be driving this trend. The second driver is increased competition. In the past, health plans found that if they underestimated their costs they could simply raise employer premiums the next year. This is no longer so easy, because other health plans are providing strong price competition. Therefore, health plans have been forced to control their costs—often through the microregulatory tools discussed earlier.

Capitation

Government should intervene in the marketplace when it can do a better job than markets in achieving social goals. But how should government's role be affected by managed care's increasing domination of the health care environment? What types of regulations—whether generated by government or markets—are likely to arise, and what impacts can we anticipate from them?

Let us consider the sorts of problems that can arise in the private managed care markets, which tend to be characterized by capitation. The term *capitation* often is used rather broadly. It is useful to consider the two different points at which capitation occurs in the system, because each has its own implications for regulatory policy.

First, health plans are capitated by employers. In general, employers pay health plans a fixed fee per enrollee per time period; plans that spend more per enrollee incur losses, whereas those spending less achieve gains. Second, providers—particularly physicians—are often capitated by health plans. These physicians are financially at risk when they provide extra services or referrals.

Capitation of Health Plans

In most urban areas, a number of health plans compete to attract enrollees. To win the competition, they must first attract employers to offer their plans; if successful, they must then attract employees to choose their particular plan.

In the past it was believed that employees were not terribly sensitive to changes in health plan premiums (Holmer, 1984). No longer: recent study shows that only a few dollars' difference in premiums can lead to substantial changes in plan choices during annual open-enrollment periods (Buchmueller and Feldstein, 1997). Plans that charge more have difficulty competing. These pressures on premiums are almost certainly most intensive in IPA/network model HMOs, which, because they often tend to have largely the same provider panel, may be viewed by consumers as interchangeable.

If health plans have to compete by providing lower prices, they must find ways to cut costs. They can attempt to do so through a variety of mechanisms: *controlling unit prices* (shifting the financial risk to providers, for example), *controlling quantities* (such as required use of primary care gatekeepers before referrals, preadmission certification of hospital stays and surgery, or pharmaceutical formularies), and *controlling expenditures* (such as directly attempting to obtain a favorable selection of patients).

It is still too early to know definitively how these capitation incentives (coupled with increased competition) are affecting overall quality of care and consumer satisfaction. Study findings vary, although one fairly common pattern is lower scores among those with chronic conditions as well as the poor (Ware et al., 1986; Ware et al., 1996). The recent outcry against HMOs and managed care suggests that the methods being used by managed care plans to control costs are becoming less tolerated by the public. As a result, in March 1997 President Clinton formed the Advisory Commission on Consumer Protection and Quality in the Health Care Industry. Later that year, the commission proposed the Consumer Bill of Rights and Responsibilities, the theme of which is that measures must be taken to overcome the natural inclination of capitated health plans to underprovide services.

In discussions regarding consumer rights and their health plans, policymakers put much emphasis on providing consumers with information about health plan performance as well as the incentives faced by the provider panel. The former includes scores on consumer satisfaction, clinical quality outcomes, and service performance such as waiting times. The latter includes disclosure of any ownership or financial arrangements between providers, provider groups, and health plans, including the method by which individual physicians are compensated and the types of financial incentives that apply.

Although requiring plans to provide this information makes sense (good information is a prerequisite for a market to operate successfully) it inevitably would result in a great deal of microregulation. Health plans, under pressure to produce "good" numbers on their quality and satisfaction scores, would be tempted to fudge (at best) or misreport their scores. Therefore, some quasi-regulatory body would have to conduct detailed audits of claims, medical records, and survey results to ensure that the information provided to consumers is accurate. Figuratively speaking, someone would have to stand over the health plan's shoulder at all times. Even more microregulation would be required to monitor the provision of services.

Capitation of Providers

The second major point at which capitation occurs in the system is capitation of providers, particularly physicians, in managed care plans. Although such capitation is not universal, the trend is in that direction. Some of the most recently published data go back to 1994, so they provide a low estimate of its prevalence. This study, by Marsha Gold and colleagues (1995), found that 84 percent of IPA/network model HMOs shared financial risk with primary care physicians and 54 percent with specialists. In two-thirds of the cases, primary care physicians were capitated by the health plan.

There is some limited evidence to indicate that putting providers at financial risk results in the provision of fewer services (Stearns, Wolfe, and Kindig, 1992; Ogden, Carlson, and Bernstein,

1990; Mooney, 1994), although no studies have directly assessed how these incentives affect quality. The incentives themselves, however, are quite worrisome. To quote Marc Rodwin (1993):

> Society makes a statement about the role of physicians when it provides incentives for them to help government or health care organizations reduce their costs. This is especially so if there are no equivalent financial incentives for physicians to improve quality of care. By using financial incentives to change the clinical practice of physicians, society calls forth self-interested behavior. In asking physicians to consider their own interest in deciding how to act, we alter the attitude we want physicians ideally to have. For if physicians act intuitively to promote their patients' interests, we will worry less that they will behave inappropriately. But if their motivation is primarily self-interest, we will want their behavior to be monitored more carefully [p. 153].

In that regard, the Consumer Bill of Rights and Responsibilities recommends that health care providers do the following:

- Discuss all treatment options with a patient in a culturally competent manner
- Discuss all current treatments and their alternatives, including risks, benefits, and consequences
- Allow patients to express preferences about future treatments
- Disclose to consumers such things as compensation methods and ownership or financial interests in health facilities by providers

Carrying out such a mandate would assure that the incentives of capitation do not lead to the underprovision of care, but it involves the kind of oversight of the interaction between the doctor and the patient that epitomizes microregulation.

Implications

The foregoing discussion has some disturbing implications, which can be summarized as follows:

- Allowing market forces to control health care has resulted in a situation where health plans and providers are at substantial financial risk if costs are not controlled.

- The predominant incentive is to underprovide services.
- Private health plans must resort to expensive and intrusive microregulation in order to ensure that providers act to control costs.
- Government must further engage in microregulatory policies to ensure that consumers receive good quality of care.

The peculiar evolution of the American medical system has resulted in a situation where both businesses and government must engage in expensive and intrusive regulation. Health plans use regulation to ensure that they compete on the basis of cost; government uses regulation to ensure that quality is not compromised through market competition. Short of wholesale reorganization of health care financing so that the underprovision of services is not rewarded, the tensions described here are only likely to escalate.

References

Abel-Smith, B. "Cost Containment and New Priorities in the European Community." *Milbank Quarterly*, 1992, *70*, 393–422.

Akerlof, G. A., and Dickens, W. T. "The Economic Consequences of Cognitive Dissonance." *American Economic Review*, 1992, *72*, 307–319.

American Heritage College Dictionary. Boston: Houghton Mifflin, 1997.

Aronson, E. *The Social Animal.* New York: Freeman, 1972.

Bator, F. M. "The Anatomy of Market Failure." *Quarterly Journal of Economics*, 1963, *53*, 351–379.

Buchmueller, T. C., and Feldstein, P. J. "The Effect of Price on Switching Among Health Plans." *Journal of Health Economics*, 1997, *16*, 231–247.

Evans, R. G. "Tension, Compression, and Shear: Directions, Stresses, and Outcomes of Health Care Cost Control." *Journal of Health Politics, Policy, and Law*, 1990, *15*, 101–128.

Goff, B. *Regulation and Macroeconomic Performance.* Norwell, Mass.: Kluwer, 1996.

Gold, M. R., Hurley, R., Lake, T., Ensor, T., and Berenson, R. "A National Survey of the Arrangements Managed-Care Plans Make with Physicians." *New England Journal of Medicine*, 1995, *333*(25), 1678–1683.

Gordon, R. L. *Regulation and Economic Analysis.* Norwell, Mass.: Kluwer, 1994.

Holmer, M. "Tax Policies and the Demand for Health Insurance." *Journal of Health Economics*, 1984, *3*, 203–221.

Jonsson, B. "What Can Americans Learn from Europeans?" *Health Care Financing Review*, 1989, *11*(supplement), 79–109.

Kuttner, R. *Everything for Sale: The Virtues and Limits of Markets.* New York: Knopf, 1997.

Levit, K. R., Lazenby, H. C., Braden, B. R., and the National Health Accounts Team. "National Health Spending Trends in 1996." *Health Affairs*, 1998, *17*(1), 35–51.

Mooney, G. *Key Issues in Health Economics.* New York: Harvester Wheatsheaf, 1994.

Nath, S. K. *A Reappraisal of Welfare Economics.* New York: Routledge, 1969.

Ogden, D., Carlson, R., and Bernstein, G. "The Effect of Primary Care Incentives." Proceedings of the 1990 Group Health Institute, Group Health Association of America, Washington, D.C., 1990.

Pollak, R. A. "Endogenous Tastes in Demand and Welfare Analysis." *American Economic Review*, 1978, *68*, 374–379.

Reinhardt, U. E. "Reflections on the Meaning of Efficiency: Can Efficiency Be Separated from Equity?" *Yale Law & Policy Review*, 1992, *10*, 302–315.

Rice, T. *The Economics of Health Reconsidered.* Chicago: Health Administration Press, 1998.

Robbins, L. "Politics and Political Economy." In *An Essay on the Nature and Significance of Economic Science.* (3rd. ed.) Old Tappan, N.J.: Macmillan, 1984.

Rodwin, M. A. *Medicine, Money, and Morals: Physicians' Conflicts of Interest.* New York: Oxford University Press, 1993.

Sen, A. *Choice, Welfare, and Measurement.* Oxford, England: Blackwell, 1982.

Sen, A. *Inequality Revisited.* Cambridge, Mass.: Harvard University Press, 1992.

Stearns, S., Wolfe, B., and Kindig, D. "Physician Responses to Fee-for-Service and Capitation Payment." *Inquiry*, 1992, *29*, 416–425.

U.S. General Accounting Office. *Health Care Spending Control: The Experience of France, Germany, and Japan.* Washington, D.C.: Author, 1991.

Ware, J. E., Jr., and others. "Comparison of Health Outcomes at a Health Maintenance Organization with Those of Fee-for-Service Care." *The Lancet*, May 3, 1986, pp. 1017–1022.

Ware, J. E., Jr., and others. "Differences in 4-Year Health Outcomes for Elderly and Poor, Chronically Ill Patients Treated in HMO and Fee-for Service Systems: Results from the Medical Outcomes Study." *Journal of the American Medical Association*, 1996, *276*, 1039–1047.

Wolfe, P. R., and Moran, D. W. "Global Budgeting in the OECD Countries." *Health Care Financing Review*, 1993, *14*(3), 55–76.

Regulatory Issues

As opposed to the broad perspective on regulation provided in Section One, this second section focuses on specific regulatory measures. Consumer choice, rights of grievance and appeal, access to services, standards of quality, and health plan liability are the topics addressed.

Uwe Reinhardt begins this section by observing that the consumer choice model of managed competition has thus far failed to emerge. He notes that a public that previously rejected government intervention in health care has now changed its mind as consumers find their choices circumscribed by "private health care regulators." In theory, he points out, purchasers were supposed to be presented with a variety of competitive health plans and sufficient information to make informed choices. But neither the choice nor the information has been made available to most consumers. Reinhardt urges public funding to support research and development of health performance measures. He suggests that government support is needed to organize the provision of information on quality measures and consumer satisfaction into a kind of farmers market similar to that envisioned by the architects of managed competition.

Advocates for consumer protection often recommend establishing an ombudsman program to help consumers deal with a complex and fast-changing health care system. William Benson is an expert on the long-term care ombudsman program and recommends it as a model for the health care industry. Benson identifies the most important features of the long-term care program, and explains why these features should be incorporated into a health industry model. He points out that an ombudsman would not substitute for a regulator, but would act as a complement to other forms of regulation. He cautions that without such a program, many patients may never avail themselves of their rights of grievance and appeal and other consumer protections discussed in this book.

Brian Biles and David Sandman address the issue of access to care for managed care patients. They cite several studies showing that managed care patients are concerned about their access to specialists and emergency room care and also about waiting times and time spent with their physicians. Pointing out that access problems have arisen from the financial incentives engendered by managed care, they recommend a three-pronged strategy to confront the problem: provision of publicly available information on measures of access; government regulation specifying minimum standards for access (such as the number, mix, and distribution of providers per enrollee); and private voluntary regulation to assure the adequacy of provider networks.

William Roper addresses the role of regulation in health care quality. He contrasts consumer protection with quality improvement and observes that although government has had a fundamental role in the former, its involvement in the latter has been somewhat rare. Roper cautions that the need for government regulation must be balanced with the necessity to encourage clinical innovation. He identifies a role for regulation in measuring and disseminating information on clinical quality, establishing and enforcing clinical standards, and encouraging internal quality improvement processes. In each area, however, he discusses a necessary but delicate balance between government and private regulation and between voluntarism and mandates.

The final two chapters in this section address managed care liability and the Employee Retirement Income Security Act of 1974, commonly known as ERISA. David Keepnews frames the general issues of whether managed care organizations (MCOs) should be held liable for their coverage and treatment decisions. He explains how the ERISA exemption has shielded MCOs from legal liability and denied remedies to some consumers. He reviews recent actions by states and proposed legislation at the federal level to broaden MCO liability. Although there are benefits that ensue,

Keepnews reasons, there are also costs of expanding a malpractice system that many consider badly flawed, and he provides a balanced view of the pros and cons.

ERISA has such a significant impact on regulation of health plans that a separate chapter is devoted to the structure and scope of this act. Craig Copeland and William Pierron provide a detailed explanation of the types of plans ERISA covers, the scope of the ERISA preemption, and the kind of remedies and regulations that currently exist under the act. Identifying the issues of concern, the authors discuss the merits and drawbacks of altering or preserving ERISA in its current form.

Chapter Five

Consumer Choice Under "Private Health Care Regulation"

Uwe E. Reinhardt

If a Martian had made the rounds of health care conferences in the United States in recent years, it would have come away with the idea that a much-celebrated "managed care revolution" had metamorphosed American patients from passive recipients of health care with limited choices into newly empowered, well-informed, rational "consumers" with "access to more choices" in a new health care market.[1]

The rhetoric at these conferences would convince the Martian that, sometime in the mid-1990s, the American people had had enough of government intrusion into their health system and had opted for a "market approach" that would put them into the driver's seat. In this new consumer-driven health system, the allocation of resources, as well as their cost and quality, are said to be governed by consumers in their local health care markets, rather than by distant bureaucrats. At the popular breakout session entitled Value Purchasing in Health Care, the Martian would hear that as a result of this revolution and uniquely in the world, the American health system henceforth will give consumers "real value" for their dollars. Real value, the Martian would learn, is arrived at by dividing "quality" by "cost." In response to the query about how quality and cost are defined and measured, the Martian would be told that "work on that problem is in progress" and likely to culminate in the giant manual *Value-Pricing & Value-Buying* that is expected to be published by Faulkner & Gray in the year 2006 (but available in galley form as early as 2005).

Eventually, between conferences, the dazzled Martian might stumble into the real world, there to talk to some real-life American health care consumers. More likely than not, these consumers would be dumbfounded by the suggestion that their health system is an answer to their fervent prayers. Far from feeling liberated and empowered by the recent revolution, they would speak of feeling increasingly like pawns in a giant financial game—a game in which what was once known as a "patient" is now viewed merely as a "biological structure yielding cash" (BSYC), with a price per BSYC that is openly quoted on Wall Street. The consumers would speak with nostalgia about the good old days (pre-1990), in which typical Americans with insurance coverage from Medicare, Medicaid, or a private employer did not ever worry about health care when they were healthy because, when they fell ill, they had free choice of doctor, hospital, and prescription drugs. Furthermore, their doctors and hospitals then had free choice on how to treat a given illness. Practice guidelines were still decried in those days as cookbook medicine, something typical of other countries.

Finally, from the media the Martian would learn that the allegedly liberated American health care consumers, far from wanting government out of their health system, are actually clamoring for ever more government regulation, and that even staunchly Republican politicians who habitually thunder against the evils of government intrusions into the private market now busily compete with one another to write new health care regulations. Evidently, when it comes to health care, America's legendary rugged individualists are not so rugged after all. "In government we trust!" they shout. "Never mind the free market."

Sources of Discontent

This chapter explores some of the sources of the current discontent over health care among the American public and its renewed trust in government regulation. It will argue that the managed care revolution was far from being a response by policymakers to yearnings at the grass roots for more choice. In the eyes of the public and the providers who care for patients, that revolution is more commonly perceived as a limit on hitherto free choice, foisted upon the bewildered grass roots by a desperate policymaking elite that has run out of patience with the mounting expense of the nation's open-ended health system. The central tenet of this cramdown revolution is that someone outside the hitherto sacrosanct doctor-patient relationship needs to monitor that relationship and occasionally say "No!" to treatments that patients and their doctors might prefer—in short, that there needs to be judicious *rationing* of health care. It follows that the managed care industry probably would have grown unpopular even if it had been staffed by angels, because to the industry fell the thankless task of destroying the long-cherished myth that rationing health care is un-American.

Lack of Respect for the Consumer

Alas, the industry complicated its task enormously by its evident lack of respect for the ultimate user of health care: the consumer. It can fairly be said that the industry has made insufficient effort so far to implement the theoretically appealing features of consumer-driven, workable competition in health care as that concept had been developed by its pioneers.[2] On the contrary, the industry seems to have obstructed the implementation of genuine competition for reasons that may be understandable but not, therefore, excusable.

Thus, it may turn out that in the end truly effective managed competition in health care, based on informed consumer choice with full transparency, will be imposed on the managed care industry from the outside. Chances are that it will be imposed by government, or at least that government will be a role model that the private sector will follow, just as it has been before in health care. This is not a normative proposition; it is merely a prediction. The conclusion seems inescapable that, by its failure to make managed competition more consumer-friendly, the health insurance industry missed a great opportunity to preclude renewed government intrusion onto its turf.

Lack of Voluntary Consumerism

In the discussions on health policy, it is useful to distinguish clearly between two quite independent developments in consumer choice that are commonly confused: voluntary consumerism and the choices forced on consumers under managed competition and managed care.

Voluntary consumerism is driven by the breathtaking progress in information technology that now can bring an enormous range of information on health and health care to the consumer with a mere click of the mouse. Already, patients adept at exploring the Internet can approach their physicians with highly sophisticated information on alternative therapies that might be suitable for their ailments. That ability is bound to grow as more and more Americans become familiar with that technology in school and at work, even those Americans without higher education. Furthermore, the media increasingly exposes consumers to new health care products and therapies, often through advertisements. There is no question that the new information technology will convert formerly passive patients into active participants in the choice of their health maintenance and therapies. Voluntary consumerism is not a uniquely American phenomenon. It is occurring worldwide, and it rides on the back of the diffusion of information technology.

Voluntary consumerism in health care is not at all the same as the consumer choice under discussion in here, namely, the new and complex set of choices that have been *forced* on consumers as part of the conversion of the American health system to managed care. *Consumerism* is not really the proper word for this consumer choice model. A more apt term would be *cram-down choice*.

From Free Choice to Cram-Down Choice

In fairness to the managed care industry, it must be said that, tactical errors notwithstanding, it came on the scene at a propitious time in the history of American health care. On balance, the industry has made a decidedly positive contribution to the American economy, because it was instrumental in putting an end to a completely unaccountable health system whose ever-growing claims on the nation's resources were neither tolerable nor defensible and whose excesses could actually be harmful to the health of Americans.

The Free Lunch

This system was built on the myth of the proverbial free lunch. The myth is not that well-insured people believe their health care to be free (to them) at the time of illness. That is not a myth; it is a fact explicitly brought about with the purchase of health insurance. Rather, the myth is the belief that health insurance, too, is free. (However, when poor Americans who are on fully subsidized, public health insurance believe that health insurance is free to them, that is not a myth either: it is free to them.) That myth, carefully nourished over the decades by the nation's corporate and union leaders, is sorely in need of destruction.

During the first three decades following World War II, more and more Americans under the age of sixty-five were taught to believe in the fairy tale that health care could be had in the form of a free lunch and, moreover, would never have to be rationed. The teachers in this instance were the members of a dubious alliance of private employers, union leaders, private health insurers, and the providers of health care, all signatories to a social contract infelicitously called *employer-provided* health insurance, although economists are convinced that it is actually paid for by the employees themselves.[3] That social contract has been the foundation of the fairy tale health system that the managed care industry now seeks to bring down to earth.

Employer-provided health insurance American-style has its accidental origin in World War II, when private employers invented it as a way around wartime wage controls. The arrangement is unique in the industrialized world and it seems incredible in retrospect, even in the United States. One may doubt that any thoughtful task force on health care would ever recommend this method of health care financing to a nation if that system had not already been in place.[4]

Under this employment-based health insurance system and until about 1990, employed Americans were taught to believe that their employer could and should assume financial responsibility for their illnesses and those of their dependent families. That belief effectively elevated the employer into the role of the employee's parent in all matters of health care, a role employers continue to play to this day. Most employers were only too happy to assume that role as a come-on in the labor market. Presumably, corporate executives knew that fringe benefits were part of the total price paid for labor and that the cost of fringe benefits normally could be shifted backward into the employees' own lower take-home pay.

Remarkably, the typical employee does not think of fringe benefits that way, for at least two reasons. First, the collectivist group health insurance policy for a firm actually does represent socialized health insurance in the sense that it redistributes the cost of ill health from sick employees to healthy ones. Second, although employers normally do deduct the average per-employee cost of group insurance from the total price of labor (the firm's total debits for labor costs to the payroll-expense account), employers do not make that deduction explicit on the employee's paycheck. There the employer deducts only what the employee believes to be his or her specific contribution to health insurance coverage (now usually less than 25 percent, but much less during the 1970s and 1980s). Both factors—the socialization of health care costs within the firm (generally viewed as a desirable feature) and the implicit (rather than explicit) deduction from gross wages of what employees' believe to be the employer's share of health insurance premium—appear to have fostered employees' belief that someone other than they (the company) paid for the great bulk of their families' health care. Thus did so many Americans come to believe in the fairy tale that health care is a free lunch.

Double-Digit Increases

Until the early 1990s the insurance carriers bore the financial risk for the group health insurance policies they sold employers only for about a year or so, because they were able to increase the insurance premiums they charged employers almost at will. During the late 1980s, for example, the annual increases in premiums for group policies reached the high double digits and yet employers paid them. Thus, effectively freed from risk themselves, private insurers felt little compulsion to control their own health care outlays. Instead, they dutifully respected the tenet that no outsider should ever intrude into the doctor-patient relationship and they passively paid the individual provider's "usual, customary, and reasonable" fees. In the process, employers and the insurance industry jointly had given the providers of health care a first claim on the paychecks of employed Americans who, as noted, generally remained unaware of that claim. Although the average total compensation of American employees rose during the 1980s, their average take-home pay languished. The health sector absorbed a large share of the difference.

Whatever one may think of this peculiar social contract, it did offer American employees and their families the most open-ended health insurance and the most luxurious health care anywhere in the world. To the chagrin of public officials, it also set the standard that had to be matched by the public sector's health insurance programs. With minimal *overt* sharing of the premiums paid by employers and very little cost sharing at the time health care was received, employees and their families enjoyed completely free choice of doctors, hospital, or prescription drugs at the time of illness. Because few if any questions were ever raised by either the private insurers or employers about the use of health care made by employees, it is not surprising that so many Americans sincerely deemed rationing of health care as un-American, something done only by the government-run health systems abroad.

This uncontrolled system of health care financing began to strain the economy as early as the mid-1970s, when the annual growth of labor productivity started to decline from over 3 percent to below 2 percent. The system stumbled at long last when double-digit increases in premiums coincided with the severe recession of the late 1980s and early 1990s. As the employers' health insurance premiums absorbed ever-larger proportions of total labor compensation, industrial relations in the labor markets turned correspondingly sour. Eventually, the increasingly desperate employers began to reevaluate the open-ended social contract they had written and supported for so long, and they looked around for an alternative deal. That deal turned out to be what is now known as *managed care.*

Private Health Care Regulator

The central driver of this new deal was a substantial *reduction* in the freedom of choice among health care providers that American employees and their families had enjoyed for so long. Instead of free choice at the time of illness, employees were forced to choose among competing private health plans, which would then have a contractual right to *regulate* the medical treatments that they and their families received at the time of illness. The preferred term in the industry for this intrusion into the doctor-patient relationship is *managing care*. From the perspective of individual patients and their physicians, however, the more illuminating term is *private health care regulators*.[5]

These private regulators differ from government regulators in several respects. First, one need not emigrate from one's own state or nation to escape a particular private health care regulator. One merely need select another, more preferred private regulator in the same locality, if that choice is available. Second, unlike government regulators, many of the private regulators are driven by the profit motive. Depending largely on their own ideology, individual consumers may view this as either a plus or a minus. Third, unlike government regulators, private health care regulators cannot ration health care through upstream limits on the overall capacity of the entire health system. Thus, they cannot prevent the delivery of care that they deem unwarranted or that they seek to subject to implicit rationing by physicians (a preferred approach to rationing in most other countries, such as in neighboring Canada and in the United Kingdom).

The private regulators can, however, refuse to *pay* for such care. In their own eyes, a mere refusal to pay for care may not appear as the withholding of the care itself or even as regulating the process of health care delivery. In the eyes of patients, health care providers, the media, and the courts, however, that refusal tends to be viewed as rationing just the same and it is now the source of much friction in American health care.

Looking back over the short history of the new managed-care industry, one of its executives recently summed up the industry's record thus: "With little fanfare, a market driven by managed care and cost-conscious employers achieved what no national health care plan ever could: access to more choices and increasingly better health care."[6]

One certainly may wonder just what the executive means by access to *more* choices. He may not realize that when they are sick, Americans often now have less choice of doctor and hospital than they had a decade ago or than do patients in countries with national health plans, such as Canada, France, or Germany, even today.[7] But the executive may well be right in regard to "increasingly better health care," if that includes both the quality of care and its cost.

Beliefs About Quality

Although the media produces anecdote after sensational anecdote pointing to a serious erosion of the quality of American health care under managed care, a detached and thorough recent review of the overall effect of managed care on the quality of American health care does not support the widespread belief that the quality has deteriorated. So far the scientific evidence is inconclusive.[8] The industry certainly can claim credit for spearheading the first systematic assault on the highly varied and inexplicable medical practice patterns of individual physicians and hospitals and of the clinical outcomes they achieve. In the process, the industry has discovered a disturbing unevenness in the quality of American health care,[9] a shortcoming that the medical profession had all but ignored in the "good old days" of complete physician autonomy and that even now organized medicine has been slow to address. To quote Michael L. Millenson, author of the influential book *Demanding Medical Excellence: Doctors and Accountability in the Information Age*,[10] "I would be willing to bet that your average HMO executive, influenced by the same capitalist incentives the AMA [American Medical Association] used to praise, eliminates more inappropriate care in a month than the cooperative effort the AMA and its partners was able to do over several years."[11]

The managed care industry also can take credit for having been instrumental in breaking at long last the intolerable upward spiral in American health spending that had been driven for decades by the old, employer-provided health insurance system. In the process, the managed care industry indirectly helped increase the take-home pay of employed Americans above the levels that would have been reached if the double-digit premium increases passively swallowed by employers in the late 1980s had persisted into the 1990s. Unfortunately, as already noted, for the most part employees do not seem to know that the so-called employer-paid premiums for their health insurance actually do come out of their own paychecks. Therefore, American workers have remained unaware of the benefits bestowed on them by the private health care regulators but are increasingly aware of the cost of managed care: the loss of the completely unfettered access they hitherto had to a luxurious, open-ended health system, with few questions asked.

A Thankless Task Today

This background on the decades-old, limitless, fairyland health care system in which most Americans had been reared since World War II highlights the difficulty of the task now faced by the managed care industry. Somehow, it must gently guide Americans through a transition from exuberant adolescence in matters of health care toward the recognition that all desirable things must be traded off against one another, which implies that all desirable things must be rationed somehow.[12] That thankless task probably would have made the managed care industry highly controversial, even if it had been directed by saints. The industry might have found the chore easier if it had made a more concerted effort to convince the media—and through it the general public—that much of the medical care provided in this country lacks a robust scientific basis and that the overall quality of care could be vastly enhanced, without added cost, if physicians and other practitioners could be held to well-researched practice guidelines. A vast and growing scientific literature on inexplicable geographic practice variations, on the delivery of unnecessary medical procedures, and on glaring gaps in the quality of American health care could have been adduced to support such claims.

Curiously, the industry so far has not engaged the public on this topic or, if it has, that effort has failed. The media and the public seem unaware that the golden age of medicine had a dark side, including the physical harm that unnecessary medical procedures (such as heart surgery and other serious surgery) can visit on patients. Indeed, the industry may have helped deflect attention from this troublesome aspect of the old health system through its heavy-handed imposition of purely mechanical practice guidelines that abstract unduly from deeply held consumer preferences and, as this author has argued elsewhere, sometimes even lack persuasive economic justification.[13]

Finally, the industry appears to have added insult to imagined injury by resisting the transparency that is called for in the theory of consumer-driven managed competition. To appreciate that proposition, it may be useful to review briefly what information infrastructure that theory required and what has been put in place so far.

Consumer Choice: The Theory

As noted, the theory of consumer choice that was to be part of the managed care revolution was not intended to be a broadening of the unlimited options Americans had hitherto enjoyed. Rather, the theory calls for the replacement of free choice among providers at the time of illness—which was thought to be ill-informed and counterproductive—with choice among a set of rival health care regulators, which would *limit* the patient's choice of doctor and hospital. It is doubtful that many consumers would view this switch as providing American consumers with "access to more choice," as the previously cited managed care executive put it in his praise for the new health care market.[14]

The ability of a health plan to limit the set of caregivers in the plan endows the latter with the power to procure health care at lower prices and, more importantly, to micromanage the care given at time of illness. Key to the theory of managed competition is that consumers should *directly* and *noticeably* experience the added cost registered by health plans that do not bargain hard with providers over prices or do not hold providers to strict practice guidelines. Also central to the theory, however, is the idea that individual consumers must have a choice from a wide roster of competing health plans. Finally, to make that choice well-informed and reasoned, the individual must be provided easy access to an information infrastructure that lists the premium charged for a standard benefit package common to all competing plans.

The following figure illustrates what such a data system might look like for an accountable, private health care regulator (health plan) on the consumer's menu of choices. In that scheme, it is assumed that the plan's performance scores on clinical and epidemiological outcomes would go, in the first place, to properly trained experts hired by a "sponsor,"[15] which might be an employer, a regional alliance of employers, or a state health department. On the basis of these data, the sponsor would decide whether a particular plan is qualified to be included in its menu of choices. Although such data would be available to individual consumers on request, it is not clear how well the untrained consumer can actually use such information. Individual consumers, however, certainly could evaluate patient satisfaction scores, especially if these were reported for enrollees with distinct chronic diseases, and other information of a less technical nature, among them the background and experience of the physicians in the plan's network and information on the financial incentives to withhold health care that may be implicit in their contract with the health plan.

Figure 5.1. Sketch of a Credible Information System for "Managed Competition."

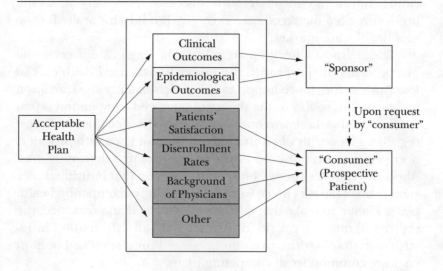

It goes almost without saying that, to be helpful for consumer choice, data presented to the consumer would have to be *credible*. In principle, the data should not be self-reported by the health plans themselves, unless that is unavoidable. To the extent that it is feasible, the data ought to be retrieved from the health plans or their enrollees by an external, detached agency, such as a single large employer. Ideally, the data for consumer-driven managed competition should be retrieved and structured by what was once known as a Health Insurance Purchasing Cooperative (HIPC) or a health alliance—that is, a well-organized analogue of a farmers market for competing private health care regulators.

Any data that by necessity would be gathered and reported by the health plans themselves would have to be subject to strict audit by an outsider, similar to the extensive audits of the self-reported financial statements issued by business corporations. Mere random spot checks of self-reported data would be no more acceptable in health care than they would be in the realm of financial accounting. As in business accounting, the self-reported data of every health plan would have to be thoroughly audited by outsiders every year. It is worth noting the huge number of auditors that would be needed in a regime of genuine managed competition if the system relied largely on self-reported data. The cost of such audits have been estimated at $15,000 to $70,000 per health plan per year for the self-reported information in the Health Plan Employers Data and Information System (HEDIS), now operated by the private, not-for-profit National Committee for Quality Assurance (NCQA).[16] These sums may seem large in the abstract, and they are cited by the managed care industry as a source of concern.[17] In fact, however, they are only a tiny percentage of the typical health plan's total revenue, and they certainly are not higher than the annual sums these plans spend on audits of their annual financial reports. It would be difficult for the plans to argue that the potential purchasers of their financial securities warrant more reliable data than do the potential purchasers of their health insurance contracts.

Ultimately, what is needed for genuine managed competition is the analogue of the business accountant—the *health care accountant*—whose training would be at the intersection of clinical science, economics, statistics, and other relevant social sciences. Health care accountants would follow generally accepted health accounting standards (like the generally accepted accounting standards now used for business accounting), and their work would be subject to strict audits. They would probably be supervised by the government through an SEC-like structure,[18] although most of their rules could be developed within the private sector. Finally, they would be devoted to making their structured information accessible to users, just as business accountants are. The latter release their information in layers of technical complexity and detail, depending on the technical competence of the users of that information. Information for consumer choice in health care would have to be similarly customized.

Consumer Choice: Current Practice

Only a small subset of families, mainly in California and in Minnesota, have access to the kind of information system sketched out in the previous section. For example, the Pacific Business Group on Health in San Francisco, the California Public Employers Retirement System (CalPERS), the Health Insurance Purchasing Cooperative for small business firms in California, the Buyers Health Care Action Group in Minnesota, and to some extent, the Federal Employees Health Benefit Program, can claim to come close to meeting the minimum requirements of a consumer choice model in health care. There may be yet other groups doing the same, but they are not in the national limelight.

For the most part, however, the typical American family does not yet experience genuine managed competition. Most employers offer their workers only limited choice among the private health care regulators that will govern their health care experience. But even when prospective enrollees are given multiple options, they often receive only sketchy information on the comportment of the competing plans and the providers associated with them.

As Etheredge, Jones, and Lewin reported in 1996, an estimated 47 percent of American working adults were given only a single health plan by their employers. Another 23 percent or so had a choice among only two health plans.[19] A more recent Kaiser-Commonwealth national survey corroborates these estimates.[20] It also revealed that 18 percent of working adults were not offered any health plan by their employers. These numbers suggest a certain irony. Having rejected as unacceptable the single-payer model of, say, Canada or its American analog—Medicare for all—millions of American families now are subjected to private, single-payer health insurance that attaches them to an unaccountable, private health care regulator not of their own choosing. That turn of events was decidedly not the idea of managed competition as it was originally proposed by its pioneers.

Lack of Information About Plans

The Kaiser-Commonwealth survey indicated that the likelihood of having insurance offered at all by an employer, or of having a choice among health plans, decreases systematically with the employee's income and with the size of the employer. Employees of firms with more than five hundred workers were more than five times as likely to have a choice of health plans than were those whose employers had twenty-five or fewer workers.[21] But many larger firms that do offer their employees a choice among health plans do not own up to the requirements of properly managed competition. Although it is difficult to gain precise data on what information about competing health plans are generally made available by American employers, anecdotal evidence on this point is not reassuring.

For example, Princeton University, with more than a thousand employees, as of this writing does not give the employees any of the information set forth in Figure 5.1 on the multiple health plans offered to employees, not even the self-reported aggregate data from HEDIS. So far, relatively few large employers or employer coalitions use HEDIS data to decide which health plans to offer their employees and even fewer make the data available to employees.[22]

One reason for this apparent lack of interest in HEDIS may be uncertainty over the accuracy of the data, which remain spotty for many health plans, and often are not rigorously audited.[23] Last year the Health Care Financing Administration (HCFA) engaged the Island Peer Review Organization (IPRO) of New York to perform a thorough audit of the HEDIS performance data submitted to the HCFA by a sample of health plans that enroll Medicare beneficiaries. That audit revealed serious flaws in the self-reported data.[24] In part, these flaws may reflect the immaturity of the HEDIS in general. However, self-reported data always are subject to the tendency among normal adults to structure information so as to maximize their own advantage. In the long run, managed competition is not well-served by self-reported data, if these data can seriously affect a health plan's popularity.

A Remarkable Notation

Surprisingly, even the Xerox Corporation, widely considered one of the more astute sponsors of multiple-choice health insurance, did not as of 1997 own up fully to the requirements of managed competition. Xerox does use HEDIS data and shares them with employees, although they are not invariably audited. Furthermore, in the *HMO Performance Report* for New Jersey that accompanied the company's otherwise excellent *1997 Benefits Decision Workbook,* there is no information on the financial incentives individual doctors face in the competing health plans to withhold care. For the four performance categories entitled Percent of Board-Certified PCPs, Percent of Board-Certified Specialists, Percent of PCPs Accepting New Patients, and Physician Turnover in Percent, there is the remarkable notation: "Oxford Plan-N.J. would not allow the publication of their data to Xerox employees." The analogous notation is shown for U.S. Healthcare N.J., another major health plan in the Northeast.

One finds the same disturbing notation, once again for both of these major health plans, for the four performance categories titled HMOs Members Satisfaction Rate, Percent of HMOs Members Who Would Recommend Plan, Wait Time for Urgent Care, and Wait Time for Emergency Care, and also for the performance standards, "Percentage of women of age fifty-two to sixty-four who have had a mammogram in the last two years" and "Percentage of women ages twenty-one to sixty-four who have had a Pap test within the last three years." For an additional five clinical or epidemiological performance standards, the relevant columns for Oxford Plan-N.J. and for US Healthcare N.J. are simply left blank. One must wonder why Xerox Corporation and its employees accept this lacuna of highly relevant consumer information.

Employees in small firms and individuals who seek to purchase single health insurance policies must make decisions with even less information. To illustrate this point, last year this author inquired of a major managed care plan in Washington, D.C., whether there existed a Web site featuring the curriculum vitae of the plan's physicians, data on patient-satisfaction scores for the individual physicians, and information on the financial incentives the network's physicians had to withhold care. Such information is fundamental for this particular plan because it is of the gatekeeper model, requiring enrollees to elect a gatekeeping primary physician at the time of enrollment. A prospective enrollee certainly would like to know something about the physician who will henceforth regulate his or her access to specialist care and other services. To the author's surprise, the response was that a Web site for the plan did not yet exist but that the plan was "working on that database." In the meantime, prospective enrollees were asked to call physicians directly for that information. To evaluate the progress made, the author repeated the inquiry at the time of this writing, about one year later. The answer was the same. Apparently, work on the database continues, but there still does not exist a Web site for the plan, nor is information available on the physician's background or on the satisfaction scores for enrolled patients (verbal communication with a representative of the George Washington University Plan, July 13, 1998.) Because the task of building such a Web site could easily be accomplished by a few bright undergraduates, one surmises that this health plan is not particularly keen on establishing the desired database.

Why the Reticence?

What can account for this disappointing state of affairs? One can think of several reasons. First, in fairness to the managed care industry, it is not yet entirely clear just what information is to be communicated to whom. The United States rushed into the theory of consumer-driven, price- and quality-competitive health care without much prior research on what kind of information individuals in different socioeconomic and demographic strata actually can interpret and use sensibly in choosing health plans and caregivers. It will probably take a decade or more before the model described in Figure 5.1 can be *fully* implemented, especially in regard to information on clinical outcomes. This circumstance is not a source of shame. By international standards the United States is ahead of every other nation in this endeavor.

In contrast, it is puzzling why the managed care industry has not made the simple and relatively cheap information on physicians and consumer satisfaction more readily available to the public. One might suspect that the industry has no interest in competing on the terms that were once envisaged by the pioneers of managed competition. It can fairly be said that any health plan that does not offer prospective enrollees a flourishing Web site containing the basic information consumers might want and could digest—such as information on enrollee satisfaction or the background of physician—is making a mockery of the theory of managed competition.

The managed care industry's cavalier attitude toward a proper information infrastructure is one reason why the American public now clamors for stricter government regulation and why politicians on both sides of the political divide see in that clamoring a field ready for harvest. In fact, the state of New Jersey already has jumped into the breach where the private sector has failed. The state's health commissioner's Office of Managed Care uses a survey research company to gather information about satisfaction directly from enrollees of all the managed care plans operating in the state, then disseminates these data in summary form, for each plan, in an easily readable format.[25] The data are also available on the Internet.[26] It is a helpful start on the road toward a genuine farmer's market for health insurance. One can expect the state to broaden this infrastructure over time, with or without the cooperation of the managed care industry.

From Catalyst to Obstacle

Finally, the disappointing performance of private employers in the practice of "managed competition" raises the question whether the employment-based health insurance system is up to the task of facilitating the difficult transition from the fairy tale health system that private employers had supported so long to a more rational one with properly managed competition and managed care. History may well record that, shortly after being the catalyst for the introduction of managed competition in the United States, the employer-based model ultimately turned out to be one of the *major obstacles* to the full implementation of the concept. In the end, state governments and the Medicare program may have to lead the way, if managed competition is ever to work properly.

Lynn Etheredge, one of the most astute observers of American health care, comes to a similar conclusion. Because it may be so startling to many readers, it is worth quoting him at length:

> Advocates for government-offered health insurance have often encountered attacks (or Harry and Louise ads) that played on fears of government. A government-run program was predicted to be one where people would be told what doctors and hospitals they could use. In contrast, a private employer-based health insurance system was held up as the model for those who valued patient freedom of choice, provider clinical freedom, and quality.
>
> The Medicare reform legislation [of 1997] confounded these predictions. With the new Medicare design, politicians provided Medicare enrollees with almost unlimited freedom of choice, not only among providers, but price-regulated fee-for-service insurance and a spectrum of private health plans. . . . There will be health plan accreditation, quality reporting and consumer rights. In contrast, most private sector employees restrict health-plan choices . . . and lack of consumer protection is a nationwide concern. . . . Our national politicians—in their new consumer choice model for Medicare's thirty-eight million enrollees and in the similar Federal Employees Health Benefits Program (FEHBP) for government officials and employees—have created insurance arrangements that are better than what is now available for most Americans with employment-based coverage.[27]

Whither Consumer Choice?

The consumer choice model is a uniquely American phenomenon, a by-product of this country's quest to extract from the providers of health care better accountability for the real resources (labor and physical capital) burned up in health care and for the ever-growing share of the gross domestic product that the providers of health care claim as their reward. That quest for better accountability, however, is *not* uniquely American; it is a worldwide quest that drives health reform efforts everywhere. The uniqueness of the American approach lies in its heavy reliance on consumers as agents of cost and quality control in health care, at least in theory.

The question is whether the theoretical models of consumer choice may not overestimate the ability of consumers to discipline as complex and powerful an enterprise as health care. For example, in their study of the use of the Consumer Guide on Cardiac Surgery by cardiac surgery patients in Pennsylvania, Schneider and Epstein found that "even among those [patients] who were aware of the Consumer Guide [on Cardiac Surgery] before surgery almost no one used it in decision making" (p. 1641).[28] Furthermore, only 12 percent of patients surveyed in the report were even aware of these data before undergoing surgery, although they are reported annually on the front pages of major newspapers in Pennsylvania. As the authors conclude: "Although the methodological barriers to reliable and valid performance measurement are substantial, delivering performance information to patients in an effective and usable format could prove even more formidable" (p. 1642).

The Economic and Social Research Institute (ESRI) recently conducted an extensive review of how report cards are used in the private and public sectors.[29] ESRI concluded from its survey of employers that many of them do care a great deal about the HEDIS performance ratings when they decide which plan to include on the menu they offer employees. However, the employers also found that report cards do not appear to have a significant impact on how employees choose among the health plans they are offered.

A similar finding is reported by Chernow and Scanlon in their econometric study of the choices among health plans made by employees in a large Fortune 100 company that structures the choice very carefully, according to the dictates of the theory of managed competition. Employees are given a fixed contribution toward the premiums charged by a variety of managed care plans offering a common benefit package. For each plan they are given the dollar amount of the premium they themselves must pay for that plan, along with a variety of nonprice attributes based on HEDIS data. The authors conclude that "employees do not appear to respond strongly to plan performance data" (p. 19). (Curiously, they also found that, other things being equal, the probability of an employee's picking a particular plan *decreased* with increases in the enrollee satisfaction score for that plan. They attribute that counterintuitive result to deficiencies in the construction of the plan's report cards.)

Robert Galvin, a physician and director of health care for General Electric, probably would not be surprised by these findings. In his response to an incisive lecture by David Eddy, a recognized authority on quality assurance, on the myriad methodological and economic problems of performance measurement in health care,[30] Galvin argues that performance measures aggregated at the level of the health plan are not interesting to the employees with whom he interacts.[31] In his words: "Because most physicians and hospitals belong to multiple plans, the relative performance of these plans are the products of essentially the same providers. Patients do not call out HMOs when they are sick; they seek doctors. They want to know who is 'the best' in treating their condition, and they cannot tell when most doctors belong to the same plans" (p. 30).

Consider Reading Levels

It may also be the case that the structure and content of the report cards simply overtax the reading skills of most employees. Citing the results from the National Adult Literacy Survey of the U.S. Bureau of the Census,[32] psychologist Mark Hochhauser argues that many reports cards issued to employees do not pass a readability test for the average employee.[33] He believes, however, that with further research on what information readers of various levels of educational attainment can digest and how consumers generally reach decisions, more readable report cards could be produced.[34] In his erudite exploration of the potential and pitfalls of Medicare+Choice, Henry Aaron cites a large body of research by psychologists, sociologists, information theorists, logicians, and experimental economists that call into the question the simplistic behavioral model that drives standard economic analysis and that also seems to drive the theory of consumer choice in managed competition.[35] Success or failure in attempts to enlist consumers effectively in the development of an accountable health care system will depend on the extent to which the architects of health policy and the leaders of the managed care industry will draw on that research and encourage its extension.

In his previously cited commentary, Galvin recommends that we learn to "understand what consumers are really interested in, and let's develop a measurement system that informs them" (p. 31).[36] It may seem that focus groups would be a logical first step in that inquiry. However, in their study of what report card information consumers claim to be salient and what information they actually use in making choices among plans, Hibbard and Jewett found that salience (stated consumer preference for information) does not coincide neatly with the information that actually drives their choices.[37] It follows that the content of report cards will have to be established iteratively, through years of experimentation with alternative formats.

Accountability as a Public Good

Even if consumers ultimately were found to be only two-bit players in the complicated market for health care, that is no reason to turn back from the worldwide quest for more accountable health systems and the performance measurements they require. Better accountability can be sought also at other levels; as noted earlier, many employers are beginning to make use of HEDIS data in selecting health plans. Medicare will do so with even greater vigor, because by law it must. As long as someone pores over performance data and can use them to make decisions that could affect the economics of health plans or providers, the latter will respond to these measurements.

Why Health Services Research Is Crucial

The development of performance measures in health care is part of health services research. If Congress were ever asked to express its appropriation for health services research as a percentage of its total appropriations for health care, it would blush. While the National Institutes of Health (NIH) are being showered with funds, the research that might help make our health system more efficient goes begging year after year. Eddy proposes that 1 percent of the NIH budget be allocated for health services research, on the logic "that all the science in the world has no effect until it is implemented properly."[38]

Government funding of research and development of health care performance measures is crucial for at least two reasons. First, much of the product from this research is in the nature of a public good. As economic theory has long established, the private sector will always underfund the production of public goods, unless its production is at least publicly funded. As Cary Sennet, executive vice president of the National Committee for Quality Assurance (NCQA) has remarked: "We [the NCQA] are not sanguine regarding the likelihood that the private purchasers of health benefits—who have been, these past few years, the clearest beneficiaries of our work—will agree to subsidize it in the future. (p. 37)"[39]

That would, indeed, be the natural posture of private sector agents in the face of production of a public good. The only method of making private purchasers of health care a stable source of support for performance-measurement development would be a government mandate to make those contributions, just as the users of the nation's interstate highway are mandated to pay user taxes for the use of that resource.

The Farmers Market

Finally, if all American consumers are ever to have choice among multiple health plans, Congress or state governments must revive one of the central ideas of managed competition—that is, the development of regional farmers markets for health insurance in which every insurance-driven or provider-driven health plan *must* exhibit its array of products with full and credible (audited) information on the cost and quality. It is not premature to conclude that only a handful of private employers will ever be able to serve this function, and even fewer will do it well.

In principle, an employee of the XYZ Corporation who is given the choice between the insurance-driven ACME Health Plan and the physician-driven Hippocrates Health Plan should not have to rely on the tidbits of information that XYZ's employee benefit manager may make available. The XYZ employees should be able to go to a state-chartered farmers market that has credible performance information on this and all other health plans doing business in the state. Such a farmers market would retrieve much of that information itself, directly from enrolled consumers, and would have the power to audit self-reported data. And its information would be available in multiple media, including on the Internet.

Notes

1. Huber, R. L. "Let the Market Remedy What Ails Health Care." *The Wall Street Journal*, July 13, 1998, p. A14. Huber is chairman and CEO of Aetna, Inc., a major managed-care company.

2. Ellwood, P. M., Enthoven, A. C., and Etheredge, L. "The Jackson Hole Initiatives for a Twenty-First Century American Health Care System." *Health Economics*, 1992, *1*, 149–168.

3. Krueger, A. B., and Reinhardt, U. E. "The Economics of Employers Versus Individual Markets." *Health Affairs*, 1994, *13*(2), 34–53.

4. United States Congress, Congressional Budget Office. *Economic Implications of Rising Health Care Costs*. Washington, D.C.: U.S. Government Printing Office, 1992.

5. For a defense of that proposition, see Reinhardt, U. E. "Employer-Based Health Insurance: R.I.P." In S. A. Altman, U. E. Reinhardt, and A. S. Shields (eds.), *The Future of the U.S. Healthcare System: Who Will Care for the Poor and the Uninsured?* Chicago: Health Administration Press, 1997.

6. Berenson, R. A. "A Physician's View of Managed Care." *Health Affairs*, 1991, *10*(4), 106–119.

7. Huber, R. L. "Market Remedy," p. A14.

8. Miller, R. H., and Luft, H. S. "Managed Care Performance: Is Quality of Care Better or Worse?" *Health Affairs*, 1997, *16*(5), 7–27.

9. Newcomer, L. N. "Perspective: Physician Health Thyself." *Health Affairs*, 1998, *17*(4), 32–35.

10. Millenson, M. L. *Medical Excellence: Doctors and Accountability in the Information Age*. Chicago: University of Chicago Press, 1997.

11. Millenson, M. L. "Miracles and Wonder: The AMA Embraces Quality Measurement." *Health Affairs*, 1997, *16*(3).

12. Reinhardt, U. E. "Spending More Through Cost Control: Our Obsessive Quest to Gut the Hospital." *Health Affairs*, 1996, *15*(2), 145–154.

13. Eddy, D. M. *Clinical Decision Making: From Theory to Practice*. Boston: Jones & Bartlett, 1996. See especially Chapter 27, "Rationing Resources While Improving Quality," pp. 279–296.

14. Huber, R. L. "Market Remedy," p. A14.
15. Enthoven, A. C. "Consumers Choice Health Plan: A National Health Insurance Based on Competition in the Private Sector." *The New England Journal of Medicine,* 1997, *320,* 29–37, 94–101.
16. Williams, S. "Growing Reliance on Self-Reported HEDIS Data Underscores Need for Auditing." *Medicine & Health Perspectives,* May 18, 1998, (newsletter).
17. Ibid., p. 4.
18. For a recent description of such a system, see Etheredge, L. "Promarket Regulation: An SEC-FASB Model." *Health Affairs,* 1997, *16*(6), 223–225.
19. Etheredge, L., Jones, S. B., and Lewin, L. "What Is Driving Health Systems Change?" *Health Affairs,* 1996, *15,* 93–101.
20. Kaiser-Commonwealth 1997 National Survey of Health Insurance. *Working Families at Risk: Coverage, Access, Costs, and Worries,* December 8, 1997, p. 40.
21. Ibid.
22. Williams, S. "Growing Reliance on Self-Reported HEDIS Data," 1.
23. Ibid.
24. Ibid., p. 2.
25. State of New Jersey, Department of Health and Senior Services. *New Jersey HMOs: Performance Report.* New Jersey: Department of Health and Senior Services, November, 1997.
26. See www.state.NJ.US/health.
27. Etheredge, L. "The Medicare Reforms of 1997: Headlines You Did Not Read." Mimeographed paper delivered at a panel on health reform sponsored by the American Political Science Association, September 27, 1997.
28. Schneider, E. C., and Epstein, A. M. "Use of Public Performance Reports: A Survey of Patients Undergoing Cardiac Surgery." *The Journal of the American Medical Association,* 1998, *279*(20), 1639–1642.
29. Meyer, J. A., Wicks, E. K., Rybowski, L. S., and Perry, M. J. *Report on Report Cards.* Washington, D.C.: Economic and Social Research Institute, 1998.
30. Eddy, D. M. "Performance Measurement: Problems and Solutions." *Health Affairs,* 1998, *17*(4), 7–25.
31. Galvin, R. S. "Are Performance Measures Relevant?" *Health Affairs,* 1998, *17*(4), 29–31.
32. Hochhauser, M. "Can Your HMO's Documents Pass the Readability Test?" *Managed Care,* September 1997, pp. 60A–60H.
33. Hochhauser, M. "Why Patients Have Little Patience for Report Cards." *Managed Care,* March 1998, pp. 31–34.

34.   Hochhauser, M. "Designing Readable Report Cards." *Managed Healthcare,* May 1998, pp. 15–21.
35.   Aaron, H. "Medicare Choice: Good, Bad, or It All Depends." Mimeographed paper delivered on June 1998. And in Saving, T. R., and Rattenmaier, A. (eds.), *Medicare Reform: Issues and Answers* (conference volume, forthcoming).
36.   Galvin, R. S. "Are Performance Measures Relevant?" 31.
37.   Hibbard, J. H., and Jewett, J. J. "Will Quality Report Cards Help Consumers?" *Health Affairs,* 1997, *16*(3), 218–228.
38.   Eddy, D. M. "Performance Measurement: Problems and Solutions." *Health Affairs* 1998, *17*(4), 25.
39.   Sennet, C. "Moving Ahead, Measure by Measure." *Health Affairs,* 1998, *17*(4), 36–37.

Chapter Six

The Long-Term Care Ombudsman Program

A Model for Health Care Consumers

William F. Benson

> *Ombudsman: (1) a government official (as in Sweden or New Zealand) appointed to receive and investigate complaints made by individuals against abuses or capricious acts of public officials; (2) one that investigates reported complaints (as from students or consumers), reports findings, and helps achieve equitable settlements.*
> —*WEBSTER'S NINTH NEW COLLEGIATE DICTIONARY*

Few would disagree that our highly complex health care world is rapidly becoming even more complex. The technology of health care is complex, as are its organizational and delivery models and its financing. For consumers, successfully navigating through a health care organization or system to obtain appropriate, timely, and high-quality health care can be a difficult if not daunting chore. At times it can be overwhelming. If the consumer is dissatisfied or unhappy with the care received or feels aggrieved in some way, the effort anticipated or expended in trying to resolve the source of discontent or to settle the grievance may be overwhelming, particularly in the absence of mechanisms for resolving problems.

In many cases, consumers may have available to them both informal and formal mechanisms for appealing what they perceive to be inappropriate or adverse decisions by health care providers and entities, as well as for voicing complaints. All states require health maintenance organizations (HMOs) to have a grievance procedure, although many do not require specific types of grievance procedures, or information about their availability (Families USA Foundation, 1996). Some states have established formal appeals and grievance procedures that are external to the health plan or provider.

Over the past several years, particularly in light of the rapid growth of managed care, policymakers and others have become increasingly concerned about how managed care plans respond to patient grievances. As a result, more attention is being paid to the importance of establishing mechanisms for consumers to voice complaints and appeal actions against health plans and providers.

A national commission appointed by President Clinton adopted as part of the Consumer Bill of Rights and Responsibilities the right to "a rigorous system of internal review and an independent system of external review" (President's Advisory Commission, 1997). But for many consumers, the availability of mechanisms for voicing complaints and filing appeals may not be enough. In many cases, even in the presence of a comprehensive set of procedures for dealing with complaints and appeals, consumers need assistance from a third party to make the complaint or appeals mechanism work for them. For a wide variety of reasons, such as feelings of intimidation, lack of knowledge or competency, and cultural, language, technical, and legalistic barriers, to name a few, consumers may need someone to help them. In the absence of meaningful mechanisms to voice or file a complaint or appeal, a knowledgeable third party to help address and resolve problems may be even more important.

Over the past several decades models of services and programs have evolved that are intended to assist consumers in their efforts to access and receive decent quality health care services and to help them redress problems that arise in obtaining and paying for their health care. Foremost among these models has been the creation of various forms of ombudsman programs, and most notably, the long-term care ombudsman program established under the Older Americans Act of 1965 (OAA), as amended.[1]

This chapter will discuss the value of consumer assistance services for health care consumers by highlighting the nationwide Long-Term Care Ombudsman Program (LTCOP). The LTCOP is described as a model for assisting consumers in other settings, including managed care. Although the ombudsman model does not generally provide a regulatory capacity over health care providers or services, it is an important component of the regulatory environment for health care.

Nursing Home Quality and the Long-Term Care Ombudsman Program

Representatives of the nursing home industry have frequently made the claim that it is among the most heavily regulated and monitored industries in the nation, and the most regulated of health care services. With regard to health care, the industry's argument is difficult to refute. As most of the nation's 16,800 nursing homes participate in either the Medicare or Medicaid programs, or both, most must operate under federal standards governing those programs. Individual states have their own standards for nursing home care that are linked to licensure standards. Each state has a legal body that licenses and governs nursing home administrators. Each state has a long-term care ombudsman program established through the OAA. And there are various other formal entities and mechanisms that have or play a role in nursing home oversight in many states (for example, certificate of need requirements, elder-abuse reporting laws, Medicaid fraud control units, and peer review organizations).

The array of laws and rules that govern nursing homes and the care provided therein are dizzying in their scope. They cover the spectrum of care and life in the facility, ranging from terms of admissions agreements, type of care provided, staffing patterns, sanitation, social services provided, individual rights of residents, management of resident funds, food and nutrition, activities, transfers and evictions, financing, construction and physical plant, and so forth.

Since its inception as a national demonstration program in 1972, the LTCOP has been firmly established as a major source of assistance in resolving the complaints and problems of residents of the nation's nursing homes and other long-term care facilities. There are statewide programs in every state, the District of Columbia, and Puerto Rico. The LTCOPs of most states include local or "substate" programs, usually located in area agencies on aging (AAAs) or community-based not-for-profit organizations, including legal aid offices. As states and the federal government debate and consider options for responding to quality problems and other consumer problems in the broader health care world, especially in managed care, there is considerable interest in developing models of consumer assistance, especially ombudsman services, for consumers. Given the size, scope, and experience of the LTCOP and its overall credibility, it seems to be a particularly important model to examine and consider for applicability in the managed care and other health care settings.

Background for the Long-Term Care Ombudsman Program

In 1972, the Department of Health, Education, and Welfare (HEW) announced a demonstration program to test the idea of nursing home ombudsman programs, awarding contracts in five states. In 1975, after responsibility for the program was shifted to the Administration on Aging (AoA), small amounts of funding were offered to each state to establish ombudsman programs. Following the establishment of the grant program, the LTCOP grew and evolved rapidly. It was formally incorporated in federal law as part of the OAA by the 1978 amendments to the act.[2]

The statutory provisions established in the 1978 OAA amendments for the LTCOP provided a common foundation for the direction of LTCOPs across the nation. The 1978 amendments included several key provisions that were crucial in forming the philosophical underpinnings of the program. First was the requirement that each state have an LTCOP and that it be operated by the state unit on aging (SUA), established pursuant to the OAA, either directly or through subcontracts with public or nonprofit agencies (Institute of Medicine, 1995). This provided a common entity with the legal responsibility for the program—the SUA. At the same time, it allowed states the option of subcontracting the day-to-day operation of the program to another entity. More significantly, it established the principle that the ombudsman program was to operate independently from the nursing home industry and from the regulators of nursing homes.

Perhaps most important among the ombudsman provisions established in the 1978 OAA amendments was language directing that LTCOPs "investigate complaints made by or on behalf of residents" of facilities. This language has firmly established the constituency of the LTCOP: the facility residents. This language reinforced the role of ombudsmen as patient or resident advocates. Although ombudsmen can and do respond to complaints from nursing home personnel, health care providers, government officials, family members, and others, they do so only when the complaint is on behalf of a resident.

One other key provision of the 1978 amendments is noteworthy. The statute required LTCOPs to use the information and knowledge about nursing homes and the problems of residents gained through their complaint investigation activities to work to improve overall conditions in facilities and to bring to the attention of other officials their observations and experiences on behalf of residents.

These roles have been a considerable source of tension, however, for many state LTCOPs. State LTC ombudsmen, who head the states' LTCOPs, are usually employees of the state, often serving at the pleasure of elected or appointed officials. Thus, the realities of politics and competing interests, coupled with traditional attitudes regarding employer-employee relations, have made it difficult for ombudsmen in many situations to openly offer their findings and observations.

Over the more than two decades that the LTCOP has been operating as a formal part of the OAA, it has proven itself to be an enduring and important source of assistance to residents of long-term care facilities, to residents' families, and to others who work on behalf of the interests of facility residents. Although not the world's oldest ombudsman program—the first was established in Sweden in 1809 (Monk, Kaye, and Litwin, 1984)—the LTCOP is no doubt the world's largest. In fiscal year 1996, the most recent year for which data are available, the program nationwide opened 126,606 new cases and closed 116,242 cases, involving 179,111 complaints. More than 72 percent of all complaints were resolved or partially resolved to the satisfaction of the resident or complainant (Administration on Aging, 1999).

Extending the Long-Term Care Ombudsman Program Model

The lengthy history of the long-term care ombudsman program, coupled with its scope (for example, numbers of individuals assisted, complaints investigated), recognition, and perceived effectiveness, has led to considerable interest in and discussion about expanding the long-term care ombudsman program into other areas. The most extensive consideration of this kind of expansion took place as part of the Institute of Medicine's (IoM) study of the effectiveness of the ombudsman program. Among the several charges given to the IoM for its ombudsman study was to examine "the need for and feasibility of providing ombudsman services to older individuals who are not residing in long-term care facilities but who are users of health and long-term care services." Although not taking a specific position on program expansion, the IoM stated that "most Committee [IoM Ombudsman Study Committee] members believe that some entity or individual—whether or not it is the current LTC ombudsman—is needed to answer questions, to provide systemic advocacy, and to intervene in problem situations for some consumers" (Institute of Medicine, 1995, p. 229).

More recently, as public concern over the behavior of managed care entities has grown and demand for greater responsiveness and accountability has increased, policymakers, analysts, and consumer advocates have stepped up their efforts in promoting various consumer protection mechanisms for health care consumers. As a result, interest in establishing formal grievance and appeals mechanisms has increased at both the federal and state levels. A national coalition of consumer and public interest groups released a "National Consumer Protection Blueprint for Managed Care." With regard to formal grievance and appeals mechanisms it states: "Current grievance and appeals mechanisms for individuals enrolled in managed care plans are not well established. . . . In the absence of regulatory standards, managed care organizations are left as judge and jury for the care they provide" (Consumer Coalition for Quality Health Care, 1997, p. 6).

Regardless of how comprehensive and accessible grievance and appeals systems are, consumers need help in accessing and using such systems, and resolving other issues they may have with their health care plans, insurers, and providers. There is considerable and growing interest in putting in place consumer assistance services, including providing independent and external avenues for voicing complaints and receiving help in addressing and resolving problems. The potential role of the ombudsman has become a substantial part of the discussion and is receiving considerable attention. The IoM's ombudsman study stated, "Even individuals who under normal circumstances have no difficulty expressing their opinions or making their needs known may need an intermediary or proponent should they fall ill or be confronted with an inadequate or nonresponsive system of care" (Institute of Medicine, 1995, p. 207).

As the LTCOP and elements of it continue to be considered as a model for use in other health care settings, from nonfacility-based long-term care (that is, home and community-based services) to managed care, LTCOP program strengths can serve to guide the development of ombudsman services, or other forms of consumer assistance, in other settings.

Several major health plans joined with two prominent national organizations, the American Association of Retired Persons (AARP) and Families USA, to embrace explicitly the principle of consumer access to an independent, external nonprofit ombudsman programs. Kaiser Permanente, Group Health Cooperative of Puget Sound, and HIP Health Insurance Plans joined with AARP and Families USA in 1997 in agreeing on this principle, adding that "health plans should cooperate with independent, external nonprofit ombudsman programs that would assist consumers in understanding plans' marketing materials and the coverage provisions of various health plans, educate members about their rights within health plans, help to identify and investigate member complaints, assist members in filing formal grievances and appeals, and report to appropriate regulatory bodies on issues of concern to consumers" (*Principles for Consumer Protection*, 1997, p. 6).

The Older Americans Act's long-term care ombudsman program provides the most comprehensive and experienced model. There is considerable variation among the LTCOP of the states, certainly in such areas as organizational structure, use of personnel (including volunteers), and approaches to complaint investigation and problem resolution (Nelson, 1995; Institute of Medicine, 1995; Benson, 1997). Nevertheless, the OAA program has a well-established statutory base that has served to build a common philosophy as a resident advocate model and to provide a foundation for a common infrastructure among the states for implementing statewide ombudsman services. Based on the experiences of the LTCOP, several features emerge as most significant for success.

Complaint Investigation and Resolution Roles

The single most important feature of any ombudsman system is its freedom to act in its complaint investigation and resolution roles, for both individual and systemic problems. In literature about the LTCOP and among ombudsmen, this is commonly categorized as having the independence necessary to carry out program responsibilities. In many respects, it can be argued that many other critical elements of the ombudsman program, such as prohibitions on conflicts of interest and confidentiality requirements, are subsets of the program independence issue.

Ombudsman services should be independent and external to the settings and services that are or may be the subject of complaints and investigations. As far back as 1981, the AoA stressed the importance of "independent judgement and freedom of action" for the "vigorous" investigation of complaints (Administration on Aging, 1981, p. 14).

Unlike regulatory and judicial bodies, ombudsmen by design have little if any formal authority that enables them to compel action by others. For example, they do not have the authority to insist on corrective action by facilities, agencies, or personnel. They do not impose sanctions or penalties for violations of residents' rights or other actions that may or do result in harm to facility residents.

The principle power of an LTCOP is its credibility and freedom to act. The greater the degree of independence to act (for example, vigorously investigate a complaint, bring problems and recommendations to the attention of government officials or the press), the greater the ability to represent fully the interests of the residents. One of the key challenges confronting the state long-term care ombudsman program today is its ability to maintain its independence in fact and in appearance in the rapidly changing world of long-term care.

Avoidance of Conflicts of Interest

Closely related to the topic of ombudsman independence is the avoidance of conflicts of interest. The initial language establishing the LTCOP in federal law recognized the importance of independence and avoiding a conflict of interest in terms of organizational placement. Some argue that to ensure independence it is best to base ombudsman programs in nonprofit rather than government settings. No doubt, in a pure sense, this could more readily guarantee that the setting is more independent (provided the nonprofit is not also associated with services or individuals that may raise their own conflicts). The set of consumer principles established by several health plans with AARP and Families USA adopted the position that consumers should have access to an independent, external nonprofit ombudsman program.

However, strong arguments can be made that not-for-profit organizations—regardless of how independent—lack the resources, access, and authority that government-based ombudsmen have in addressing and resolving complaints (Park, 1997). Moreover, the not-for-profit-based ombudsman is a substantial deviation from the traditional role of the ombudsman—which is based in either the executive or legislative branches. This is particularly true when much of the complaint subject matter brought to the ombudsman either concerns or directly involves government, as does the long-term care ombudsman program (for example, Medicaid financing, licensure, and certification requirements).

As a practical matter, governments, whether federal, state, or local, will establish ombudsman services and locate them in a variety of organizational settings that operate within a political context. This is inherent in the legislative and public appropriation of funds processes. The most important lesson from the long-term care ombudsman program experience is the importance of striving to make the office of the ombudsman as independent as possible and ensure the greatest degree of freedom to vigorously and fully investigate complaints, resolve problems, and otherwise act on behalf of program clients. Moreover, it is imperative that the program's client community and the public at large perceive the ombudsman as independent in fulfilling its duties and public promise.

Confidential Investigation and Resolution of Complaints

The ability of the ombudsman to ensure the confidential investigation and resolution of complaints is another key feature of the long-term care ombudsman program. The assurance of confidential treatment of the information provided has been essential in establishing the trust necessary for residents of facilities and others acting on their behalf to file complaints and provide information to the ombudsman. Primarily, this has been necessary to provide complainants with respect for their privacy in sharing intimate information about their fears and details of their treatment and condition. Beyond privacy considerations, fear of retaliation or reprisal can be a powerful disincentive for residents and family members to detail their problems and grievances.

The guarantee of confidentiality is paramount to the work of the ombudsman. The OAA has clear and strong language governing confidentiality and assures that identities of complainants or residents may only occur with those individuals' written consent. The confidentiality and disclosure provisions governing the long-term care ombudsman program have created practical and political difficulties for the ombudsman at times. Officials that have authority over the ombudsman but are not part of the ombudsman program, such as a director of a state agency on aging, have not always been comfortable with the notion of subordinates having information they cannot reveal, particularly in cases that receive public attention. At times, the federal standards on confidentiality have also put the ombudsman program at odds with other state policy objectives, particularly in the area of mandatory abuse-reporting laws. Although the ombudsman is ultimately protected by the supremacy of federal law over state law when refusing to submit to the abuse-reporting mandate, the ombudsman is not protected from the discomfort and other problems created by resistance to complying with state law.

Protection Against Retaliation or Discrimination

An important corollary to the confidentiality issue is protecting complainants and informants against retaliation or discrimination for having made a complaint or provided information in good faith. The OAA provides for such protections, and they would be an important ingredient of ombudsman services in other health care settings. In situations in which there is not an equal balance of power or authority, those with less power or authority may be fearful to complain or provide information if they are concerned about the potential to be harmed by such expression. Clearly, if a health care consumer believes that he or she risks adverse decisions regarding approval for services or treatment, there may be a legitimate fear of taking a complaint to a third party, particularly if it is an externally based party, including government-sanctioned individuals.

Positive Change for Residents on a Collective Basis

If investigating and resolving the individual complaints is the daily "bread and butter" of long-term care ombudsmen, then it could be argued that their efforts to effectuate positive change for residents on a group or collective basis are their "meat and potatoes." Since the outset of the LTC ombudsman program, there has been emphasis on both individual advocacy for residents and systemic advocacy for residents collectively. Individual complaint processing underlies the overall structural, functional, and programmatic development and orientation of the LTC ombudsman program. The complaint-handling process is the key ingredient in informing ombudsmen about the broader issues that would be more appropriately addressed through systems advocacy.

Ombudsmen played a key role in the nationwide effort to achieve reform of the rules and systems governing nursing home care under Medicare and Medicaid that resulted in the landmark nursing home reform provisions of the Omnibus Budget Reconciliation Act of 1987.[3] Today, ombudsmen continue to have an important and effective voice with Congress in providing relevant and timely information on matters concerning long-term care that are under consideration by Congress. Similarly, they have been crucial to state-based efforts to enact nursing home–related legislation by providing real life examples of poor care, harmed residents, conditions of facilities and residents, and the need for specific improvements.

In writing about the role of ombudsmen in managed care, Frank states that "systems advocacy has proactive and reactive elements. Effective ombudsman programs recognize when an individual's problem is rooted in the way the system is designed or functioning, and work to resolve the problem at its root. Ombudsman programs need to establish means of communication with the leadership of the plans, the state oversight agencies, and legislative bodies responsible for the managed care programs, so that there is a forum for bringing these systemic problems forward and working out solutions" (Frank, 1997, p. 13).

Although long-term care ombudsmen toil daily in thousands of nursing homes to respond to the problems that residents face, they make their greatest impact in their systems advocacy, which is based largely on the daily resident complaints. The daily hassles and problems dealt with by ombudsmen are the seeds for many administrative, regulatory, legislative, and judicial changes that ultimately are crucial to the direction and overall condition of life in nursing homes. An ombudsman program that only responds to individual complaints lives up to, at best, half the potential impact of the program, and is likely consigned to respond to many of the same problems over and over.

Accessibility and Availability

An ombudsman's success depends on accessibility and availability. In the long-term care setting, the ombudsman should not sit and wait for the phone to ring when it comes to their caseload. There is a clear need for the LTC ombudsman to make himself or herself truly available to the residents and others interacting with LTC facilities. An ombudsman poster on the wall near the facility's administrator's office or the nurses' station is an inadequate way to demonstrate availability and accessibility. The presence of local designated offices and representatives of the ombudsman are in many states the key to ensuring the program is in fact accessible and available.

Similarly, ombudsmen for other populations and other health care settings will need to be sensitive to, and have strategies for, ensuring they are truly available and accessible. The more vulnerable the population—whether because of impairment or diagnoses, education or income levels, cultural issues, or other factors—the more necessary it will be for ombudsmen to assert themselves not only to their client population but also to the entities (for example, health plans, Medicaid officials, providers) with whom they are likely to initiate complaint resolution activities on behalf of their clients.

Nonregulatory Role

An ombudsman should serve in a nonregulatory role, seeking to work on behalf of the consumer with providers, plans, and others to get problems resolved as quickly as possible, thereby avoiding longer, costlier formal proceedings in most cases. In the majority of cases in the LTC ombudsman experience, problems are resolved without formal proceedings such as hearings or litigation. The role of the ombudsman in essence is to get others to do their jobs—to "do right" by the client. In other words, the ombudsman's mission very often is to convince or persuade the provider, the payer, the bureaucrat, the regulator, and others not to do harm to the well-being or interests of the resident-complainant and, if harm has been done, to ameliorate, reverse, or remedy that harm. The process of convincing or persuading is accomplished through an arsenal of tools or skills, ranging from the ombudsman's knowledge of the law, rules, and regulations governing the setting or service that is at issue to the use of the media or public opinion to reverse or remedy adverse decisions to the ability to assist the complainant in obtaining legal counsel and representation when necessary.

There is no reason to think that these same functions and skills would not be as important for an ombudsman in the managed care or other health care setting.

Consideration of Program Funding Needs

A final lesson from the long-term care ombudsman experience that is invaluable to ombudsman programs for other constituencies is to consider the funding needs of the program. An ombudsman program needs a stable and sufficient funding stream to provide resources for adequate programming. The LTC ombudsman program has been plagued by inadequate funding from both federal and state sources. Funded primarily through the OAA, many states have augmented the funding through state resources. In Ohio, the state legislature established a statutory "bed tax" paid by nursing facilities to augment other funding sources for the ombudsman program. Other states have provided minimal, if any, nonfederal resources.

Although an ombudsman program is arguably considerably less expensive than a regulatory system of oversight, it is not cost-free. Nor can it be considered as an alternative to a regulatory system or service for budgetary purposes. The ombudsman performs a much different role than the regulator does. The ombudsman is not a substitute for the regulator. In fact, the ombudsman strives to get the regulator to do a more consistent and more responsive job. Even if volunteers are to be used, as they are in the LTC ombudsman program, as previously indicated, there are clearly associated costs. Volunteers must have the skills and resources to investigate complaints vigorously and fully and to seek to resolve them. Ombudsmen, especially volunteers, must be recruited, trained, and adequately supervised for both complaint investigation and casework.

Adopting the Ombudsman Model

For more than two decades the long-term care ombudsman program has continued to expand and refine its legislative foundation to reflect the day-to-day experience of its thousands of paid and volunteer ombudsman in representing the interests of facility residents, on both an individual and a collective basis. The most important structural and programmatic features have continued to be identified and reinforced over the same period. This is not to suggest that these features are not subject to debate and that there are not issues related to them yet to be to resolved. Yet, collectively, most ombudsmen and analysts would agree that the features described here are essential to the development and effectiveness of the long-term care ombudsman program. Similarly, these key features ought to be included in any ombudsman program designed for other health care settings, such as managed care.

As already mentioned, there is considerable and growing interest in adopting the ombudsman model, including the long-term care ombudsman program model, for consumers of other health care services. The model has expanded in a number of states into other areas of long-term care, particularly in-home care. In fact, the ombudsman concept has made inroads into other parts of the health care system, especially Medicaid managed care. Some fourteen states have established ombudsman or ombudsman-like consumer assistance programs for Medicaid managed care (Lee and Scott, 1996; Families USA Foundation, 1998).

Unfortunately, it appears that many of these new programs do not adopt the identified critical features that are part of the long-term care ombudsman program. For example, a number of them are operated by the Medicaid agency, which, of course, is ultimately responsible for decisions made and actions taken affecting Medicaid beneficiaries. Florida did establish an independent agency but provided no funding, consequently it operates solely with volunteers (Families USA Foundation, 1998). In 1998, according to Families USA, Vermont became the first state to establish "an independent consumer assistance program by requiring the state to contract with a nonprofit organization that will fulfill this function" (Families USA Foundation, 1998, p. 22). Among other functions, the program is designed to help consumers understand their rights and responsibilities; identify, investigate, and resolve complaints on behalf of consumers; and assist consumers in filing and pursuing complaints.

Several model statutes have been developed to guide states and others in considering and drafting laws to create ombudsmen or other forms of independent consumer assistance for health care consumers (for example, those developed by the National Health Law Project and the Consumers Coalition for Quality Health Care). The Consumers Coalition model bill, a comprehensive managed care model statute, contains a "managed care ombudsman program" section, as well as a section for an "independent quality monitoring and improvement program." It was distributed to all states for consideration as they craft legislation related to managed care quality.

As this volume goes to press, Congress is considering consumer protection legislation for health care consumers, as are a number of states. Some of the proposals under consideration include mechanisms for consumers to voice complaints, obtain assistance in filing grievances and appeals, and engage in systems advocacy. For example, S. 6, the Patients' Bill of Rights of 1999 introduced by Senator Tom Daschle, Democrat of South Dakota, and its House companion legislation, H.R. 358, the Democratic leadership's Patients' Bill of Rights Act of 1998 (PBRA), would establish an independent external appeals process and would provide an independent consumer assistance program (Families USA Foundation, 1999). Such a program would complement other forms of government oversight or regulatory mechanisms to ensure quality or consumer protection.

In today's complex health care system, the availability of an ombudsman or other independent party to address problems may not only be beneficial to the consumer but also necessary—even at times life-saving. Consumer rights and avenues for redress of grievances mean nothing without a way to enforce those rights, and they may mean nothing without someone to help in the exercise of those rights, in questioning a plan or provider, for example, much less filing and acting on an appeal.

The LTCOP coupled with other independent consumer assistance models provide a wealth of features that have served the elderly well in addressing many individual problems as well as systemic issues. As consumer protection measures are considered and enacted, policymakers, advocates, and health care representatives would benefit from a thorough examination of the experience and lessons learned from the considerable history associated with the long-term care ombudsman and other consumer assistance models.

Notes

1. The Older Americans Act of 1965 (OAA) was enacted into law as Public Law 98–73 and has subsequently been amended numerous times. The Long-Term Care Ombudsman Program was incorporated into the OAA as part of the 1978 amendments to the Act under P.L. 95–478. For full text of current OAA provisions governing the ombudsman program, see Title VII, especially Chapter Two—Ombudsman Programs—of Subtitle A, *Compilation of the Older Americans Act of 1965, as Amended Through December 31, 1992,* Committee Print, Serial No. 103-E, June 15, 1993.
2. Public Law 95–478 enacted the Older Americans Act Amendments of 1978.
3. Public Law 100–203, the Omnibus Budget Reconciliation Act of 1987 (OBRA), establishing the nursing home patient protection provisions, was signed into law on December 22, 1987.

References

Administration on Aging. *Supplemental Guidance in Implementation of Long-Term Care Ombudsman Program Requirement of the Older Americans Act, as Amended.* AoA-Program Instruction 81–8. Washington, D.C.: Author, Jan. 19, 1981.

Administration on Aging. "Executive Summary." *Fiscal Year 1996 Long-Term Care Ombudsman Report.* Washington, D.C.: Author, Jan. 1999.

Benson, W. F. Testimony given before the Subcommittee on Consumer Rights, Protections, and Responsibilities of the President's Advisory Commission on Consumer Protection and Quality in the Health Care Industry, on behalf of the U.S. Administration on Aging, Washington, D.C., 1997a.

Benson, W. F. Remarks presented to the Consumer Advisory Council of the American Association of Health Plans, on behalf of the U.S. Administration on Aging, Washington, D.C., 1997b.

Consumer Coalition for Quality Health Care. *National Consumer Protection Blueprint for Managed Care.* Washington, D.C.: Author, 1997.

Families USA Foundation. *HMO Consumers at Risk, States to the Rescue.* Washington, D.C.: Author, July 1996.

Families USA Foundation. *ASAP! UPDATE: Grassroots Action for Health & Long Term Care. Special Report: Health Care Consumer Assistance Programs.* Washington, D.C.: Author, 1998a.

Families USA Foundation. *Hit and Miss: State Managed Care Laws.* (Report funded by the Henry J. Kaiser Family Foundation.) Washington, D.C.: Author, 1998b.

Families USA Foundation. *Basic Consumer Protections: How the Federal Bills Compare.* Washington, D.C.: Author, 1999.

Frank, B. "Managed Care Ombudsman for Medicare and Medicaid Beneficiaries: Advocacy in the Medical Marketplace for Consumers Who Cannot Vote With Their Feet." A paper for the State of Connecticut Department of Social Services, 1115 Waiver Development Committee, Subcommittee on Quality. Unpublished executive masters thesis, Rensselaer Polytechnic Institute, 1997.

Institute of Medicine. *Real People, Real Problems: An Evaluation of the Long-Term Care Ombudsman Programs of the Older Americans Act.* Washington, D.C.: National Academy of Sciences, 1995.

Lee, P. V., and Scott, C. *Managed Care Ombudsman Programs: New Approaches To Assist Consumers and Improve the Health Care Systems.* Los Angeles: Center for Health Care Rights, 1996.

Monk, A., Kaye, L. W., and Litwin, H. *Resolving Grievances in the Nursing Home: A Study of the Ombudsman Program.* New York: Columbia University Press, 1984.

Nelson, H. W. "Long-Term Care Volunteer Roles on Trial: Ombudsman Effectiveness Revisited." *Journal of Gerontological Social Work,* 1995, *23*(3–4).

Park, M. Draft paper prepared for Subcommittee on Consumer Rights, Protections, and Responsibilities of the Advisory Commission on Consumer Protection and Quality in the Health Care Industry, Washington, D.C., 1997.

The President's Advisory Commission on Consumer Protection and Quality in the Health Care Industry. "Consumer Bill of Rights and Responsibilities," Report to the President of the United States, 1997.

The President's Advisory Commission on Consumer Protection and Quality in the Health Care Industry. "Quality First: Better Health Care for All Americans," Final Report to the President of the United States, March 1998.

Principles for Consumer Protection: Preliminary Statement of Principles for Consumer Protection. American Association of Retired Persons, Families USA Foundation, Group Health Cooperative of Puget Sound, HIP Health Plans, Kaiser Permanente, 1997.

Chapter Seven

Ensuring Equal Access to Care

Brian Biles and David Sandman

Access to health care—that is, an individual's ability to obtain services when needed—is a slippery concept, but one that lies at the heart of any health care system. Access is a by-product of thousands of decisions that range from policy judgments at the highest levels of government to choices made by individual patients on a daily basis. It depends on factors as diverse as insurance status, financing and delivery arrangements, availability of trained medical personnel, transportation, consumer information, and patient preferences. The many aspects of access to care have been categorized into those that predispose patients to use health services, those that depend on patients' level of illness and need for health care, and those that enable patients to get services on demand.[1]

Growing Concern About Access

Changes occurring in the nation's health care system have placed concerns about access high on the list of priorities of both policymakers and the public. For Americans with insurance, the health care system they confront today is very different from that of the past. In particular, the rapid growth of managed care has brought renewed concern over patients' ability to access appropriate, high-quality services when needed.

Managed care enrollment is increasing in every insurance market. Among employees of firms with two hundred or more workers,

135

81 percent belonged to a managed care plan in 1997, compared with just 29 percent in 1988.[2] Similarly, 48 percent of Medicaid beneficiaries[3] and 14 percent of Medicare beneficiaries were enrolled in managed care by 1997.[4]

A Nagging Problem

Although concerns over access to care have gained greater urgency in recent years, the issue is not a new one. As early as 1952, the President's Commission on the Health Needs of the Nation declared that "access to the means for attainment and preservation of health is a basic human right."

Under the now-vanishing fee-for-service system, access to care was often considered in terms of the ratio of physicians to population in a given geographic area. The reasoning was based on fundamental principles of supply and demand. In most cases, lower physician-population ratios were found in rural areas and distressed inner-city areas. The response to such shortages was increased emphasis on the development of safety-net providers and programs. The National Community Health Center Program and the National Health Service Corps were specifically designed to improve access to care in underserved areas.

Concerns about access to care then extended to the support of primary care physicians. Since 1965, most of the increase in physicians per capita has occurred in the medical specialties, rising from 56 per 100,000 people in 1965 to 123 per 100,000 in 1992.[5] Policymakers feared that an undersupply of generalists could contribute to problems with access to primary care. A number of physician training programs were established in the Health Professions Education Assistance Act of 1976 to expand the training of family physicians and primary care internists and pediatricians.

Incentives to Skim and Skimp

Such access problems were recognized when the nation began its transition to a health care system based on managed care. The HMO Act of 1973 acknowledged early on that health plans would have incentives both to "skim" by enrolling only healthier members and avoiding patients with serious and chronic illnesses, as well to "skimp" by limiting access to services for plan members. As a result, it declared that "basic health services shall within the area serviced by the HMO be available and accessible to each of its members with reasonable promptness and in a manner that assures continuity."[6]

Concerns over access in managed care derives from the financial incentives and administrative constraints that are often present. Under capitation arrangements, health plans and providers can potentially increase their profit margins by limiting medical services, including diagnostic tests and procedures, specialty care, and hospitalizations. Similarly, organizational features of managed care—like closed provider panels and primary care gatekeeping—can limit a patient's ability to access appropriate care.

Warning Signs

Today, a quarter of a century later, it appears that the HMO Act of 1973 was prescient in its concern about barriers to accessing care in a managed care environment. Although our ability to monitor the impact of managed care on access lags behind the restructuring of the industry, warning signs have emerged indicating that patients may encounter problems obtaining the health care they need.

The 1994 Commonwealth Fund Survey of Patient Experiences with Managed Care interviewed 3,347 working adults in Boston, Miami, and Los Angeles with employee- or union-sponsored health insurance coverage regarding their health care and their experiences with their health plan.[7] This survey found that managed care enrollees reported greater difficulty accessing health care services. For example, managed care enrollees were almost three times more likely than those in fee-for-service arrangements to rate their access to specialty care as fair or poor (23 percent of managed care enrollees versus 8 percent of those in fee-for-service programs). Similarly, managed care participants were more than twice as likely as those in fee-for-service to give fair or poor ratings to their access to emergency care (12 percent of the former versus 5 percent of the latter). Those in managed care plans also were far more likely than their fee-for-service counterparts to rate their waiting times for medical appointments as fair or poor (28 percent of managed care enrollees did versus 11 percent of those in fee-for-service programs).

Other studies have found that vulnerable populations—the chronically ill, elderly, and low-income—may face particular difficulties accessing care in a managed care setting. Patients with health problems have reported greater difficulty obtaining a continuum of care and less satisfaction with their care in managed care plans than have similar patients in fee-for-service arrangements.[8] A longitudinal study suggests also that elderly and low-income patients with chronic illnesses in managed care plans experience worse health outcomes than similar patients in traditional fee-for-service plans.[9]

Consumer Anxiety

Studies that document patients' experiences with access barriers are complemented by those that reveal substantial anxiety among patients over their current and future ability to obtain needed services. The Kaiser-Commonwealth 1997 National Survey of Health Insurance found that 30 percent of all adults of working age (eighteen to sixty-four) worried "a great deal" or "a lot" that they would be denied a necessary medical procedure. An even higher proportion—40 percent—reported being worried that they wouldn't be able to get needed specialty care.

Other surveys of patients have also revealed significant concern over managed care's impact on access to high-quality care. The Kaiser-Harvard National Survey of Americans' Views on Consumer Protections in Managed Care found that solid majorities of the public believe managed care poses threats to health care access: 59 percent reported that health maintenance organizations and other managed care plans have made it harder for sick patients to see medical specialists, and 61 percent stated that managed care has decreased the amount of time that doctors spend with patients.[10] Allowing patients with serious medical conditions direct access to specialists without the approval of a primary care physician topped the list of provisions that consumers would most like to see enacted into law.

Three Types of Remedies

The extent of patient anxiety over access to care is reflected in the volume of proposals to strengthen consumer protection. Numerous remedies have been proposed to assure access to care. They include information-oriented approaches, increased regulation of the managed care industry, and private voluntary initiatives.

Information-Oriented Strategies

In addition to raising concerns about access, managed care has also created opportunities that were unavailable in a fee-for-service-based system to measure access to care and hold health plans accountable. The past decade has witnessed strides made in the ability to measure and compare the performance of health plans in terms of access for their members.[11] Collecting reliable information and developing effective methods of disseminating it to purchasers and consumers are essential to assuring access to care.

The National Committee for Quality Assurance

The National Committee for Quality Assurance (NCQA) has emerged as the leader in efforts to assess, measure, and report on the performance of managed care organizations. Its accreditation process reviews how well health plans manage all parts of their care delivery systems, including access to care for their members in areas such as utilization and grievance and appeals procedures when access to services has been denied. Since 1991, more than half of the nation's HMOs, representing approximately 75 percent of all HMO enrollees, have voluntarily sought NCQA accreditation.

Health Plan Employer Data and Information Set

NCQA's accreditation efforts are complemented by its Health Plan Employer Data and Information Set (HEDIS), a group of more than seventy standardized performance measures for comparing health plans. The latest version—HEDIS 3.0—contains ten measures that address access and availability of care explicitly, including the availability of primary care providers; children's access to primary care providers; availability of mental health-chemical dependency providers; annual dental visits; availability of dentists;

adults' access to preventive-ambulatory health services; initiation of prenatal care; availability of obstetrical-prenatal care providers; low birth-weight deliveries at facilities for high-risk deliveries and neonates; and availability of language interpretation services. An additional measure of access—problems with obtaining care—is currently in the development and testing stage.

Consumer Assessment of Health Plans Survey

Patient reports of access to care experiences are important complements to HEDIS measures, which are based largely on administrative data. Pioneering work by the Picker Institute has demonstrated that consumers may be able to provide more accurate data than medical records in regards to access to care. The Consumer Assessment of Health Plans Survey (CAHPS) project is the leading effort to measure and assess access from the patient's perspective. This state-of-the-art survey was developed by a consortium of researchers with support from the federal Agency for Health Care Policy and Research. Although designed to be applicable to all patient populations, CAHPS will receive its first large-scale demonstration among the Medicare population because the Health Care Financing Administration plans to use the survey with approximately 140,000 beneficiaries enrolled in some 235 managed care plans across the country. In combination with administrative measures, the newly available CAHPS will significantly advance the nation's ability to measure and monitor access to care.

Regulatory Strategies

Policymakers have responded to consumer worries about access with a host of proposals to increase regulation of the managed care industry. A number of proposals under consideration by Congress would increase federal or state oversight of health plans.[12] More than a thousand proposals to regulate managed care were introduced in state legislatures in 1997, and in excess of two hundred have become law. At least twenty-one states have enacted comprehensive consumer rights bills that include provisions designed to assure both access to care and quality of care.

Some of these proposals focus on specific aspects of care delivery, such as requiring access to a minimum length of stay in a hospital following either a birth or a mastectomy. Other provisions address a broad range of consumer and provider concerns, including direct access to obstetricians and pediatricians as primary care physicians, and a "prudent layperson" rule regarding access to emergency care. Some proposals include a mandatory point-of-service option that would allow access to physicians not in the plan network, with the payment of additional amounts.

But the broader access provisions in these proposals tend to be vague and subject to differing interpretations. For example, some proposals require that patients have access to a sufficient number, mix, and distribution of providers, but they do not specify actual physician-patient ratios or require that a specific proportion of a network's providers accept new patients. Similarly, some proposals require that access standards may not be relaxed in rural areas, but they do not establish specific access thresholds for such regions.

Access provisions often hinge on undefined terms such as "timely and proximate" or "reasonable promptness," which discourage enforcement because it is difficult to document failure. As a result, these proposals generally do not include the graduated enforcement provisions that have been used in other health care sectors, such as the nursing home industry. With a few notable exceptions, current proposals do not provide for the use of intermediate sanctions, including freezing new enrollment, consent agreements, civil money penalties, and other steps that could be taken to strengthen access provisions.

Efforts to regulate access to care by managed care plans, always a complicated and difficult task, might be strengthened by developing more specific standards for access and mandating that plans measure and report indicators of access. Incentives such as higher payments for plans with exemplary records of assuring access to care could improve the performance of plans. Graduated sanctions for plans that fail to meet standards could also increase the effectiveness of a regulatory program.

Voluntary Initiatives

Although considerable public support exists for increased regulation of aspects of managed care, there is less consensus on the proper locus of responsibility to assure access and quality. A large proportion of the public would prefer to see managed care regulated by private voluntary organizations than by federal or state government.[13] The President's Advisory Commission on Consumer Protection and Quality in the Health Care Industry reflected this divide in its recommendations on how quality standards should be implemented and enforced. It recommended the creation of two bodies—one public and one private—to continue efforts to assure access and quality.[14]

The American Association of Health Plans (AAHP), which represents managed care plans, has responded to concerns over access and quality with an initiative entitled Putting Patients First. It calls for AAHP member plans to pledge their responsiveness to patient needs and embrace specific access-related provisions such as a prudent layperson standard for emergency care.[15] This initiative's principles have been adopted by more than a thousand health plans serving at least 120 million Americans. Since its introduction, AAHP has continued to adopt policies designed to ensure access, such as ensuring the adequacy of physician network supply relative to plan membership size. Skeptics, however, contend that such voluntary, industry-led efforts to assure access and quality are inadequate in the absence of legal liability for the care delivered by industry members.[16]

Conclusion

Assuring access to health care is an ongoing process. The rapid growth of managed care enrollment has simultaneously raised new concerns over barriers to care and increased the ability to track plan members' access. Managed care holds the promise of improving access to primary and preventive care, as well as coordinating a spectrum of services for patients with complex medical needs. But managed care also poses risks to access, particularly for chronically ill and other vulnerable patient groups. Preserving access in a managed care environment will require a mixture of public and private efforts, as well as independent and reliable information with which to inform decision making and monitor future trends.

Notes

1. Aday, L. A., and Andersen, R. "A Framework for the Study of Access to Medical Care." *Health Services Research,* 1974, *9,* 208–220.
2. KPMG Peat Marwick. *Health Benefits in 1997.* Arlington, Va.: Author, 1997.
3. Health Care Financing Administration. *Medicaid Managed Care Enrollment Report.* Washington, D.C.: Author, 1997.
4. Christensen, S. *Memorandum on Medicare+Choice Provisions in the Balanced Budget Act of 1997.* Washington, D.C.: Congressional Budget Office, 1997.
5. Kindig, D. A. "Federal Regulation and Market Forces in Physician Workforce Management." In M. Osterweis, C. J. McLaughlin, H. R. Manasse, Jr., and C. L. Hoppes, *The U.S. Health Workforce: Power, Politics, and Policy.* Washington, D.C.: Association of Academic Health Centers, 1996.
6. Public Health Service Act, section 1301(a)(4).
7. Davis, K., Scott Collins, K., Schoen, C., and Morris, C. "Choice Matters: Enrollees' Views of Their Health Plans." *Health Affairs,* Summer 1995, 99–112.
8. Davis, K., and Schoen, C. "Changing Health Care Systems and Access to Care for the Chronically Ill." In F. J. Manning and J. A. Barondess (eds.), *Changing Health Care Systems and Rheumatic Disease.* Washington, D.C.: Institute of Medicine, National Academy Press, 1996; and Robert Wood Johnson Foundation. "Sick People in Managed Care Have Difficulty Getting Services and Treatment, New Survey Reports" (press release). June 28, 1994.
9. Ware, J. E., Jr., Bayliss, M. S., Rogers, W. H., Kosinski, M., Taylor, A. R. "Differences in 4-Year Health Outcomes for Elderly and Poor, Chronically Ill Patients Treated in HMO and Fee-for-Service Systems: Results from the Medical Outcomes Study." *Journal of the American Medical Association,* 1996, *276,* 1039–1047.
10. "Henry J. Kaiser Family Foundation–Harvard University National Survey of Americans' Views on Consumer Protections in Managed Care." Menlo Park, Calif.: Henry J. Kaiser Family Foundation, 1998.
11. Epstein, A. M. "Rolling Down the Runway: The Challenges Ahead for Quality Report Cards." *Journal of the American Medical Association,* 1998, *279*(21), 1691–1696.
12. Tapay, N., Pollitz, K., and Curtis, J. "Consumer Protection in Managed Care Plans: A Side-by-Side Comparison of Proposed Federal Legislation." Menlo Park, Calif.: Henry J. Kaiser Family Foundation, 1998.

13. "Henry J. Kaiser Family Foundation–Harvard University National Survey of Americans' Views on Consumer Protections in Managed Care." Menlo Park, Calif.: Henry J. Kaiser Family Foundation, 1997.

14. The President's Advisory Commission on Consumer Protection and Quality in the Health Care Industry. "Quality First: Better Health Care for All Americans." Final report to the President of the United States, March 1998.

15. Jones, D. A. "Putting Patients First: A Philosophy in Practice." *Health Affairs,* 1997, *16*(6), 115–120.

16. Havighurst, C. C. "Putting Patients First: Promise or Smoke Screen." *Health Affairs,* 1997, *16*(6), 123–125.

Chapter Eight

Regulating Quality and Clinical Practice

William L. Roper

Striking a balance between the often-competing objectives of efficiency, accessibility, and quality in health care requires governmental intervention. The challenge lies in identifying the *appropriate* role for government—a challenge that is particularly daunting in the area of health care quality.

Traditional Approaches to Health Care Regulation

Historically, our nation has relied primarily on industry self-regulation rather than government intervention for assuring clinical quality (Brennan and Berwick, 1996). It has long been argued that only health care professionals and organizations themselves have the necessary expertise to develop and enforce rules for such highly specialized and rapidly evolving fields of practice. By contrast, governmental roles in financing health services have become widely accepted and practiced, both in purchasing health care through public programs such as Medicare and Medicaid and in regulating the health insurance industry. Federal and state governments have proven to be relatively effective in making eligibility and coverage decisions for public programs, as well as in establishing standards for the private insurance industry in areas such as financial solvency, benefit determination, and consumer grievance processes.

Health Plans Influence Care

Managed care creates a wrinkle in these traditional approaches to health care regulation because it provides for a single organization to assume responsibility for the delivery and financing of health services to defined groups of individuals. It therefore becomes possible to regulate not only the insurance practices of health plans but also their delivery practices. Health plans are able to affect the quality of care delivered to their enrolled members through the administrative and financial arrangements they develop with their affiliated physicians, hospitals, and other health care providers.

Indeed, plans employ a variety of utilization management strategies to influence how patients seek care and how providers deliver it. These strategies include establishing clinical practice guidelines to encourage providers to use the most effective and efficient practices for preventing, diagnosing, and treating common medical conditions; using primary care case management models to ensure the coordination of health services delivered to members; establishing precertification and referral requirements for specialized medical services to discourage the delivery of medically unnecessary or inappropriate care; and using selective contracting practices to ensure that enrolled members receive care from the most effective and efficient providers.

Health plans also influence the delivery of care through an expanding array of provider payment methodologies and financial incentives designed to encourage efficiency and quality in service delivery. These methods include capitated payment arrangements as well as financial withholds and bonuses tied to performance in specific clinical areas such as reduced hospital and emergency room visits and enhanced delivery of clinical preventive services.

An Easier Target for Regulation

In the past, regulating the clinical practices of individual physicians and groups has not been administratively or politically feasible for governments at any level. Strong professional opposition combined with high enforcement costs have precluded substantial governmental involvement in this area (Starr, 1982). Regulation of health plan practices, however, appears much more feasible and politically acceptable in the current health care environment. By assuming responsibility for delivering a continuum of health services to a defined population, managed care plans represent a much easier target for governmental regulation than do individual physicians and groups. Moreover, mounting public concern about health plan operations is contributing to a political environment that is highly supportive of regulation (Moran, 1997). In truth, however, most of the popular concerns about managed care have relatively little to do with clinical quality, and much to do with issues of consumer protection and choice.

Defining Clinical Quality

To assess the prospects for regulation of clinical quality, we need to start with a workable definition of the concept. According to the widely recognized Institute of Medicine definition, quality is "the degree to which health services for individuals and populations increase the likelihood of desired health outcomes and are consistent with current professional knowledge" (Institute of Medicine, 1990).

Three Concepts

At least three concepts implicit in this definition invite consideration from a regulatory perspective:

- Quality is realized at both the individual and the population level. Individual clinicians historically have assumed responsibility for quality at the single-patient level. By comparison, the managed care systems now emerging are structured to manage quality at the population level, across defined groups of health plan members. Therefore, clinical quality may be delivered, measured, regulated, and improved both at the individual level *and* at the population level.
- It is important that health outcomes be valued and "desired" by health care consumers. Judgments of clinical quality must be based on the effects that health services have on health status, and these effects must be evaluated from the perspective of the individuals and populations experiencing them.

- Professional knowledge and judgment have the central role in determining clinical quality. Clinical knowledge and technology are evolving rapidly, and so too must the mechanisms for assuring clinical quality. Consequently, these mechanisms depend heavily on the expertise of physicians and other health care professionals.

Five Dimensions

Clinical quality is a multidimensional concept. Systems for assuring quality must therefore address the various ways in which quality is realized by individuals and populations. A recent review of the scientific literature by the U.S. Congressional Research Service identifies five separate dimensions that are commonly used to assess the quality of clinical services (Congressional Research Service, 1997). Quality depends on:

Effectiveness of the service in producing a desired diagnostic, therapeutic, or preventive effect on health status. Despite continual advances in clinical knowledge, many of the health care services and products administered to patients today offer limited or uncertain medical benefits.

Appropriateness of the service for a given individual or population group. This dimension accounts for the fact that effective clinical services and products must be targeted at the appropriate health conditions and patient populations in order to achieve optimal health outcomes.

Technical skill in delivering a service to an individual or population. Technical skill can have a profound effect on health outcomes for services ranging from surgical procedures to immunizations.

Accessibility of services to individuals and populations in need of them. Accessibility may depend on factors such as geographic location, appointment availability, waiting times, referral relationships, and health insurance coverage. These structural and operational characteristics may have profound effects on health outcomes through their impact on the timing of service delivery in the context of disease progression.

Acceptability of health services to the individuals and populations receiving care. For many health conditions, an array of potential interventions offer different mixes of costs and benefits to patients. To achieve health outcomes that are desired by their patients, providers must be able to offer objective information on risks and benefits, identify patient preferences, and share the medical decision-making responsibilities with their patients. These skills represent an important component of clinical quality.

Consumer Protection Versus Quality Improvement

When considering regulatory options in health care, one must make a distinction between the regulatory goals of consumer protection and quality improvement. Much of the recent public debate over managed care involves issues of consumer protection rather than quality improvement.

Consumer Protection Issues

Consumer protection issues involve the safety of services and products; the proper labeling, advertising, and marketing of these products; and the existence of appropriate appeal rights regarding consumer dissatisfaction with products. In the case of insurance, several additional consumer protection issues emerge, such as the financial stability of the carrier and the benefit determination processes it uses. The need for direct, explicit governmental regulation in these areas is widely accepted and relatively noncontroversial.

Having taken the lead historically in establishing consumer protection regulations for health insurance organizations, state governments are heading the movement toward managed care plan regulations. These regulations include provisions for assuring that health plans exercise due diligence in monitoring the safety and competency of their providers; requiring public disclosure of key information regarding covered benefits, choice of providers, and consumer cost-sharing requirements; limiting health plan marketing practices to ensure unrestricted consumer decision making; and requiring an acceptable process for consumers to appeal the coverage decisions made by health plans.

These provisions offer important protections to consumers in choosing an appropriate health plan and using it to cover needed services. However, they offer relatively few assurances about clinical quality, which remains an outcome of the decisions and actions of individual health care providers and their interactions with patients. Assuring clinical quality necessarily entails influencing provider knowledge, decision making, and practices.

What is needed, therefore, are systems that encourage clinicians to provide the right services, to the right patients, at the right time, using the best possible techniques. In contrast to consumer protection provisions, these systems focus on achieving improvements in clinical quality, acknowledging that clinical knowledge, services, technologies, and skills are continually evolving with advances in medical science.

Quality Improvement Techniques

Many health care organizations are using techniques borrowed from the fields of industrial management and operations research to achieve quality improvement goals. Known alternatively as continuous quality improvement (CQI) and total quality management (TQM), these techniques are applied as part of a continuous, cyclical process to measure quality and implement improvements in clinical practice. In an ideal application, organizations base their quality improvement initiatives on targeted studies of health care processes and outcomes. Results from these studies are then used to identify best practices that produce optimal health outcomes.

To facilitate implementation of these practices among affiliated providers, health care organizations develop clinical practice guidelines detailing when and how they should be applied. Organizations use an expanding array of strategies for disseminating these guidelines and encouraging their adoption. Systems for monitoring provider practices are then used to track adherence to guidelines and to encourage improvements in practice using periodic provider feedback. Finally, organizations compare their overall levels of clinical performance with those of competing organizations in order to identify clinical areas needing further improvement.

Ideally, this cyclical process of improvement is supported by the public availability of comparative information on health care quality within organizations. This information can then be used by health care purchasers and consumers in making decisions among competing organizations, and perhaps among individual physicians and groups as well.

Regulatory Options for Assuring Clinical Quality

Regulatory approaches for assuring quality in health care differ, depending on whether the regulatory goals involve consumer protection or clinical quality improvement.

Consumer Protection Goals

A precedent exists for direct, explicit governmental regulation regarding consumer protection issues. Historically, state governments have taken the lead on consumer protection regulations in health care—especially those involving health insurance organizations and managed care plans. Many state regulations have followed the model statutes developed by the National Association of Insurance Commissioners (NAIC) that were reviewed in Chapter Two.

Despite notable state regulatory action in these areas, proposals in Congress would give the federal government an enhanced role in setting minimum consumer protection requirements in health care. There is some support in the health care industry for federal consumer protection regulations, which potentially would reduce the effort and expense currently required to meet fifty different state requirements for information disclosure. However, this reduction in compliance costs would occur only if federal legislation preempted similar state regulations.

The need for governmental regulation to ensure consumer protection in health care is clear. The remaining challenge is to strike an appropriate balance between state and federal regulation.

Quality Improvement Goals

Governmental regulation in the area of clinical quality improvement is much less straightforward. Historically, assuring the clinical quality of health care professionals and organizations has been left largely to private organizations. State medical societies and national specialty boards maintain responsibilities for licensing and certifying physicians. Recently, the American Medical Association announced plans for a national quality assessment system for physicians, which would include measures of health outcomes and practice statistics. Other state and national professional associations perform similar licensing and certification functions for other types of health professionals. The Joint Commission on Accreditation of Healthcare Organizations (JCAHO) holds responsibility for reviewing and accrediting hospitals, nursing homes, and other health care facilities. Similarly, the National Committee for Quality Assurance (NCQA), the most widely recognized accrediting body for managed care plans, maintains a performance assessment system—the Health Plan Employer Data and Information Set (HEDIS)—which generates comparative information in specific areas of plan performance, including clinical quality and consumer satisfaction. A number of other industry-based associations maintain accreditation and quality assurance processes for health care organizations.

Direct governmental involvement in clinical quality has been somewhat rare until recently. But growing public concern about quality in managed care has motivated legislative activity at both the state and federal levels. Many of these initiatives target the utilization management strategies and clinical practice guidelines used by health plans to encourage efficient resource use. A prominent example is the 1996 provision included in the federal Health Insurance Portability and Accountability Act, which requires health plans to offer a minimum forty-eight-hour length of hospital stay for patients after childbirth ("Interim Rules," 1997).

Such an approach represents only one of several regulatory strategies that governments may use in attempting to assure clinical quality. Regulatory options under consideration at federal and state levels generally involve one or more of three basic strategies: measuring and disseminating information on clinical quality, establishing and enforcing standards of clinical quality, and encouraging internal quality improvement processes.

Measuring and Disseminating Information

Regulatory options that focus on quality measurement and dissemination are based on the premise that health care purchasers and consumers *will use* relevant information on quality to inform their decisions. Such options, then, potentially promote quality improvement by encouraging quality-based competition among health plans and providers. However, the success of this approach depends on several factors: the widespread availability of comparative information on quality at the health plan level; the use of this information by purchasers and consumers in making choices among competing plans and providers; and the existence of competitive markets in which multiple health plans and providers vie to assume responsibility for providing health services to individuals and groups.

A central policy question that emerges from this discussion is whether government or industry-based groups should assume primary responsibility for measuring and disseminating information on clinical quality.

Federal Government Entity

One approach, which is reflected in several legislative proposals, gives the federal government a leading role in establishing a reporting system for health plans and in identifying the measures of quality to be included. This approach would be carried out either by vesting authority for quality measurement and dissemination in an existing federal health agency such as the Health Care Financing Administration or by creating a new, independent federal agency to assume this authority. An advisory council of health care industry representatives would be appointed to provide guidance in selecting quality measures, operating a reporting system, and disseminating information on quality to consumers and purchasers.

Industry-Based Entity

An alternative to the federal approach places greater reliance the quality measurement systems that are already developing within the health care industry, such as the NCQA's HEDIS system, the JCAHO's Project Oryx, and the performance measurement activities of the Foundation for Accountability (FAcct). Using this approach, an industry-based entity or collection of entities would assume authority for establishing and maintaining a quality measurement and reporting system for health plans. It would select quality measures, ensure that they are reported in a reliable and timely manner, and disseminate information to consumers and purchasers. The rationale underlying this approach is that quality measurement systems need to remain optimally responsive to changes in clinical practice and technology, and that such responsiveness is more likely to be found in the health care marketplace than in governmental regulatory bureaucracies.

Mandatory or Voluntary?

A key policy question that emerges from this discussion is whether participation in a quality measurement and reporting system should be mandatory or voluntary for health plans and other providers. A mandatory system would impose substantial compliance costs on the health care industry, which potentially could pose barriers to market entry for new health plans and providers. But reporting systems cannot be useful to consumers and purchasers unless they achieve full or nearly full participation. Unless large numbers of consumers and purchasers base their health care decisions on the quality measures produced by the reporting system, there is little chance of such a system having a meaningful effect on clinical quality. This rationale serves as a compelling argument for the use of strong participation incentives, if not participation requirements.

The federal government has several regulatory and policy tools for assuring the participation of health plans and providers in a quality measurement system. As an effective alternative to an explicit legislative mandate, it may use its market power as a monopsony health care purchaser to encourage participation by health plans and other providers. The federal government is by far the single largest purchaser of health services, having Medicare, Medicaid, the Federal Employee Health Benefits Program, and the Civilian Health and Medical Program for the Uniformed Services under its auspices. Requiring health plans and providers that participate in these federal programs also to participate in a quality measurement and reporting system may prove to be an efficient means of achieving a critical mass.

Establishing Standards for Clinical Quality

Another set of regulatory options facing policymakers involves setting clinical quality standards for health plans and providers to achieve. Quality standards may take a variety of forms, ranging from rules about specific clinical practices that should or should not be performed, to established targets for health care processes and outcomes such as rates of vaccine-preventable childhood diseases or cancer screening rates for age-appropriate adults.

The former type of standard, involving clinical practice regulations, was almost unheard of as a governmental action until recently. The 1996 federal regulation on minimum hospital stays for childbirth was unprecedented. A number of state governments have also adopted clinical practice regulations of this type in recent years (Fuchs, 1997). Virtually all such regulatory activity is emerging in response to managed care—to counter the utilization management strategies and clinical practice guidelines used by many plans (American Association of Health Plans, 1998).

In addition, many state governments are now regulating the referral practices and provider networks that are established and maintained by health plans. Twenty-eight states require plans to allow direct patient access to obstetricians and gynecologists. Twenty-four states require health plans to allow their enrollees freedom of choice in selecting providers within their network. A similar number of states have "any willing provider" laws requiring health plans to contract with any providers who accept the plans' contractual terms and conditions. Such regulations substantially limit the ability of plans to manage the quality and efficiency of health services through case management and selective contracting mechanisms.

A Public-Private Partnership

Despite its growing prevalence at federal and state levels, direct governmental involvement in establishing standards of clinical practice and quality create several problems from the perspective of quality improvement. First and foremost, this strategy can never hope to evolve into a comprehensive regulatory framework that includes all major areas of clinical practice. Legislative and regulatory bodies have neither the time nor the expertise to create rules to govern all clinical areas where quality problems exist. Similarly, governmental agencies cannot begin to keep pace with the changes occurring in clinical practice and medical technology, which will make existing regulations obsolete in a matter of years, if not months. Unresponsive regulatory systems will only serve to retard the pace of medical innovation and adoption, ultimately slowing progress toward quality improvement.

These arguments suggest that the authority for establishing standards for clinical quality should lie with the health care industry rather than with the legislative and regulatory machinery of federal and state governments. An industry-based authority would have an enhanced ability to track changes in practice and technology and ensure that performance standards keep pace.

A public-private partnership approach may offer a strategy for capturing the responsiveness of an industry-based authority with the enforcement powers of a governmental agency. The approach used in regulating the financial industry has been suggested as a promising model for quality measurement systems in health care (Etheredge, 1997). This model includes an independent, nonpartisan federal regulatory agency (the Securities and Exchange Commission) linked with an industry-based board for setting performance standards (The Financial Accounting Standards Board).

The trade-off between voluntary and mandatory compliance with clinical quality standards is another important policy consideration. A voluntary compliance system would allow quality standards to be used as "best practices" and benchmarks for encouraging continuous improvement among health plans and providers. Publicly available report cards could enable consumers and purchasers to compare health plan performance with established quality standards, and thereby motivate quality-based competition. This approach is used in voluntary accreditation systems such as those maintained by NCQA and JCAHO.

By comparison, a mandatory compliance system would require health plans and providers to meet or exceed specified quality standards, which would then serve as minimum performance requirements rather than as best practices or benchmarking tools. Mandatory compliance systems cannot offer strong incentives for continuous improvement in quality once minimum standards are met. Further, they entail higher enforcement costs by necessitating periodic efforts to identify and respond to those organizations not meeting the quality standards. And as with the clinical practice standards already implemented at federal and state levels, mandatory compliance systems run the risk of inhibiting the development and dissemination of innovations in clinical practice.

Encouraging Internal Processes

Another regulatory option is to encourage health care organizations to adopt their own internal quality improvement processes. This approach recognizes that the most powerful strategies for improving clinical quality must occur at the organization level and be tailored to the specific capacities, skills, and environments of individual organizations. Following the model legislation created by the National Association of Insurance Commissioners, a number of states now require health plans to operate internal quality improvement programs. Similarly, industry-based accreditation entities such as JCAHO and NCQA require organizations to maintain these programs. Under these laws and accreditation programs, health care organizations usually are required to have clinical records and information systems that are adequate to support their quality improvement processes and to show evidence of quality goals, improvement strategies, and active interventions.

As with other regulatory options, a key policy question is whether to use voluntary or mandatory adoption requirements for internal quality improvement processes. Given the importance of an active quality improvement process to overall clinical quality, policymakers may be inclined to mandate the adoption of these processes. The problem lies in the fact that the science of internal quality improvement is still young. Mandates for adopting specific components of a quality improvement process may discourage organizations from developing and testing innovations in quality improvement, such as new information systems, planning processes, implementation mechanisms, and dissemination strategies. Mandates may also dampen enthusiasm for improvement processes among clinicians and other staff. In this light, flexible regulations for the adoption of internal quality improvement processes appear advantageous.

One approach under consideration at the federal level involves developing an accreditation program for the internal quality improvement processes maintained by health care organizations. An industry-based organization such as NCQA could assume responsibility for reviewing and accrediting quality improvement processes on a periodic basis. As an incentive for organizations to obtain and maintain accreditation, the accreditation status of health care organizations could be widely disseminated to consumers and purchasers to help inform their decisions.

Clinical Studies

Governments have another role to play in encouraging internal quality improvement processes. The primary driver of quality improvement processes is knowledge about the effectiveness of alternative health care practices, and governments have an important responsibility in financing clinical studies of health care processes and outcomes and in disseminating the results. Academic health centers, which traditionally have served as the backbone of the nation's clinical research infrastructure, face an increasingly daunting challenge of financing these activities while remaining viable as health care providers within competitive markets. A key federal government responsibility lies in assuring consistent and equitable systems for financing the development and dissemination of clinical innovations through outcomes research and clinical training programs. This responsibility cannot be understated in the policy discussions surrounding quality improvement.

Finding the Right Balance

As we consider policy options to support quality in health care, we must recognize that both governmental regulatory tools and private market incentives offer opportunities for improving clinical quality. The key to sustainable improvement lies in finding the right balance between regulation and market incentives in order to avoid impeding the progress of clinical innovation. The most promising regulatory options combine the strengths of existing governmental authority with the power of emerging competitive health care markets.

We should not underestimate the challenges that must be faced in moving to a more market-based regulatory framework for assuring quality, especially in view of current public opinion about the health care system. Such an approach runs counter to the traditional bureaucratic culture within our governmental agencies as well as our political process that favors incrementalism at federal, state, and local levels. Nonetheless, the progress already under way within the health care industry is substantial, suggesting that we are within reach of realizing sustained quality improvement through the synergies of market dynamics and responsible government leadership.

References

American Association of Health Plans. *The Regulation of Health Plans.* Washington, D.C.: Author, 1998.

Brennan, T. A., and Berwick, D. M. *New Rules: Regulation, Markets, and the Quality of American Health Care.* San Francisco: Jossey-Bass, 1996.

Congressional Research Service. Unpublished memorandum. Washington, D.C.: Author, 1997.

Etheredge, L. "Promarket Regulation: An SEC-FASB Model." *Health Affairs,* 1997, *16*(6), 22–25.

Fuchs, B. C. *Managed Health Care: Federal and State Regulation.* Washington, D.C.: Congressional Research Service, 1997.

Institute of Medicine. *Effectiveness and Outcomes in Health Care: Proceedings of an Invitational Conference by the Institute of Medicine.* Washington, D.C.: National Academy Press, 1990.

"Interim Rules for Health Insurance Portability for Group Health." *Federal Register,* 1997, *62*(67).

Moran, D. W. "Federal Regulation of Managed Care: An Impulse in Search of a Theory." *Health Affairs,* 1997, *16*(6), 7–33.

Starr, P. *The Social Transformation of American Medicine.* New York: Basic Books, 1982.

Chapter Nine

The Scope of Managed Care Liability

David M. Keepnews

As public attention has focused on managed care organizations (MCOs) and their role in the delivery, financing, and management of health care services, liability issues also have drawn growing interest. Efforts to specify liability for MCOs raise a number of important legal and policy issues about the relative responsibility and accountability of provider and payer, the role of the MCO in making treatment-related decisions, and basic questions about balancing financial and legal risk. In the following discussion, we examine some of the factual, legal, and policy issues related to MCO liability and identify some of the unresolved issues raised by extending liability for medical injury to MCOs.

The question of when MCOs are, or should be, liable for harm caused to patients has been the subject of court cases, public discussion, and policy initiatives. A proposal to establish enterprise liability for health plans (whereby plans would be solely liable for the malpractice of employed or affiliated health professions) was floated by President Clinton's health care reform task force in 1993, and a modified proposal—to pilot its use—was included in the administration's Health Security Act. State legislative proposals to establish or clarify MCO liability have been debated in several states, and in 1997, Texas and Missouri enacted laws to address

The author wishes to thank the following colleagues for their invaluable comments on earlier drafts of this chapter: Patricia Butler, Alice Gosfield, Karl Polzer, and David Shactman.

managed care liability. Other states considered similar legislation in 1997, and many are continuing to debate such proposals. Congressional efforts to eliminate the federal Employee Retirement Income Security Act of 1974 (ERISA) preemption of state lawsuits against MCOs became a focus of sharp debate in the second half of the 105th Congress and can be expected to be a continued subject of debate among policymakers.

In the eyes of some observers, establishment of clear parameters for MCO liability could provide an alternative to creating extensive regulatory processes for MCO accountability that may, in the opinion of some, limit the evolution of new approaches to care represented by the growth of MCOs (Havighurst, 1997).

Any discussion of MCO liability is complicated by a number of issues. The evolution of case law has been stymied to a large extent by the fact that many courts never reach the substantive issues posed by claims against MCOs (and, presumably, many claims are never filed) because so many of these claims are preempted by ERISA. The lingering "corporate practice of medicine" doctrine in some states has provided some ammunition for MCOs to resist liability for medical malpractice, based on the premise that they could not have practiced medicine negligently because they are legally barred from practicing medicine at all.[1] The varied nature of MCOs—which range from relatively simple financing or utilization review structures to fully integrated, staff-model HMO-type entities—makes developing a single standard for MCO conduct complex. Similarly, the presence of larger issues about how providers and insurers are to weigh cost and patient risk—issues on which the health system, policymakers, and the general public have yet to reach anything approaching consensus—may make a standard for allocation of legal risk difficult to achieve.

The Evolution of Medical Liability

The system of tort liability as applied to health care malpractice is commonly (if not universally) viewed as a means of establishing and enforcing accountability for health care professionals and for most institutional and organizational providers. Poor practice—largely defined as failure to meet professional standards of care—is sanctionable through imposing legal liability, usually consisting of monetary damages, on providers.

The Growing Reach of Liability

For some time, physicians were the chief, and usually the only, targets of malpractice claims. Physicians were seen as the primary (or sole) source of professional judgment in health care decision making. But the liability of health care institutions (as well as non-physician professionals) has evolved considerably. The increasingly prominent role of the hospital came to be reflected more clearly in accountability for medical errors through a variety of mechanisms. The once-common doctrine of charitable immunity, through which many hospitals were shielded from liability, has largely disappeared. The legal doctrine of *respondeat superior* ("let the master answer"), through which an employer can be held vicariously liable for the actions of an employee, came to be applied to physician employees as well as to nurses, other professionals, and technicians.

Traditionally, however, the relationship between hospital and physician has not been that of employer and employee. Because physicians have functioned essentially as independent contractors, the law for some time provided no mechanism by which to hold hospitals liable for physicians' negligence, except in the minority of instances in which physicians were in fact employees.

In the past two decades, however, the hospital's liability for physician malpractice, even in the absence of an employment relationship, has become well established. For instance, hospitals have been found negligent for failing to select and screen physicians adequately in granting staff privileges. (Notably, although this may achieve the same effect as finding a hospital *vicariously* liable for the actions of a physician-employee, negligent selection and screening is a means for finding the hospital *directly* liable for its failure to exercise due care.) The theory of "ostensible agency" also has been used to find a hospital liable for its physicians' negligence, where the institution has acted in such a way as to lead a patient to believe that the physician was acting on the hospital's behalf.

Thus, although no hard and fast rule has been established through which hospitals are uniformly and consistently held liable for professional malpractice, they commonly are found liable for the actions of both employed and affiliated practitioners.

Liability Beyond Physicians and Hospitals?

The extension of malpractice liability to hospitals came about in large part as a result of their growing role as the center of health care delivery. Similarly, the increasing dominance of MCOs makes the question of whether and how these organizations are to be held accountable for malpractice more important.

This may appear to be a simple question. The law expects everyone to act "reasonably," with prudent care, and to face liability when failure to do so is the cause of injury to another (or more precisely, to an individual to whom a duty of care is owed). Absent the interference of obstacles such as ERISA, is there anything complicated about the proposition that MCOs should be treated like any other business entity in determining liability?

In a limited sense, the answer is no. If an HMO employs a physician who negligently causes injury, the HMO may be found liable for his or her actions, just as any other employer could be found negligent for harm caused by an employee. And it is not a far stretch to suggest that some of the same legal theories that have been used to find hospitals liable for the actions of independent contractors—such as negligent selection and screening, or ostensible agency—can be applied to MCOs. In fact, such approaches have been attempted, with some success.

Regarding other approaches—most particularly failure to authorize treatment—the picture may be less clear. An MCO may be expected to act in a reasonably prudent manner, like any other person or entity. But what is it that an MCO *does?* Does it merely make recommendations to physicians and hospitals? Does it make decisions about financing care, does it make administrative decisions implementing a plan agreement, or does it make medical decisions? How can these be distinguished? To what standards is it held in balancing its cost, and utilization, control priorities against possible risk to the patient? In what ways does it share legal risk with its practitioners and providers?[2]

Part of the answer to these questions, of course, is that there is wide variability in how MCOs function—from tightly organized, fully integrated staff-model HMOs to entities that limit their role to negotiating capitated payment agreements with physician networks. MCOs' role (if any) in treatment-related decisions is thus itself quite varied, making answers to most of the foregoing questions difficult.

But another reason why many answers have not been forthcoming is that the courts have been largely unable to reach them because of the role of ERISA in preempting state court actions.

The Reach of the ERISA Preemption

The ability of the states to regulate MCOs and the ability of plan participants to seek redress in state courts has been profoundly affected by ERISA. As Chapter Ten describes in some detail, ERISA was enacted to promote and protect the interests of participants in employee benefit plans, including any "plan, fund, or program . . . established or maintained by an employer . . . for the purpose of providing its participants and beneficiaries, through the purchase of insurance or otherwise, . . . medical, surgical or hospital care." The act specifically preempts "any and all state laws insofar as they may now or hereafter relate to any employee benefit plan" that falls under ERISA. The broad preemption protects many plans from the widely varying regulatory requirements (including coverage mandates) that states may seek to impose on plans operating within their borders. ERISA applies to employees of private businesses; government-sponsored benefits plans, including health plans, are not affected by the act or its preemption of state regulation. Likewise, ERISA does not apply to individuals who purchase their own health care coverage.

A series of federal cases, beginning with *Metropolitan Life Ins. Co. v. Massachusetts,* clarify the effect of the ERISA preemption on state regulation of employee health plans. The act's "savings clause" (section 514[b][2][A]) ensures that states generally retain their traditional power to regulate the "business of insurance." This power does not reach to every activity conducted by an insurer, however, and an important exception is the noninsurance activities of third-party administrators (Butler, 1998, citing *Group Life & Health v. Royal Drug Co.* [1987]), *Insurance Bd. of Bethlehem Steel Corp. v. Muir* [1987], and *Powell v. Chesapeake & Potomac Telephone Co. of Virginia* [1985]).

ERISA also bars states from deeming employee health plans to be insurers in order that the state can regulate it (section 514[b][2][B]; Butler, 1998). Thus, self-insured plans (in which employers bear their own insurance risk directly, often contracting with a third-party administrator to provide for services) are generally exempt from state regulation because of the ERISA preemption. This is important, because a significant minority of private-sector employees are covered through self-insured plans. The distinction between self-insured and other employee health plans is critical in terms of the power of the state to regulate: "A business can operate without state oversight if it is self-insured, but any insured product it buys, such as one offered through an indemnity plan or HMO, is subject to state regulation" (Butler, 1998, p. 5).

No such distinction is made, however, for state lawsuits for damages arising from administration of an employee health plan. Largely as a result of the Supreme Court's ruling in *Pilot Life v. Dedeaux* (1987), such lawsuits—regardless of whether the plan is self-insured—are preempted by ERISA; thus, the only remedies available to an employee are those offered in the statute itself.

ERISA does not regulate the content of employer-provided health care plans. Rather, it relies on disclosure, administrative requirements, and fiduciary obligations to prevent abusive practices (Farrell, 1997). Its substantive provisions focus on requirements for pension plans. Standards for plan administration and rights of plan participants are developed in further detail in regulations issued by the Department of Labor (DoL).

Limited remedies for an employee who has been denied benefits under an employee benefit plan are included. Section 502(a) allows a participant to recover the cost of the denied benefits or to seek an injunction against the denial of benefits. Of course, this is a far cry from what a typical malpractice plaintiff could seek in a state court, because it does not allow for substantially more expansive forms of damages, such as compensation for additional health care costs, lost wages, and noneconomic damages (pain and suffering, punitive damages). Nor does it provide any remedy for a delay in providing benefits, as opposed to an outright denial.

New federal rules proposed by the DoL on September 9, 1998 would significantly revamp current requirements for processing of claims submitted by plan participants and beneficiaries. The goal of these proposed rules is to "ensure more timely benefit determinations, improved access to information on which a benefit determination is made, and greater assurance that participants and beneficiaries will be afforded a full and fair review of denied claims" ("Employee Retirement . . . , 1998, p. 48390). At the time this chapter was written, no final action had been taken by DoL on these proposed rules.

To Preempt . . .

MCOs have been largely successful in removing suits against them from state to federal courts, where the potential remedy is limited to those offered by section 502(a) of ERISA. Malpractice claims, like other negligence claims, generally are governed by state law (usually common, or court-made, law). Taking lawsuits against MCOs out of state court, and out of the reach of state law, is thus not merely an inconvenience. In view of the substantially limited damages available under ERISA, proponents of repealing or modifying the preemption hold that it effectively means that the plaintiff is without a remedy.

A long line of federal court decisions has found that ERISA preempts state courts from hearing claims arising from a failure to provide benefits under an employee health plan—in other words, a refusal to treat or to authorize treatment. As noted earlier, the U.S. Supreme Court's 1987 decision in *Pilot Life Insurance Co. v. Dedeaux* provided a broad application of the ERISA preemption of state lawsuits for damages based on administration of employee health plans. Following *Pilot Life,* the federal courts have produced a number of decisions finding that state lawsuits for damages arising from improper administration of a plan (including denial of benefits) were preempted by ERISA. One of the best known is *Corcoran v. United HealthCare, Inc.,* a 1992 case in which a managed care plan refused to authorize hospitalization for a high-risk pregnant woman whose fetus subsequently went into distress and died. (The woman's obstetrician had ordered her hospitalization. The plan authorized ten hours a day of home nursing care instead. The fetus went into distress during a time when no nurse was on duty.) The woman sued in state court, alleging that the plan's refusal to authorize her hospitalization was wrongful and caused the death of the fetus. The Fifth Circuit Court of Appeals found that her claim was preempted by ERISA.

This case continues to stand as a significant example of the sweep of the ERISA preemption. A continuing line of cases has applied the preemption to malpractice suits based on a refusal to approve or authorize treatment. These include *Spain v. Aetna Life Insurance Co.*, a 1993 decision in the Ninth Circuit; *Kuhl v. Lincoln National Health Plan of Kansas City, Inc.*, a 1993 Eighth Circuit decision; *Tolton v. America Biodyne, Inc.*, a 1995 Sixth Circuit decision; and *Bast v. Prudential Insurance*, a 1998 Ninth Circuit decision.

The federal courts have not always come to their preemption decisions gladly. The court in *Corcoran* noted that the lack of a state or federal remedy "eliminates an important check on thousands of medical decisions made in the burgeoning medical review system." A similar lament has been voiced by courts around the country that have noted the lack of a remedy for similar cases (Pear, 1998). In *Bast*, a plan administrator had refused to authorize a bone marrow transplant for a woman with cancer. The administrator subsequently reversed the decision and authorized the procedure, but the cancer had already metastasized and Bast died several months later. Her survivors sued in state court. In upholding a federal district court decision granting summary judgment to the plan administrator, Judge David Thompson of the Ninth Circuit wrote: "The Basts' state law claims are preempted by ERISA, and ERISA provides no remedy. Unfortunately, without action by Congress, there is nothing we can do to help the Basts and others who may find themselves in this same unfortunate situation."

. . . Or Not to Preempt

Despite the brick wall encountered by many who have tried to sue MCOs, the last few years have seen a new line of cases in which federal courts have found some state claims *not* to be preempted by ERISA. The full significance of this apparent evolution—whether it represents an erosion of the ERISA preemption or merely a clarification of it—remains to be seen.

In *Dukes v. U.S. Health Care Systems of Pennsylvania* (1995), the Third Circuit rejected the application of the ERISA preemption in two cases based on negligence in providing health care services. The court found that "the plaintiffs' claims . . . merely attack the quality of the benefits they received: The plaintiffs here simply do not claim that the plans erroneously withheld benefits due. Nor do they ask the state courts to enforce their rights under the terms of their respective plans or to clarify their rights to future benefits." Instead, the court characterized both claims as an attack on the quality of the benefits received under the plan.

The court stressed that the role of the health plans in *Dukes* involved "arranging for medical treatment," rather than the "utilization review role" played by the plan in *Corcoran*. It noted that "only in a utilization review role is an entity in a position to deny benefits due under an ERISA welfare plan," a denial that would trigger the ERISA preemption as it had in *Corcoran*. The court explained that "Congress sought to assure that promised benefits would be available when plan participants had need of them and section 502 [of ERISA] was intended to provide each individual participant with a remedy in the event that promises made by the plan were not kept. We find nothing in the legislative history suggesting that section 502 was intended as a part of a federal scheme to control the quality of the benefits received by plan participants. *Quality control of benefits, such as the health care benefits provided here, is a field traditionally occupied by state regulation and we interpret the silence of Congress as reflecting an intent that it remain such*" (emphasis added).

In making this observation, *Dukes* cited the Supreme Court's decision in *New York State Conference of Blue Cross & Blue Shield Plans v. Travelers Insurance Co.* (1995), which rejected federal preemption of New York's surcharge on hospital fees as applied to ERISA plans. In *Travelers,* Justice Souter wrote that "nothing in the language of [ERISA] or the context of its passage indicates that Congress chose to displace general health care regulations, which historically has been an area of general local concern." In other words, as *Dukes* concluded, it is a field traditionally occupied by state regulation.

For its part, the Department of Labor, in an *amicus curiae* (friend of the court) brief, had urged the court in *Dukes* to find that suits based on malpractice for care delivered under the plan are not preempted (U.S. Department of Labor, 1994). It has maintained this position in other *amicus* briefs filed in similar cases. In the wake of *Dukes,* a number of other federal courts have found that malpractice claims against MCOs based on the quality of care delivered are not preempted by ERISA. These include *Pacificare of Oklahoma, Inc. v. Burrage* (1995) in the Tenth Circuit and *Rice v. Panchal* in the Seventh Circuit (1995).

Will the Distinction Hold?

Whether the line between these two categories of cases—those based on a denial of benefits and those based on quality of care provided—can survive has been questioned by some commentators, one of whom labels this an "unsatisfactory distinction" and suggests that "it is likely to be superseded by events" (Mariner, 1996). She notes the Third Circuit's observation in *Dukes* that

> The distinction between the quantity of benefits due under a welfare plan and the quality of those benefits will not always be clear in situations . . . where the benefit contracted for is health care services rather than money to pay for such services. There may well be cases in which the quality of a patient's medical care or the skills of the personnel provided to administer that care will be so low that the treatment received simply will not qualify as health care at all. In such a case, it well may be appropriate to conclude that the plan participant or beneficiary has been denied benefits due under the plan.

This observation is potentially significant because it suggests that a neat division of cases into those in which no care has been provided (preempted as a "denial of benefits" under ERISA) and those in which care has been provided negligently (not based on denial of benefits and therefore not preempted) may not hold. The idea that a continuum exists between "poor care" and "no care" is not a difficult one to appreciate. What might strike some as troubling, however, is its application in a legal context in which cases alleging a denial of benefits are preempted: if care is bad, the MCO may face liability, but if the care is *extremely* bad (as the *Dukes* court described it, "so low that . . . [it] simply will not qualify as health care at all"), it may not. What kind of impact such a continuum may have, and whether it will confound the lines between cases in which the ERISA preemption does and does not apply (as the Third Circuit suggests it might) remains to be seen.

Theories of MCO Liability

Many courts have examined issues of MCO liability apart from the overarching issue of ERISA preemption. The liability of MCOs for the negligence of employee physicians and other professionals (under traditional tort law principles)—such as in staff-model HMOs—is well established (Mariner, 1996). Other approaches predicated on the relationship between the MCO and the health care provider have been put forward (Gosfield, 1997) and generally mirror the range of legal theories used to hold hospitals liable for the negligence of affiliated physicians (Bearden and Maedgen, 1995; Randall, 1993; Kilcullen, 1996; Perdue and Baxley, 1995). These include the theory of ostensible agency, in which the actions of the physician, even though he or she is not an employee of the MCO, is nonetheless imputed to it. Generally, ostensible agency applies where the physician is seen by the patient as the MCO's agent, the patient would not have been harmed but for the action of the physician, and the plan both selected the physician and then limited patient choice to the physicians it selected (Gosfield, 1996). One often-cited case illustrating the application of ostensible agency to MCO liability is *Boyd v. Einstein,* a 1988 case involving an IPA-model HMO.

One author suggests that this theory of liability "has gained a significant foothold in the industry and drives plans to be far more stringent in both their selection of physicians and in the process of reviewing physicians' performance throughout the term of their relationship with the MCO" (Gosfield, 1996). The same author also points to potential liability for MCOs in negligently credentialing their physicians. Under this approach, hospitals have been found to have an ongoing obligation to monitor the care provided by those physicians, and to take appropriate action where care is found wanting. In at least one case, a similar duty has been found for MCOs *(McLellan v. HMO of Pa.,* 1992).

Other approaches, more tailored to the characteristics of MCOs, have also been attempted. These include direct attacks on utilization review decisions. One of the earliest and most prominent cases is *Wickline v. State of California* (1986), in which a patient sued the state Medicaid program for her premature discharge from the hospital, which occurred despite her physician's recommendation for continued hospitalization. Complications that became evident after discharge resulted in amputation of her lower leg. A jury verdict in her favor was subsequently overturned, based primarily on her physician's failure to appeal the utilization review decision. The court noted that the physician bore ultimate responsibility for the decision to discharge a patient, but found that

> The patient who requires treatment and who is harmed when care which should have been provided is not provided should recover for the injuries suffered from all those responsible for the deprivation of such care, including, when appropriate, health care payers. Third party payers of health care services can be held legally accountable when medically inappropriate decisions result from defects in the design or implementation of cost containment mechanisms as, for example, when appeals made on a patient's behalf for medical or hospital care are arbitrarily ignored or unreasonably disregarded or overridden.

In another case, *Wilson v. Blue Cross of Southern California* (1990), a patient hospitalized for depression committed suicide after discharge. His insurer, following a utilization reviewer's recommendation, had refused to pay for further hospital care, finding it medically unnecessary. A California appellate court said an insurer could be found liable when its conduct is a substantial factor in a patient's injury although, as in *Wickline*, no damages were imposed. Other actions have challenged financial incentives inherent in managed care but have generally either been unsuccessful or have been settled before a verdict has been reached (Gosfield, 1997).

Arguably the most important issue in MCO litigation is liability for failure to authorize or provide treatment. As noted earlier, however, this is precisely the issue to which federal courts continue to apply the ERISA preemption consistently, leaving little in the way of case law on this question.

Cases based on theories other than negligence have also drawn some attention. Possibly the best known is *Fox v. HealthNet* (1993), in which an MCO denied authorization for bone marrow treatment to a breast cancer patient based on its position that this treatment was "investigational" and thus not covered under the plan agreement. The plaintiff sued the health plan based on breach of contract, bad faith, and intentional infliction of emotional distress. A jury awarded $89 million in damages. The case was settled for $5 million before it reached review by an appellate court. (In this case the plan was a government benefits program and thus was not preempted by ERISA.) Cases like *Fox* and *Ching v. Gaines* (1995), which resulted in a $3 million award, have drawn much public attention, although whether their legal significance matches their visibility has been questioned (Gosfield, 1997).

Notably, state law claims against MCOs may be brought by individuals other than plan participants—providers, contractors, vendors, employees of the MCO—under state law. ERISA preempts claims by plan participants, which leads to the anomalous result that the individuals whom ERISA was designed to protect may be barred from relief whereas other claimants are not (Fredel, 1995; Mariner, 1996).

Legislative Efforts to Expand Liability

Faced with an uncertain body of case law and difficult legal obstacles, proponents of MCO liability have turned to the legislatures to attempt to establish patients' ability to sue MCOs for malpractice.

State-Level Initiatives

During the 1997 and 1998 legislative years, a number of states considered proposals on MCO liability. A much-watched Texas bill, Senate Bill 386, was passed in 1997 by both houses of the state legislature, after which Texas's Governor Bush allowed the bill to pass into law without his signature. In part, S.B. 386 provided that a "health insurance carrier, health maintenance organization, or other managed care entity for a health care plan has the duty to exercise ordinary care when making health care treatment decisions and is liable for damages for harm to an insured or enrollee proximately caused by its failure to exercise such ordinary care."

The bill also provided that employees, agents, "ostensible agents," and representatives can similarly be found liable. A "health care treatment decision" is defined as "a determination made when medical services are actually provided by the health care plan and a decision which affects the quality of the diagnosis, care, or treatment provided to the plan's insured or enrollees."

Further, "'Ordinary care' means, in the case of a health insurance carrier, health maintenance organization, or managed care entity, that degree of care that a health maintenance organization, or managed care entity of ordinary prudence would use under the same or similar circumstances."

In its broad definition of health care treatment decisions, the Texas law potentially reaches most actions an MCO may take with regard to authorization or delivery of care. In its definition of ordinary care, it invokes the language of traditional negligence doctrine. A legal challenge to the new Texas law was announced by Aetna almost as soon as it was enacted. Aetna's suit in federal court against the state of Texas alleges that the bill violates not only ERISA but, by casting its net widely enough to include health plans that provide benefits to federal employees, the Federal Employees Health Benefit Act as well. A federal district court upheld the Texas law's provision regarding the right to sue, while striking down the independent appeal rights granted under that law (*Corporate Health Insurance, et al. v. Texas Department of Insurance, et al.*, 1998).

Missouri also enacted legislation in 1997 aimed, in part, to expand liability of managed care plans. Missouri's House Bill 335 was a more comprehensive managed care reform initiative. It included two provisions relevant to managed care liability: one that repealed the corporate practice of medicine doctrine as applied to HMOs, and one that prohibits HMOs from requiring physicians with whom they contract to indemnify the plan. The Missouri legislation was much more limited in its approach than the Texas bill. The Missouri law is specific to HMOs. It prevents HMOs from invoking the corporate practice of medicine as protection against damages suits but does not actually establish a new cause of action or set forth the extent of liability HMOs may face as a result of treatment decisions. These questions will be left to the Missouri courts to determine (Butler, 1997).

Other states witnessed unsuccessful attempts in 1997 to enact legislation expanding MCO liability, including New York, California, and Florida (where legislation approved by the legislature was subsequently vetoed by the governor). In these and other states, efforts to win expanded MCO liability are ongoing.

Federal-Level Initiatives

The issue of MCO liability—particularly the threshold issue of removing or modifying the ERISA preemption of state lawsuits and
state tort remedies—has been a focus of increasing attention in
federal efforts to regulate managed care. Two legislative vehicles
that sought to address this issue gained notable support in the
105th Congress, but both ultimately failed. The Patient Access to
Responsible Care Act (PARCA), an early managed care regulation
proposal cosponsored by Congressman Charlie Norwood (R-GA)
and then-Senator Alfonse D'Amato (R-NY) was notable for the
broad bipartisan support it gathered during the 105th Congress.
That bill would have amended section 514(b) of ERISA by providing that ERISA's preemption provisions would not "be construed to preclude any State cause of action to recover damages
for personal injury or wrongful death against any person that provides insurance or administrative services to or for an employee
welfare benefit plan maintained to provide health care benefits."

Subsequently, the Democratic leadership's Patients' Bill of
Rights Act of 1998 (PBRA) in the same Congress proposed amend-
ing ERISA such that it not "be construed to invalidate, impair, or
supersede" most suits under state law arising "out of the arrangement by such person for the provision of . . . insurance, administrative services, or medical services by other persons." Efforts to
eliminate or change the ERISA preemption were, of course, ultimately unsuccessful in the 105th Congress. Whether these approaches are reflected in legislative efforts in the 106th Congress
(or subsequently) is unclear as of this writing.

Employers' Opposition to Expanded MCO Liability

Employer groups represent the most significant force in opposition to expanded MCO liability—and in particular, to elimination
or relaxation of the ERISA preemption. Organizations such as the
National Association of Manufacturers (NAM) and the ERISA Industry Committee (ERIC), made up of large employers, have been
outspoken in their opposition to changes in ERISA.[3]

Employers are concerned that the added legal exposure for
MCOs would trigger higher insurance premiums, discourage employers from offering coverage, and lead employers to reduce or

eliminate health care coverage in order to shield themselves from liability (National Association of Manufacturers, 1997; see also ERISA Industry Committee, 1997a).

Higher Costs

Opponents of expanded MCO liability point to an April 1998 study by the Barents Group that predicted sharply increased liability costs as a result of proposals contained in an early federal bill that would have established the right to sue ERISA plans and in Texas's S.B. 386. That study, commissioned by the American Association of Health Plans, estimated both "direct costs" and "indirect costs" that would be incurred by health plans from 1999–2003. Direct costs related to an increase in the number of plans covered by malpractice insurance, increase in liability costs of plans currently covered by malpractice insurance, and administrative costs related to conducting additional utilization review and maintaining records on treatment decisions (Barents Group, 1998). Indirect costs primarily consisted of "the increased provision of services to reduce the probability of suit (defensive medicine)" (p. 21). The study estimated the total increased costs as ranging between 2.7 percent and 8.6 percent of plan premiums. It also projected considerable increased household costs, job loss, and wage loss as a result.

Subsequently, the Congressional Budget Office (CBO) scored the Democratic leadership's managed care reform legislation in the 105th Congress, including its proposal to lift the preemption of lawsuits against ERISA plans. The CBO estimated that ending the preemption would increase liability costs by 60.0 to 75.0 percent, representing about 1.4 percent of ERISA plan premiums and about 1.2 percent of the premiums of all employer-sponsored plan (Congressional Budget Office, 1998).

A June 1998 study conducted by Coopers & Lybrand for the Kaiser Family Foundation offers some additional data regarding potential costs of expanded MCO liability resulting from changes in the ERISA preemption (Hunt, Saari, and Traw, 1998). This study examined three large government entities that sponsor group health insurance coverage: the California Public Employees Retirement System (CalPERS), the Los Angeles Unified School District (LAUDS), and the State of Colorado Employee Benefit Plan. Because the ERISA preemption does not apply to government-sponsored plans, state lawsuits against them are not barred as they are for private employee health plans. The Coopers & Lybrand study noted that the government-sponsored programs included very specific administrative appeals procedures (along with the requirement that individuals exhaust available administrative remedies before seeking redress in court).

The study found that rates of litigation against the government-sponsored health plans it examined ranged from 0.3 to 1.4 cases per one hundred thousand enrollees per year, and (for CalPERS) 0.9 grievances per one hundred thousand enrollees per year who reached the administrative hearing stage. Based on these figures, the study estimated the direct monthly cost per enrollee related to litigation to range between $0.03 and $0.13 (Hunt, Saari, and Traw, 1998).

In addition, the study compared the litigation experience of one large health insurer and HMO in California prior to and following the U.S. Supreme Court's 1987 decision in *Pilot Life v. Dedeaux,* the case that established the broad sweep of the ERISA preemption of state lawsuits. From 1985 to 1988, this carrier reported an average of 3.2 suits per one hundred thousand members; after 1988, the number dropped to 2.4 per one hundred thousand (this figure includes both group coverage cases and individual coverage cases—the latter remaining outside the reach of the ERISA preemption). The higher rate, which presumably might be replicated or surpassed if the ERISA preemption of state lawsuits were eliminated or scaled back, represented $0.27 per member per month, or 0.25 percent of premiums. The study authors acknowledge that their findings regarding both government-sponsored plans and the private carrier in their study are illustrative, and not necessarily predictive of future experience following a possible change in ERISA. Opponents of expanded MCO liability also suggested that the study failed to take into account the cost of defensive medicine, which the Barents Group research had identified in its discussion of projected indirect costs.

Avoiding Inconsistent State Laws

Employer representatives also argue that use of ERISA to prevent plans from having to comply with a "patchwork" of state-imposed standards and rules to be applied in state-court malpractice suits is precisely in line with what the preemption was intended to do—in part, to ensure that plans had a set of uniform, consistent rules to deal with—rather than an unintended effect of that preemption.[4] The argument that the ERISA preemption has promoted uniformity in health plan regulation is part of an overall objection to subjecting MCOs to state regulation (ERISA Industry Committee, 1997b). Indeed, as one author notes, "the sparse legislative history of [ERISA's] preemption clause indicates that the objective of preemption was to avoid subjecting employee plans operated by large interstate firms to inconsistent and varying state laws" (Butler, 1998).

Implicating Employers

Employer groups have also warned that plans' malpractice liability would most likely not be limited to the MCOs who administer them but will ultimately reach the sponsors of those plans, opening them up to liability for harm attributed to those plans (National Association of Manufacturers, 1997). The issue of potential employer liability provides a focal point for employer opposition to PARCA. Congressman Norwood responded to these criticisms by introducing an additional measure, the Responsibility in Managed Care Act (H.R. 2960 in the 105th Congress), which would remove the ERISA preemption as it applies to state lawsuits but would generally exempt employers and other plan sponsors from liability. The Patients' Bill of Rights also seeks to address the issue of potential employer liability, but providing that its modification of the ERISA preemption against state damages lawsuits does not apply to employers or other plan sponsors unless "such action is based on the employer's or plan sponsor's exercise of discretionary authority to make a decision on a claim for benefits covered under the plan or health insurance coverage in the case at issue" and "the exercise . . . of such authority resulted in personal injury or wrongful death" (section 302[a], proposed section 514[e][2] of ERISA).

Arguments About Expanded Liability

Employers have not been the only group to oppose expanded MCO liability. Health plans and other insurers have echoed employers' predictions of higher premiums and the likelihood of employers dropping coverage. Some have also argued that expanded liability for MCOs is simply unnecessary in light of existing and potential means for redressing consumers' grievances (American

Association of Health Plans, 1997; Health Insurance Association of America, 1997; Self-Insurance Institute of America, 1997).

Organized medicine's reaction has been different. Some state medical societies have supported state legislative efforts to expand MCO liability, including the successful efforts in Texas and Missouri. The American Medical Association has indicated support for "hold[ing] health plans liable for medical treatment decisions" ("Legislation '98," 1998). The AMA is a vocal supporter of the Patients' Bill of Rights, as are other health professional groups.

But whether expanding MCO liability operates entirely in physicians' interests is not clear. Greater MCO liability would most likely draw heightened attention by MCOs to reducing risk. Optimally, this could mean emphasis on identifying and reducing risk in collaboration with its providers. It could also mean, however, greater MCO involvement in physician practice, possibly including an increased focus on provider selection and exclusion in an attempt to identify those who are seen as posing a higher legal risk. On what bases and how effectively or equitably this might be achieved may prove a source of concern for physicians. In testimony on the PARCA bill, the National Association of Manufacturers suggested that "creating plan liability for treatment may bring the very result that physicians are trying to avoid—an increased role for administrators and lawyers in medical decision making" (National Association of Manufacturers, 1997). This admonition was echoed in stronger terms by the leading managed care industry group in its testimony against PARCA: "[PARCA] creates the strongest possible incentive for plans to completely restructure their relationships with physicians. Under the bill, plans would find it essential to become directly involved in physician practices and treatment decisions. Ironically, then, a bill intended to promote physician autonomy would eliminate the very considerable autonomy that physicians have today" (American Association of Health Plans, 1997).

Enterprise Liability as an Earlier Attempt to Address MCO Liability

A previous, highly visible initiative to address liability of MCOs came through the malpractice reform group of President Clinton's health care reform task force in 1993. This group proposed a form of enterprise liability through which health plans would have sole legal accountability for care provided by them and their affiliated providers. When this proposal was first floated as a likely part of the Clinton health plan, it drew rapid, strong opposition from many quarters, including organized medicine. Physician groups, unpersuaded by the prospect of reducing their members' legal exposure and costs, feared the loss of autonomy that they believed enterprise liability would represent. The administration's Health Security Act eventually included a far less ambitious proposal—namely, to fund pilot projects to test and to evaluate the use of enterprise liability. With the demise of the Health Security Act in 1994, the enterprise liability proposal faded from active consideration, at least for the time being. It continues to enjoy support among some legal scholars (Havighurst, 1997), and it is not inconceivable that it, or some elements of it, may reappear as issues of MCO liability continue to be considered.

The concept of enterprise liability had its roots in product liability law. Proposals to extend it to medical malpractice were made by professors Kenneth Abraham of the University of Virginia and Paul Weiler of Harvard (Abraham and Weiler, 1994a; Abraham and Weiler, 1994b). These proposals were reflected in the American Law Institute's 1991 report on *Enterprise Liability for Personal Injury*. They center on the hospital as the responsible entity in a plan for enterprise liability for medical malpractice—the idea being that the hospital, as the locus of health care services, is the logical enterprise on which to center legal accountability for health care practice. The Clinton task force's malpractice reform working group adapted this proposal to one in which the health plan would be the responsible enterprise.

The cochairs of that working group provided an explanation and discussion of their vision of enterprise liability in a 1994 article. The principle features included liability of each health plan for negligent injury to its enrollees caused by the health plan's affiliated practitioners and providers; immunity from suit for physicians and other health professionals employed by, or under contract with, the health plan; encouragement of alternative dispute resolution procedures; and limits on damages (Sage, Hastings, and Berenson, 1994).

Outstanding Policy Questions

Efforts to establish and to expand liability of MCOs raise a number of policy questions. Although a full exploration of these issues is beyond the scope of this chapter, it is helpful to take note of some of the more prominent ones.

Expanding a Flawed System?

MCO liability for medical malpractice means bringing a new group of actors into a system that has been under fire for some years. Critics have long faulted the medical malpractice system as a burdensome, costly one that adds expense to health care services through high malpractice premiums, costly damage awards, and encouragement of the practice of "defensive medicine." These critics have pushed for various tort reform proposals, including caps on damages, use of alternative dispute resolution procedures, review of malpractice claims before they are allowed to proceed to court, and other means. Such proposals have been heard in state legislatures and in Congress for the past two decades, meeting with varying degrees of success. Not surprisingly, physician and other provider groups have been among the leading proponents of medical malpractice "reform" initiatives, while (also not surprisingly) strong opposition has come from trial lawyers and some organized consumer groups who argue against limiting access to the courts and stress the role of malpractice suits in ensuring accountability from health care providers.

At the same time, a body of literature raises questions about the current system's ability to address the extent of medical negligence. The Harvard medical practice study, which focused on hospitalized patients in New York State, suggested that 1 percent of hospitalized patients suffered adverse events attributable to negligence (Brennan and others, 1991), with only one in eight such incidents resulting in a suit for malpractice and half of those suits resulting in some degree of compensation. Is this the system—attacked on one side for being costly and overreaching, and on the other for failing to take account of the scope of medical injuries or of their cause—the one to which MCO liability should be grafted?

An alternative approach to medical error focuses on the need to look at systems of care and systems failures in addressing and reducing adverse events. Proponents deemphasize individual failings and stress "looking on errors as evidence of system failures and concentrating the efforts of all affected parties to develop ways to minimize these failures" (Leape, Lawthers, Brennan, and Johnson, 1993). Such an approach takes account of the increasingly systems-based nature of health care delivery. To the extent that MCO liability represents accountability by an organized system for errors committed under its auspices, it may provide some promise of a more systems-based approach not just to post hoc liability for negligence, but—by effecting systemwide accountability—to reducing medical error.

Are Authorization Decisions "Medical" Decisions?

An area of serious debate related to MCO liability focuses on whether and when MCOs make medical decisions in deciding when to authorize care. Are MCOs merely implementing the provisions of an insurance plan, as payers have done for decades, or are they making actual medical decisions about a patient's health care needs?

This is not an easy question to answer in a system that integrates financing, organization, and delivery of health care services. But in such an integrated system, the precise character of an authorization decision may not be so significant. Whether medical *or* administrative in nature, an MCO's decision to authorize or deny care has a direct relationship to the patient's ability to obtain it.

The availability of appeal rights—both by the patient and the physician—may be of some significance here. The *Wickline* court posed the responsibility of the treating physician to utilize available appeals procedures. The existence of adequate appeal rights, the treating practitioner's actions in utilizing them, and the time-sensitivity of the patient's condition (was it so urgent as to make any appeal useless?), are all issues that should be examined in determining who holds, or shares, accountability for a failure to treat.

The availability of appropriate appeal rights for MCO beneficiaries has, most logically, been a focus of many policy proposals at the state and federal levels. It is important that professional and institutional providers be able to appeal denials of treatment authorization as well. This gives the patient the advantage of an advocate with sufficient professional knowledge to challenge an authorization decision, but it also may ensure that, assuming MCO liability for failure to authorize treatment is more firmly established, the provider's own accountability is not eliminated or abdicated the moment an MCO refuses to authorize a service.

This issue of fixing accountability on the provider and the MCO is also an important one in assessing the role of financial incentives in managed care. In any capitated system, providers stand to gain from spending less on care. Many would argue that such incentives can inspire an interest in long-term preventive measures and other approaches that seek to keep medical costs down over time. Others suggest that it creates a perverse incentive to undertreat and thereby corrupts medical decision making.

Hospitals have lived with capped payments in the form of the Medicare prospective payment system for a decade and a half. Although today's health care environment may be less amenable to cost-shifting practices that arguably mitigated the impact of the Medicare PPS, it is difficult to argue that a shift from fee-for-service payment is a new or radical development in the health care system. What lessons can be drawn from hospitals' experience? Have changes in treatment patterns operated to patients' benefit or detriment? Strong arguments can be heard on both sides of this question. But would it be logical to argue that hospitals should no longer be accountable for injury caused by (for instance) premature discharge or unavailability of professional staff because they are operating under a capitated payment system?

The question may very well be when, if ever, a provider's hand is "forced" by the nature of the payment mechanism. Is it a matter of the mere *existence* of financial incentives or of the *degree* of the financial incentive? When is professional judgment overridden by financial considerations, and who is accountable for the adverse results (if any): the one who offers the financial reward or the one who accepts it? And how should that accountability be enforced: through legal action by an injured patient, through regulatory sanctions, or through criminal prosecution?

Whether the answers to these questions—whatever they may be—argue for a continued focus on individual accountability or a sharper focus on improving systems (or some of each) is a matter for continued debate. Such discussion would necessarily address whether proposed changes in liability, such as instituting a system of enterprise liability, would help to resolve these issues of fixing accountability.

Fairness and the Right to Sue

The ability, or right, of employees to seek adequate remedies in court when they have been (allegedly) harmed by the acts or omissions of their MCOs has emerged as a significant focus of legislative efforts to address managed care. Clearly, expanding MCO liability would not by itself provide answers to many questions about the parameters of plans' liability. Nor would it address any of the perceived flaws in the current malpractice system. But the importance of the (seemingly) simple, threshold issue of the right of individuals covered by employee health plans to seek redress in court when harm has occurred cannot be overlooked or easily dismissed. It presents basic issues of equity and fairness that have proved compelling as members of the public, policymakers, and even appellate court judges decry employees' lack of access to the courts (or to seek adequate remedies in court) as a result of the ERISA preemption.

The argument by spokespersons for health plans and employer groups that the existence of the right to appeal plan decisions renders lawsuits unnecessary has proved a largely unpersuasive response to the argument that private-sector, insured employees should have the right to sue their plans (particularly considering that the ERISA preemption that prevents these employees' lawsuits does not apply to individuals covered by government-sponsored plans). Proposals for enhanced appeal rights, including the right to an external appeal, have emerged as an alternative or a counter to proposals to eliminate or modify the ERISA preemption. Of course, much depends on the specifics of any such proposals. Their ability to resolve many Americans' uneasiness about their inability to sue their managed care plans may be questionable.

But the availability of strong, expeditious, external appeal processes may prove most effective, not as an *alternative* to the right to sue health plans but as a *complement* to it. This is an area in which careful study of the experience of government-sponsored plans may prove helpful. Recall that the June 1998 Coopers & Lybrand study performed for the Kaiser Family Foundation noted the existence of appeal rights in California and Colorado, along with a requirement that individuals exhaust these administrative remedies prior to initiating litigation (Hunt, Saari, and Traw, 1998). A number of other states have considered and enacted legislation providing external appeal rights for participants in non-ERISA plan, and as noted earlier, the U.S. Department of Labor has also proposed substantially more detailed requirements for ERISA plans to follow in processing appeals by plan participants and beneficiaries, including, in some cases, review by an independent medical professional. Aside from the other compelling reasons to establish and enforce strong, timely appeals procedures, the use of such procedures—like the use of other alternative dispute resolution mechanisms—without abrogating individuals' right to sue may ultimately prove to be an effective means of quelling fears about an explosion in litigation, while simultaneously ensuring that MCOs can be held accountable for their actions.

Balancing Cost and Risk

A more fundamental question in examining MCO liability may be whether a balance can be found between financial risk and legal risk in the American health care system. Managed systems of care are based in large part on controlling utilization and thus reducing cost. Utilization may be controlled through various means other than outright denial of services—by emphasizing preventive services over the long term, by providing for earlier intervention, and by substituting less costly but still effective services. (For instance, had Ms. Corcoran been given twenty-four-hour-a-day home nursing care instead of the ten hours a day her MCO authorized as an alternative to hospitalization, the outcome for her and her fetus might very well have been different). Presumably, reducing utilization by denying a service will almost always involve *some* degree of risk, even if sometimes a slight one.

What level of risk are we willing to tolerate in order to reduce health care spending? What marginal increases in risk are tolerable, and how should they be measured? How should liability for injury based on failure to provide a service, which is necessarily a retrospective determination, mesh with treatment decisions based on prospective payment mechanisms? Will expanded MCO liability actually encourage more defensive medicine by MCOs and their providers—and how will a capitated system that strives to reduce unnecessary care deal with this pressure?

Can traditional approaches to liability coexist with organized cost containment—and if so, how? Some may believe (or hope) that they cannot. Others may believe that the courts, given the opportunity, will provide answers to these questions. Or that the "market" will eventually iron out whatever thorny problems consumers and their attorneys may throw at MCOs. Still others may prefer that these issues be the province of policy analysts and legislators who may (some will argue) be better able to shape a coherent, conscious, and systematic response to what are ultimately policy, as well as legal, questions.

The answers to these questions will depend on a continued assessment and debate about how health care is delivered, financed, and organized. Most importantly, those answers must be based on a determination of which policy, regulatory, and legal approaches can best assure and protect patients' interests in a rapidly changing health care system.

Notes

1. The "corporate practice of medicine doctrine" refers to state laws, originating in the early 1930s, that "ban unlicensed individuals and companies from engaging in the practice of medicine, and thus controlling patient care, by employing licensed professionals such as doctors or dentists. Its intent was to assure that only persons with medical licenses could actually deliver medical care and that lay persons would not influence professional decisions regarding treatment" (National Health Lawyers Association–American Academy of Hospital Attorneys, 1997, 5). Most states currently do not have such statutes; those that have them may interpret their specific applications differently. The existence of these statutes has prevented (and often continues to prevent) hospitals and other nonphysician employers in some states, but not all, from directly employing physicians.

2. Another question in examining allocation of legal risk and accountability for managed care plans is whether *employers* who contract with health plans to administer benefits to employees can be

held accountable for harm caused by the plan or its practitioners or providers. This question has surfaced in arguments against the repeal of the ERISA preemption of state lawsuits against employee health plans, as is discussed later in this chapter.

3. ERISA Industry Committee describes itself as the "association of more than 130 of the nation's largest employers concerned with national retirement and welfare benefit issues."

4. This objection might apply to PARCA and to the Democrats' Patients' Bill of Rights Act but would presumably be answered by Congressman Stark's proposal to create a more comprehensive federal remedy for harm attributed to MCOs.

References

Abraham, K. S., and Weiler, P. C. "Enterprise Medical Liability and the Evolution of the American Health Care System." *Harvard Law Review*, 1994a, *108*, 381–136.

Abraham, K. S., and Weiler, P. C. "Enterprise Medical Liability and the Choice of the Responsible Enterprise." *American Journal of Law & Medicine*, 1994b, *20*, 29–36.

American Association of Health Plans (AAHP). Statement before the United States House of Representatives Committee on Commerce, Subcommittee on Health and Environment, on the Patient Access to Responsible Care Act of 1997, H.R. 1415, the Health Insurance Bill of Rights Act of 1997, H.R. 820, Oct. 28, 1997.

Barents Group. *Impact of Four Legislative Provisions on Managed Care Consumers: 1999–2003*. Washington, D.C.: Author, 1998.

Bearden, D. J., and Maedgen, B. J. "Emerging Theories of Liability in the Managed Health Care Industry." *Baylor Law Review*, 1995, *47*, 285–356.

Brennan, T. A., and others. "Incidence of Adverse Events and Negligence in Hospitalized Patients." *New England Journal of Medicine*, 1991, *324*, 370–376.

Butler, P. A. *Managed Care Plan Liability: An Analysis of Texas and Missouri Legislation*. Menlo Park, Calif.: Kaiser Family Foundation, 1997.

Butler, P. A. *Policy Implications of Recent ERISA Court Decisions*. Washington, D.C.: National Governors' Association, 1998.

Congressional Budget Office. *Cost Estimate: H.R. 3605/S. 1890, Patients' Bill of Rights Act of 1998*. Washington, D.C.: Author, 1998.

"Employee Retirement Income Security Act of 1974; Rules and Regulations for Administration and Enforcement; Claims Procedure; Proposed Rule." *Federal Register*, Sept. 9, 1998, *63*, p. 48390.

ERISA Industry Committee. Written statement before Subcommittee on Employer–Employee Relations, Committee on Education and the Workforce, U.S. House of Representatives, on Patient Access to Responsible Care Act, H.R. 1415, Oct. 28, 1997a.

ERISA Industry Committee. *National Uniformity Issue Brief #2: Costly, Overlapping, and Inconsistent Regulation Is Reduced by Nationally Uniform Standards.* Washington, D.C.: Author, 1997b.

Farrell, M. G. "ERISA Preemption and Regulation of Managed Health Care: The Case for Managed Federalism." *American Journal of Law & Medicine,* 1997, *23,* 251–289.

Fredel, E. A. "ERISA and Managed Care: What the Courts Are Saying." *Benefits Law Journal,* 1995, *8,* 105–118.

Gosfield, A. G. "Who's Responsible? Liability in Managed Care Caselaw." In *Guide to Key Legal Issues in Managed Care Quality.* New York: Faulkner & Gray, 1996.

Gosfield, A. G. "Who Is Holding Whom Accountable for Quality?" *Health Affairs,* 1997, *16,* 26–40.

Havighurst, C. C. "Making Health Plans Accountable for the Quality of Care." *Georgia Law Review,* 1997, *31,* 587–647.

Health Insurance Association of America (HIAA). Statement on Managed Care before the Subcommittee on Health and the Environment of the Commerce Committee, U.S. House of Representatives, Oct. 27, 1997.

Hunt, S., Saari, J., and Traw, K. *Impact of Potential Change to ERISA: Litigation and Appeal Experience of CalPERS, Other Large Public Employers and a Large California Health Plan.* Menlo Park, Calif.: Kaiser Family Foundation, June 1998.

Kilcullen, J. "Groping for the Reins: ERISA, HMO Malpractice, and Enterprise Liability." *American Journal of Law & Medicine,* 1996, *12,* 7–50.

Leape, L. L., Lawthers, A. G., Brennan, T. A., and Johnson, W. G. "Preventing Medical Injury." *Quality Review Bulletin,* May 1993, 144–149.

"Legislation '98: From Patient Rights to Medicare Reform Fights" (editorial). *American Medical News,* Feb. 23, 1998, p. 21.

Mariner, W. K. "Liability for Managed Care Decisions: The Employee Retirement Security Income Act (ERISA) and the Uneven Playing Field." *American Journal of Public Health,* 1996, *86,* 863–869.

National Association of Manufacturers (NAM). Testimony before the Health and the Environment Subcommittee of the Commerce Committee, U.S. House of Representatives on the Patient Access to Responsible Care Act, H.R. 1415, Oct. 28, 1997.

National Health Lawyers Association–American Academy of Hospital Attorneys (NHLA-AAHA). *Patient Care and Personal Responsibility: Impact of the Corporate Practice of Medicine Doctrine and Related Laws and Regulations.* Washington, D.C.: Author, 1997.

Pear, R. "Hands Tied, Judges Rue Law That Limits HMO Liability." *The New York Times,* July 11, 1998, pp. A1, 1.

Perdue, J., and Baxley, S. R. "Cutting Costs—Cutting Care: Can Texas Managed Health Care Systems and HMOs Be Liable for the Medical Malpractice of Physicians?" *St. Mary's Law Journal,* 1995, *27,* 23–67.

Randall, V. R. "Managed Care, Utilization Review, and Financial Risk Shifting: Compensating Patients for Health Care Cost Containment Injuries." *University of Puget Sound Law Review,* 1993, *17,* 1–86.

Sage, W. M., Hastings, K. E., and Berenson, R. A. "Enterprise Liability for Medical Malpractice and Health Care Quality Improvement." *American Journal of Law & Medicine,* 1994, *20,* 1–28.

Self-Insurance Institute of America (SIIA). Statement before the Subcommittee on Health and Environment, Committee on Commerce, U.S. House of Representatives, on the Patient Access to Responsible Care Act of 1997, H.R. 1415, Oct. 28, 1997.

U.S. Department of Labor. Reply brief of Secretary of Labor as amicus curiae, Dukes v. United HealthCare, Inc., no. 941373, 1994.

Chapter Ten

ERISA and the Regulation of Group Health Plans

Craig Copeland and William L. Pierron

About 73 percent of nonelderly Americans with private health insurance are covered by plans under the aegis of the Employee Retirement Income Security Act of 1974 (ERISA). Still, much confusion and misconception surround the act. Because of ERISA's tremendous impact on Americans' health insurance coverage, policymakers and other concerned individuals need to understand how ERISA regulates group health plans.[1]

Why ERISA Was Enacted

The regulation of private-sector employee benefit plans became primarily the responsibility of the federal government with the passage of ERISA. Specifically, ERISA sets forth standards on reporting and information disclosure, claims and appeals procedures, remedies for wrongfully denied benefits, and fiduciary standards: the "backbone" of the act.

Prior to its enactment, employee benefit plans were regulated mainly by the states while receiving preferential tax treatment at the federal level. However, state oversight of employee benefits varied considerably, and because of the lack of consistent legal protections that state regulations afforded pension plans, retirees in some well-publicized cases received fewer benefits than anticipated.[2] Such incidents raised congressional concerns about the solvency and security of employment-based pension plans, which was the primary force behind the passage of ERISA (Employee Benefit Research Institute, 1979). Even though the regulation of health and other employee benefit plans was not as central as pension issues in the formation of the act (and early draft versions of the legislation addressed *only* pensions), all employee benefit plans, including group health plans, were factors in the passage of the final version (Copeland and Pierron, 1998; Shay, 1993; Butler, 1994).

Regulation of Insured and Self-Insured Group Plans

To understand ERISA regulation it is necessary to distinguish between a *group health plan* and a *health plan*. The former is a benefit plan, a contractual promise to provide benefits. This is different from a health insurance policy or a managed care organization (MCO) contract—commonly referred to as a *health plan*—that is the actual mechanism providing benefits.

Sponsors implement their group health plan by using one of two loosely named arrangements: a self-insured or an insured plan. A self-insured (or self-funded) plan is one in which an employer pays for the health care claims of its participants directly out of its own income or assets. Such programs are usually funded on a pay-as-you-go basis, with claims paid by the sponsor as they arise. However, a third-party administrator (TPA), such as an insurance company or other claims-processing organization, generally administers these plans; a relatively small number of plan sponsors self-administer them.

In contrast, an insured plan is one in which a plan sponsor pays premiums to buy a health insurance contract, including an MCO contract, from an insurer or MCO to cover the claims of the plan's participants. (A health insurance contract or MCO contract in this context of an insured plan would include any health plan—health maintenance organization, preferred provider organization, or indemnity plan—that a state has regulatory authority over, whether through insurance regulation or HMO regulation.) A sponsor can use both arrangements to implement the benefit plan and can offer different forms of each arrangement. Thus, within a group health plan, a sponsor can offer several variations of both insured and self-insured plans. Generally, large plan sponsors offer self-insured plans, whereas small sponsors purchase coverage for participants.

Savings Clause and Deemer Clause

ERISA preempts *all* state laws that "relate to" employee benefit plans (section 514[a]). Thus states may not, for example, require group health plans offered by private-sector employers or unions to include specified benefits or follow mandated procedures. There is an important exception, though, to this general principle. The act specifically preserves the states' right to regulate the "business of insurance" under what is commonly called the "savings" clause (section 514[b][2][A]), which reinforces states' authority to regulate insurance that the McCarran-Fergurson Act of 1945 had previously established. Under the savings clause, states can regulate the offerings of firms that cover their workers through an insured plan. However, there is a limit to the savings clause exception. ERISA includes another provision, commonly called the "deemer" clause (section 514[b][2][B]), which prevents states from deeming employee welfare plans to be in the business of insurance for the purposes of state regulation. This prevents states from regulating self-funded plans under the theory that they function as if they were insured plans.

As a result of these provisions, states are able to regulate the content of insurance contracts purchased by benefit plans by virtue of their ability to regulate the business of insurance.[3] But states are preempted from regulating the content of self-insured (self-funded) plans, because these are not considered to be in the business of insurance. Consequently, sponsors that self-insure their plans are not subject to state benefit mandates, other state health insurance regulations, or direct taxes on insurance premiums, whereas insured plans are subject to these types of regulation indirectly through the state's regulation of the health insurance policy or MCO contract.

Thus, state legislators face a major obstacle when they attempt to regulate managed care. Residents who are covered by self-insured plans are not covered by all regulations promulgated at the state level.

Stop-Loss Insurance

Some policymakers have attempted to get around this restriction by attempting to regulate the stop-loss insurance that many sponsors of self-insured plans purchase. Plan sponsors use stop-loss policies to protect the plan from unusually large claims; if claims surpass a certain dollar limit, the stop-loss insurer will reimburse the plan sponsor for any additional claims. The dollar limits can be either on a per person basis or on a total claim basis. Although stop-loss insurance is seen as an important safety valve by the sponsors of self-insured plans, some state regulators are concerned that when such coverage begins reimbursement at relatively low dollar levels the line between stop-loss coverage and full insurance is blurred (Butler and Polzer, 1996).

Regulation of stop-loss insurance has not been a successful strategy. Courts have ruled that states have very limited ability to regulate when stop-loss coverage becomes primary insurance as a result of previous court rulings regarding ERISA and stop-loss coverage.[4] In one recent case, *American Medical Security, Inc. v. Bartlett* (1997), the Fourth Circuit U.S. Court of Appeals affirmed a lower court's ruling that Maryland's attempted regulation was preempted by ERISA. The regulation required stop-loss policies with an attachment point below $10,000 to offer state-mandated benefits.[5] The ruling went on to reject the idea that a low attachment point could turn stop-loss coverage into full insurance, because by doing so it would treat self-funded plans as insurers, a violation of the deemer clause in ERISA. This decision was unlike those in previous cases,[6] in which courts suggested that a sufficiently low (say, $500) attachment point on a stop-loss plan may exist that would turn that coverage into a fully insured plan (Butler, 1994). Thus, it appears that as long as the plan sponsor maintains a reasonably high attachment point on its stop-loss insurance, the plan will be considered immune from state benefit mandates (Employee Benefit Research Institute, 1995; Liston and Patterson, 1996).

Scope of ERISA's Preemption

The Supreme Court appears to have altered its view on the scope of ERISA's preemption. Up to and including the 1992 ruling in *Dis-*

trict of Columbia v. Greater Washington Board of Trade, the Court consistently ruled that the preemption of state laws was broad and sweeping. It held that "relates to" in section 514 means "having a connection with or referring to" and was "conspicuous in its breadth."[7] However, in *New York State Conference of Blue Cross & Blue Shield Plans v. Travelers Ins. Co.* (1995) and subsequent rulings, the Court has moved from the broad, expansive, and literal interpretation of ERISA preemption to a somewhat more narrow view of what Congress's objectives were when it passed the act.[8] In *Travelers,* the Court held that a New York statute imposing a surcharge on hospital bills paid by insurers, MCOs, *or* self-insured plans (except for Blue Cross) was not preempted by ERISA because it only had an "indirect" effect on health plans.

Consequently, it appears that if the law in question does not have an explicit reference to an ERISA plan or does not specifically require or prohibit actions by plans, a law of general applicability that imposes burdens of administration on ERISA plans may survive an ERISA preemption challenge. Thus, some observers suggest that the states will have more flexibility to impose laws of general applicability even if they have an impact on employee benefit plans—whether self-funded or insured (U.S. General Accounting Office, 1995; Butler, 1998).

The Savings and Deemer Clauses

In addition to the ambiguities of the preemption clause, the Supreme Court also has had to interpret the "savings" and "deemer" clauses in order to help pinpoint the limits of ERISA preemption.

Metropolitan Life Insurance v. Massachusetts (1985) was the defining case on the savings clause. In it, the Supreme Court considered a Massachusetts mental health benefit mandate for group health policies. The Court held that the mandate did "relate to" employee benefit plans, but the law regulated the terms of an insurance contract because the benefit mandate (and benefit mandates in general) meet the criteria of the "business of insurance" test outlined in *Union Labor Life Ins. v. Pireno.*[9] Thus, mandated benefit laws are exempt from preemption. However, the Court acknowledged that its ruling created a distinction between plans that are insured and "uninsured" (self-funded), because the deemer clause would immunize an uninsured plan from state mandated benefit laws.

The Supreme Court specifically ruled on the application of the deemer clause to self-funded ERISA plans in *FMC Corporation v. Holliday* (1990). A woman injured in an automobile accident had her medical expenses paid for by her employer's self-funded health plan. Under its provisions, the plan attempted to get reimbursed from funds the woman collected from the driver of the other car. This conflicted with a Pennsylvania law that did not allow anyone else to be reimbursed out of auto injury recoveries. The Court stated that the law in question did come under the savings clause as a law that regulated the business of insurance, but ruled that state insurance laws "do not reach self-funded employee benefit plans because the plans may not be deemed to be insurance companies, other insurers, or engaged in the business of insurance for purposes of such state laws." Therefore, the Court exempted self-funded ERISA plans from state insurance regulation under the deemer clause, and the health plan was able to collect the reimbursement.

The Supreme Court further refined its analysis of the savings clause in *Pilot Life Ins. v. Dedeaux* (1987). Here, it determined that implicit in the language of the clause is the requirement that "in order to regulate insurance, a law must not just have an impact on the insurance industry, but must be specifically directed toward that industry." Because the law in question—a claim for fraud and breach of contract—had *general* applicability, not specific applicability to the insurance industry, it did not meet the test. In addition, the Court found that the civil enforcement provisions of ERISA were intended to be the "exclusive vehicle for action by ERISA-plan participants and beneficiaries asserting improper processing of a claim for benefits." Consequently, the Court held that the act would be undermined if the savings clause were applied to allow causes of action that might vary from state to state, something Congress explicitly rejected when drafting the statute. Thus, under this interpretation, a state law that does not directly regulate the business of insurance is not exempted under the savings clause from preemption, and ERISA's remedies are the sole method for causes of action.

It is clear that preemption of state law remains broad as it relates to specific requirements of ERISA plans, despite the holdings in *Travelers* and subsequent rulings. However, state laws of general applicability that do not single out employee benefit plans may avoid being preempted by ERISA or be saved under ERISA if the courts find that the law does not frustrate the purposes of ERISA and does not create a substantial negative economic impact on plans. As is obvious from this brief overview, the case law on preemption including the savings and deemer clauses has tended to be fact-specific and is subject to continuing evolution.

Disclosure Rules

Disclosure is mandated in a number of ways. ERISA requires that each participant receive a summary plan description (SPD) that must include information on the name and type of administration of the plan, the name and address of administrators, requirements for eligibility, explanations of situations that may result in denial or loss of benefits, source of the plan's financing, identity of any organization through which benefits are provided, methods of presenting claims, and remedies available to redress denied claims. The SPD also must contain a statement of participants' rights under ERISA. A safe harbor provision under federal regulations recommends that an SPD include a description of the administrator's fiduciary duty to administer the plan prudently and in the sole interests of the participants.

Department of Labor (DoL) regulations require that the SPD contain a description of benefits. And under the Health Insurance Portability and Accountability Act of 1996 (HIPAA), an ERISA group health plan sponsor has up to sixty days or at regular intervals of not more than ninety days after any "material reductions in covered services or benefits" to provide participants with a summary description of the reduction. Although the Balanced Budget Act of 1997 eliminated the requirement that the SPD must be filed with the DoL, it must be supplied by the plan if requested by the department. Last, participants have the right to see insurance contracts and trustee reports. Financial penalties apply to any plan administrators who refuse to comply with such a request.

Appeals Procedures

ERISA states that every plan must "afford a reasonable opportunity to any participant whose claim for benefits has been denied for a full and fair review by the appropriate named fiduciary of the decision denying the claim."

Under DoL regulations defining the claims and appeals procedure, a plan has 90 days to make a determination of a submitted claim by a participant. A claim denial must be explained in writing and must include references from the plan to support the decision. The plan must then allow at least 60 days for the claimant to appeal. A decision is ordinarily made within 60 days after the request for a review to the appropriate fiduciary or designee, but under special circumstances it can take up to 120 days.[10] (Group health plans that use an insured plan generally also adhere to the state insurance law appeal rules.[11])

The appeals procedures under ERISA were widely discussed in the 1997–98 congressional session. The length of time allowed for a plan to make claims decisions and appeal decisions has been questioned by numerous consumer advocates. In a managed care environment, claims decisions in many instances are made prior to the care being given, which potentially can hinder the timeliness of care. The DoL, therefore, is proposing to alter its regulations to shorten substantially the time allowed before a decision must be made, and also require an expedited review for medical emergency claims and appeals.

Independent Review

The use of independent external review of appeal decisions is receiving widespread attention. ERISA does not require the use of external review, and the DoL claims it does not have the regulatory authority to require group health plans to implement one. Therefore, the appeal of a claim decision potentially may be returned to the same administrator or committee who initially ruled on it. Some consider this to be procedurally inadequate. In addition, because employees of the plan frequently serve as the administrator or committee making the claims and appeals decisions, and because the plan may benefit from a delay or denial of care, the potential for conflict of interest could exist. However, ERISA holds that an administrator of the plan who acts as fiduciary is obligated to administer the plan in the sole interest of the participants and can be held personally liable for any breach of that duty.

Under an independent external review, an entity outside of the plan would rule on an appeal that has not been resolved through the internal appeals process. This entity could be a government-created agency or a certified private organization with no financial interest in the outcome of the decision. However, many issues would have to be resolved during the implementation of an external review system. For example, who will pay for the review? What kind of claims can be appealed? What are the necessary qualifications external review boards must have? Will a system be modeled on arbitration or mediation? What is the enforcement mechanism of the external appeal?[12] Will uniform benefits for multistate employers be preserved?

We can see that although requiring independent external review under ERISA appears to be fairer for consumers, it still faces tough questions about implementation and the potential cost impact on health care coverage.

ERISA Plan Participants

In order to estimate the cost impact of amendments to ERISA, one must first determine the number and percentage of participants in plans governed by the act on a state-by-state basis. In states having regulations similar to those being proposed for ERISA, or with a low percentage of participants in self-funded plans, the cost impact of any amendments would be lower than in states with less regulation or higher percentages of participants in self-funded plans. However, for issues such as remedies where ERISA provides the exclusive vehicle of action,[13] a breakdown of participants by plan arrangement across states is not important; only the total number of participants in plans governed by ERISA is important for cost estimates.

The March 1997 Current Population Survey (CPS) allows for an estimation of the number of participants in all plans governed by ERISA on a state-by-state basis. These data reveal whether an individual has employment-based coverage, and the sector (public or private) of the person's employer. Furthermore, individuals with dependent coverage can be matched to the policyholder of the health insurance policy (or MCO contract). The total participants in plans governed by ERISA can be determined from this match, although the data do not distinguish between self-funded and insured plan arrangements.[14]

The CPS indicates that between 117.2 million and 122.6 million nonelderly people were in plans governed by ERISA in 1996. California had the highest number, with 12.7 to 13.2 million participants in plans governed by ERISA, whereas Wyoming had the lowest number, with approximately 200,000.[15] Currently, no other data set provides a complete breakdown by state of participants in the different plan arrangements. However, Copeland and Pierron (1998) estimated a national figure of 48 million people enrolled in self-funded ERISA plans in 1995. This represents about 39 percent of the individuals covered by such plans that year.[16]

What Advocates and Critics Say

Many large employers claim that ERISA is crucial to their ability to provide employee health benefits, despite the sometimes confusing interplay between the act and state law. ERISA allows multistate employers and unions to provide uniform coverage across all states, which may be critical to their ability to provide health benefits cost-effectively (Atkins and Bass, 1995). This uniformity reduces problems with employee relations,[17] lowers the administrative costs of having to conform to many different state regulations, and allows for national collective bargaining.[18] Employers and unions or workers, therefore, can negotiate the level of health benefits relative to other benefits and wages, instead of having a mandated health benefit package.

Employers and unions that self-fund find that the ERISA preemption allows them to control their costs better.[19] They are able to negotiate with specific providers and be flexible with the type of coverage they offer. Thus, the plan sponsor is able to identify more efficient providers and ensure that they meet certain quality standards. Also, employers and unions are not subject to direct state excise taxes on insurance premiums. (Employee Benefit Research Institute, 1984).

Finally, ERISA allows plan sponsors to tailor their benefit package to their participants instead of providing the package defined by individual state governments. Some employers argue that if it were not for this ability to control or limit costs and the flexibility to define their own health benefit packages under ERISA's framework, they might provide much less generous benefits or none at all.

In contrast, critics of ERISA push for more appeal rights and increased liability for health plans. They believe there is inadequate regulation of self-funded plans, creating uneven regulations for participants in insured plans and self-funded ones (Butler and Polzer, 1996). They maintain that this is unfair and that participants of self-funded plans are at risk for harm under ERISA's present structure. Specifically, they assert that participants in self-funded plans do not have the protections of solvency standards, do not have the specific benefit mandates and protections against managed care practices that those in insured plans do, and do not receive the information and assistance with complaints that participants in insured plans have access to. Further, ERISA critics argue that state governments should be able to fully regulate health care in their jurisdictions.

Should It Be Altered or Preserved?

There are strong arguments for both altering and preserving ERISA. Anecdotes, some arising out of court cases surrounding the ERISA debate, make a compelling case for greater liability of health plans. However, anecdotes do not paint an adequate picture of the problems or the successes of the health care system. Thus, when policymakers look to amend ERISA, they should consider whether any change to the act will provide a higher level of quality for consumers in the future than is being provided under the present system.

Policymakers also must decide whether quality of care would be better enhanced by health plans' greater exposure to liability or market forces. If increased exposure to liability is the route to go, will it enable consumers to enjoy any potential improvement in quality or will more individuals end up uninsured because of increased costs? It is clear that additional mandates and regulations on health plans will increase costs, but it is not known by how much.[20] Therefore, it is impossible to predict the extent to which employers and unions would stop providing benefits if faced with more regulations.

The central question is this: Can the present marketplace force a higher quality of health care, or will regulation better serve consumers? And if regulation is chosen, will many potentially innovative ways to finance health care be lost, as employers assert, because strict regulations limit experimentation?

Notes

1. The term group health plan is used in ERISA to describe "an employee welfare benefit plan providing medical care (as defined in section 213[d] of Title 26) to participants or beneficiaries directly or through insurance, reimbursement, or otherwise."

2. For example, in the early 1960s, when the Studebaker automobile company collapsed, thousands of vested workers too young to retire were left with substantially reduced pension benefits.

3. Recent court rulings appear to have placed a limit on the states' ability to regulate completely the design of an insured plan. For instance, some states' any willing provider laws have been ruled to be preempted by ERISA. For example, in *Texas Pharmacy Association v. Prudential Insurance Company,* the Fifth Circuit Court of Appeals ruled that any willing provider law was preempted by ERISA.

4. States are able to regulate the solvency and other basic insurance aspects of stop-loss insurers but cannot mandate health benefits for stop-loss insurance plans.

5. An attachment point is the maximum amount a self-funded plan must pay on a total cost or per employee per benefit year basis before the stop-loss insurer assumes liability.

6. For example, see *Brown v. Granatelli* (1990).

7. *Shaw v. Delta Air Lines* (1983).

8. *Debuono v. NYSA-ILA Medical Services Fund* (1997), *California Division of Labor Standards Enforcement v. Dillingham Construction, N.A., Inc.* (1997), and *Boggs v. Boggs* (1997).

9. The test contained the following three parts: the activity must spread risk, the relationship between insured and insurer must be an inte-

gral part of the activity, and it is limited to entities in the traditional insurance industry (*Union Labor Life Ins. Co. v. Pireno*, 1982).

10. ERISA allows for the use of an injunction (section 502 [a][3]) to force the provision of benefits, but it is rarely used because it is costly and is not a final decision. Ordinarily, claims and appeals decisions do not take the total amount of time allowed under ERISA regulations.

11. Insured plans do appear to be following the state laws on appeal procedures. However, the limited case law on state appeal laws lead to virtually no guidance on whether these laws are preempted for insured or self-insured plans. In fact, a Texas managed care law's provision of appeals and external review was ruled to be preempted by ERISA (*Corporate Health Insurance, Inc. v. Texas Department of Insurance.*)

12. Some observers have suggested that without the proper remedies external review cannot guarantee that wrongly denied benefits will be corrected.

13. ERISA appears to provide the exclusive remedies for the quantity of benefits provided but not necessarily the quality of benefits provided. Nevertheless, both plan arrangements are treated equally for remedies.

14. The CPS data has two weaknesses in this estimation. First, church plan enrollees are included in the estimate even though they are not governed by ERISA. This is done because it is not clear when a person is in a church plan or a private plan from the CPS, and the number in these plans is known to be small relative to the number in private sector plans. Second, the sector of the policyholder's employer is recorded for the employer of the longest duration during the reference period. This employer may not be the employer providing the coverage due to job change and the possibility of receiving continued coverage under COBRA.

15. The estimates have a range due to some dependents not matching and others who are no longer working but received employment-based coverage. However, the nonworkers do not have employer data that can be attributed to them to determine the sector of the employer. The smaller state estimates should be used with caution because of the small sample size.

16. Copeland and Pierron followed the method that the U.S. General Accounting Office (GAO, 1995) used in order to show the trend in self-funded plan enrollment. GAO found that 39 percent of participants or forty-four million in plans governed by ERISA were in

self-funded plans in 1993. Consequently, the percentage in self-funded plans remained unchanged. Other authors have suggested that there may be an increased use of self-funding, particularly by small employers as a result of the greater availability of stop-loss insurance products (Gabel, Ginsburg, and Hunt, 1997). Furthermore, the creation of creative risk arrangements, especially among managed care plans, could lead to increases in self-funding. Yet the data now available reveal that the percentage of ERISA plan participants in self-funded plans is holding relatively constant.

17. Employees in all states may not have the same benefits without ERISA preemption, which could create strife among employees because employees in states with a large number of benefit mandates could have more generous benefits just due to where the employee resides. In addition, employees who transfer can expect to have same benefit package upon arrival in the new location, so the employee would not be upset over any change in benefits due to the move.

18. Unions consider this to be important in that unions are able to bargain for certain benefits without being constrained by differing state regulations on required benefit levels. However, many unions have supported the various patient bill of rights proposals that would amend ERISA to impose requirement on self-funded plans offered to unionized employees.

19. There appear to be no solid data on the average cost savings for employers who self-fund health benefits. However, a 1996 GAO study looked at the costs of various state mandates. It concluded that mandates do increase costs, but many self-funded plans provide the mandated benefits. The GAO did point out that, on average, self-funded plans save 2 percent by not having to pay premium taxes. Thus, the GAO concludes that cost savings are gained by self-funding because mandates do increase cost, but in some cases the savings is small because self-funded plans already provide the mandated benefits.

20. The impact has been estimated to be relatively negligible to substantial, depending on the interpretation of the mandates and assumptions from that interpretation. Despite the wide range, any increases in costs for health benefits could have potentially serious implications for the likelihood of small businesses offering health benefits. For instance, Feldman, Dowd, Leitz, and Blewett (1997) estimated that for small establishments (with fewer than fifty employees) in the state of Minnesota, an increase of one dollar in monthly premiums would lead to approximately a 2 percent reduction in the proportion of small establishments offering health

insurance. In addition, The Lewin Group estimates that a 1 percent increase in employer premiums would lead to an additional four hundred thousand individuals being uninsured, later revised to three hundred thousand being uninsured. Consequently, if these regulations raise the costs of health insurance significantly, a potentially significant number of individuals could be without health insurance, especially employees of small businesses.

References

Atkins, G. L., and Bass, K. *ERISA Preemption: The Key to Market Innovation in Health Care.* Washington, D.C.: Corporate Health Care Coalition, 1995.

Butler, P. *Roadblock to Reform: ERISA Implications for State Health Care Initiatives.* Washington, D.C.: National Governors' Association, 1994.

Butler, P. *Policy Implications of Recent ERISA Court Decisions.* Washington, D.C.: National Governors' Association, 1998.

Butler, P., and Polzer, K. *Private-Sector Health Coverage: Variation in Consumer Protections Under ERISA and State Law.* Washington, D.C.: George Washington University, 1996.

Copeland, C., and Pierron, W. "Implications of ERISA for Health Plans and the Number of Self-Funded Plans." EBRI Issue Brief, no. 193. Washington, D.C.: Employee Benefit Research Institute, 1998.

Employee Benefit Research Institute. *The Employee Retirement Income Security Act* (pamphlet). Washington, D.C.: Author, 1979.

Employee Benefit Research Institute. "ERISA and Health Plans." EBRI Issue Brief, no. 167. Washington, D.C.: Author, 1995.

Employee Benefit Research Institute. "Regulating Employee Health and Welfare Plans." EBRI Issue Brief, no. 36. Washington, D.C.: Author, 1984.

Feldman, R., Dowd, B., Leitz, S., and Blewett, L. A. "The Effect of Premiums on the Small Firm's Decision to Offer Health Insurance." *Journal of Human Resources,* Fall 1997, pp. 635–658.

Gabel, J. R., Ginsburg, P. B., and Hunt, K. A. "Small Employers and Their Health Benefits, 1988–1996: An Awkward Adolescence." *Health Affairs,* Sept.–Oct. 1997, pp. 103–110.

Liston, P., and Patterson, M. P. "Analysis of the Number of Workers Covered by Self-Insured Health Plans Under the Employee Retirement Income Security Act of 1974 and 1995." KPMG Peat Marwick, report to the Henry J. Kaiser Foundation, 1996.

Shay, E. F. "Regulation of Employment-Based Health Benefits: The Intersection of State and Federal Law." In M. J. Field and H. T. Shapiro (eds.), *Employment and Health Benefits: A Connection at Risk.* Washington, D.C.: National Academy Press, 1993.

U.S. General Accounting Office. *Employer-Based Health Plans: Issues, Trends, and Challenges Posed by ERISA.* HEHS publication no. 95–167. Washington, D.C.: Author, 1995.

U.S. General Accounting Office. *Health Insurance Regulation: Varying State Requirements Affect Cost of Insurance.* HEHS publication no. 96–161. Washington, D.C.: Author, 1996.

Perspectives on Regulation

The purpose of the third section in this collection is to provide a variety of perspectives on regulation from some of the major stakeholders inside and outside the health care industry. The first stakeholder we hear from is the consumer, as Robert Blendon and his colleagues report on the sources of the managed care backlash. Their research reveals that managed care enrollees are less satisfied with their health coverage than those enrolled in fee-for-service plans. They also conclude that media reports of threatening but rare medical events involving denial of care or catastrophic errors have raised the public's anxiety about managed care.

Karen Davis, the president of the Commonwealth Fund and a longtime health care advocate, writes with David Sandman about the need to ensure quality through regulation. The authors commend the President's Advisory Commission on Consumer Protection and Quality in the Health Care Industry that produced the Consumer Bill of Rights and Responsibilities (CBRR), and they recommend many of its provisions. Emphasizing the importance of adequate insurance coverage, choice of health plan, disclosure of information, and rights of grievance and appeal, they contend that these regulations should be adopted at the national level. Davis and Sandman also recommend adoption of the commission's recommendations for the establishment of a quality advisory council, possibly similar to the Medical Payment Advisory Commission (MedPAC), and a private, independent forum for the establishment of national quality standards.

The next perspective is provided by Karen Ignagni, the president of the American Association of Health Plans. A reasoned and articulate advocate for the largest managed care industry trade organization, Ignagni calls for a balance between regulation and market forces. She contends that regulatory policy should be formulated in the context of objective data from benchmarking and outcomes studies and not as a result of anecdotes or subjective criteria. The ideal regulatory model, she suggests, is at a balance point between public and private regulatory responsibility and on a continuum between general guidance and micromanagement.

A contrasting perspective is provided by Ronald Pollack, the president of Families USA, the nation's largest consumer health organization. Pollack begins by recognizing the positive potential of prepaid managed care plans but claims that they have not lived up to their promise. As a member of the President's Commission that issued the CBRR, Pollack insists that regulatory oversight is needed at the national level to establish a number of basic procedural rights. He also advocates for changes in ERISA so that patients have adequate recourse when they are wrongfully denied care. In addition, he recommends that an independent, nonprofit, ombudsman program be established and supported by public funds to help consumers navigate the changing health care marketplace.

As strongly as Pollack advocates for regulation, Bill Gradison, president of the Health Insurance Association of America (HIAA), praises the efficiency of the free market in meeting consumer demand. Gradison points out that consumer demands for a wider choice of plans, a greater choice of physicians, and the right to see any provider have resulted in a proliferation of PPOs, POSs, and other fast-growing segments of a market that is responding to consumer needs. He praises the industry for meeting the demand for more affordable health insurance. And cautioning that regulation can be a two-edged sword, Gradison claims that stringent regulation could result in fewer people with insurance coverage who will be paying higher premiums.

The final chapter in this section is a wake-up call to advocates on both sides of the regulation debate. Larry Gage, president of the National Association of Public Hospitals, admonishes both sides, claiming that the question of regulating managed care misses the essential problem confronting consumers of health care in

America: the plight of the forty-three million uninsured. Gage explains that lower reimbursement by private health plans in addition to government cutbacks threaten the financial stability of safety-net providers that care for the uninsured. He argues that resources must be contributed by the entire health system, including managed care plans, to sustain the institutional health safety net. He specifically recommends that disproportionate share payments be included in Medicare managed care premiums, and he calls for the creation of a national indigent care trust fund. Gage concludes that with a health care system that leaves forty-three million uninsured, we do not have the luxury of limiting our policy debate to protecting those who already have insurance.

Chapter Eleven

The Public

Understanding the Managed Care Backlash

*Robert J. Blendon, Mollyann Brodie, John M. Benson,
Drew E. Altman, Larry Levitt, Tina Hoff, Larry Hugick*

Managed care has grown rapidly over the past decade, to become
the dominant way Americans get their health insurance and health
care. During this period managed care has been credited with
being one of the main factors in slowing the growth of employer
health premiums. However, the nation's transition into these new
types of health plans has not been free of controversy. Criticisms
of managed care have led to the introduction both in Congress
and in state legislatures of more than a thousand bills dealing with
consumer protection in managed care, as well as the establishment
of a presidential commission to examine the need for future guidelines in this rapidly growing industry.[1]

Advocates for these measures believe that they are responding
to a broad public "backlash" against managed care. They point to
surveys that show the public favoring some type of regulation of
managed care plans. Those who oppose regulation point to other
opinion surveys showing that most Americans today are satisfied

This chapter originally appeared as Blendon, R. J., Brodie, M., Benson, J. M., Altman, D. E., Levitt, L., Hoff, T., and Hugick, L. "Understanding the Managed Care
Backlash." *Health Affairs*, 1998, *17*(4), 80–94, copyright © 1998 by The People-to-
People Health Foundation, Inc., Bethesda, Md. The chapter is reprinted here
with permission from The People-to-People Health Foundation, Inc.

with their own managed care plans. Thus, opponents see no need for government regulation.

This chapter seeks to explain the underlying issues that drive what has been called a backlash against managed care and the seemingly contradictory findings between surveys showing support for regulation and surveys showing satisfied consumers. The focus here on public opinion relates to its likely relevance to the outcome of policy debates in areas such as these. Over the past two decades a substantial body of research has emerged showing that public opinion has a major influence on many public policy decisions.[2] In addition, studies of the 1993–1994 debate over the Clinton health care reform plan show members of Congress listing changes in public opinion as a major reason for the plan's demise.[3]

Data and Methods

The data presented here were derived primarily from two sources.

Sources of Data

The first source is a survey designed by researchers at the Henry J. Kaiser Family Foundation and Harvard University. The interviews were conducted via telephone by Princeton Survey Research Associates (PSRA) between August 22 and September 23, 1997, with randomly selected samples of 1,204 adults nationwide and 500 adults in California.[4] The second data source consists of specific results drawn from twenty other surveys conducted nationwide between 1995 and 1997. We compiled these data from the Public Opinion Location Library (POLL) database at the Roper Center for Public Opinion Research in Storrs, Connecticut, and from the Louis Harris subscription service. These polls involved telephone interviews with between 500 and 2,000 randomly selected adults.[5]

Response Rates

Response rates in the Kaiser–Harvard–PSRA survey were 49 percent for the national sample and 51 percent for California. Completion rates among contacted households were 67 percent for the national sample and 71 percent for California.

A recent methodological experiment has shown that nonresponse at the level encountered in opinion polls as they are normally conducted by reputable firms does not underestimate the
views of particular segments of the American public.[6] Also, published research has shown that the techniques usually used in opinion polling have helped prominent polling firms to achieve a high
level of accuracy on the outcome measure for which actual public
opinion can be measured with considerable precision: voter choice
in elections.[7]

Determination of Type of Health Care Coverage

Because many people are unsure about what kind of health insurance they have, insured respondents under age sixty-five in the
national sample of the Kaiser–Harvard–PSRA survey (778 respondents) were asked a series of four questions to establish their type
of coverage. They were asked if they were required to do any of the
following by their health plan: choose doctors from a list and pay
more for doctors not on the list; select a primary care doctor or
medical group; or obtain a referral before seeing a medical specialist or a doctor outside the plan. Respondents were listed as
being in "heavy" managed care if they reported that their plan had
all of the characteristics described (34 percent of insured respondents under age sixty-five). They were listed as being in "light"
managed care if they reported that their plan had at least one but
not all of the characteristics listed above (45 percent). Finally,
respondents were listed as having "traditional" insurance if they reported that their plans had none of the characteristics (21 percent).[8] This distribution mirrors direct estimates of enrollment by
type of plan.[9]

Is There Evidence of a Managed Care Backlash?

Confirming the findings of a number of earlier studies, the
Kaiser–Harvard–PSRA survey found that most insured Americans,
regardless of whether they have managed care or traditional coverage, are satisfied with their own health insurance plan.[10] Two-
thirds (66 percent) of adults under age sixty-five in managed care
and three-fourths (76 percent) of adults under age sixty-five in

traditional plans give their own health plan a letter grade of B or better.[11]

However, the same survey also confirmed earlier findings that a majority of Americans favor government regulation of managed care, even if it raises costs.[12] A slight majority (52 percent) believe that the government should protect consumers of managed care, whereas 40 percent say that such intervention is not worth the increased costs that would result. The groups most in favor of government regulation are those who describe their own health as poor, only fair, or good (the lowest three of five categories offered); those who have some college education but not a college degree; and Democrats (see Exhibit 11.1). The groups least in favor of such regulation are Republicans, those from households with an annual income of $30,000 to $49,999, those ages fifty to sixty-four, and those in self-described excellent or very good health.[13] Other surveys have raised the issue of regulating managed care without mentioning concerns about increasing the cost of benefits. These surveys find public support for such policies at 75 percent or higher.[14]

Exhibit 11.1. Americans' Views About Governmental Regulation of Managed Care, 1997.

Group	Percent favoring government regulation
All American adults	52%
Most in favor of government regulation	
Respondents in only fair or poor health	65
Respondents in good health	58
Respondents with some college training but not a college degree	57
Democrats	57
Least in favor of government regulation	
Republicans	40
$30,000–$49,999 household income	42
Ages 50-64	46
Respondents in excellent or very good health	47

Source: Kaiser–Harvard–Princeton Survey Research Associates poll, 1997.

This support for regulation appears to reflect public concerns that managed care is hurting the quality of care available to patients, and that this sector is not doing as good a job for patients as are other professions and institutions in health care.

A plurality (45 percent) of Americans believe that during the past few years managed care has decreased the quality of health care for patients, whereas only 32 percent believe that managed care has improved quality.[15] In addition, 54 percent believe that in the future the trend toward more managed care will harm the quality of medical care that people like themselves will receive; 33 percent think that the trend will improve quality.[16]

A majority of Americans express concern that in managed care plans, people may not receive the services they need when they are very sick. Six in ten (59 percent) say that managed care plans have made it harder for people who are sick to see medical specialists; 25 percent say that managed care makes it easier. Half (51 percent) say that managed care has decreased the quality of care for people who are sick; 32 percent say that quality is increased. A majority (55 percent) of people in managed care say that they are at least "somewhat worried" that if they were sick, their health plan would be more concerned about saving money than about what is the best medical treatment; 34 percent of those with traditional health insurance feel this way.[17]

When asked about specific examples taken from news stories of dramatic events that might be considered statistical outliers, the public's perception is that these are fairly common occurrences. For example, two-thirds of Americans believe that a health maintenance organization (HMO) holding back on a child's cancer treatment is something that happens "often" (26 percent) or "sometimes" (40 percent); only 23 percent think that this happens "rarely." Two in five (39 percent) think that newborn babies are often sent home after just one day because of a managed care plan's policy in spite of mothers' concerns about their children's health; another third (34 percent) think that this occurs "sometimes"; only 18 percent think that this happens "rarely."[18]

These perceptions of managed care are reflected in the ratings of the industry compared with other health care groups. Other health care groups and many other industries are viewed far more favorably than managed care plans are (see Exhibit 11.2). Solid majorities of Americans think that nurses, doctors, pharmaceutical companies, and hospitals generally do a "good job." More people do think that managed care plans do a "good job" than a "bad job" serving health care consumers, but their comparative rating is lower than any other health care group and lower even than oil companies, a traditionally unpopular industry among the public. However, for many people the jury is still out: the two surveys show that many people have no opinion about the kind of job managed care plans are doing.[19]

Four in ten (39 percent) of those in the Kaiser–Harvard–PSRA survey who think that managed care plans generally do a "bad job" serving health care consumers (21 percent of all Americans) report that the main reason they feel this way is their own direct personal experience; 22 percent say that they have been mainly influenced by what they have seen or heard on television, in newspapers, or in other media. One in three (32 percent) say that the main reason they feel that managed care plans do a "bad job" is what they have heard from family or friends.[20]

Public perceptions about the managed care industry are not merely the product of a rapidly changing health care marketplace, where many Americans are experiencing managed care for the first time. In California, with its long history of managed care, support for regulation and concerns about being denied care are comparable to findings nationwide (see Exhibit 11.3).[21]

Are Americans Worried About Their Own Health Plans?

In this study we wanted to test a phenomenon observed in public opinion about other institutions: people are distrustful of large systems but not of the individuals with whom they have contact within the system. One example can be cited from the field of medicine. Although two-thirds of Americans (68 percent) reported in the mid-1980s that they were increasingly losing faith in physicians, this did not affect the high level of satisfaction most people had with their most recent physician encounter (83 percent) or their positive feelings about their own physician (80 percent).[22] A frequently cited example concerns Congress: Americans generally give rather low performance ratings to Congress as a whole but express a much higher opinion of the job being done by their own representatives in Congress.[23]

Exhibit 11.2. Ratings of Groups or Industries on Service to Consumers, 1997 and 1998.

Group or Industry	Ratings of groups on service to health care consumers[a]		Ratings of industries on service to their consumers[b]	
	Good	Bad	Good	Bad
Nurses	83%	4%	–[c]	–[c]
Doctors	69	12	–[c]	–[c]
Computer software companies	–[c]	–[c]	78%	7%
Telephone companies	–[c]	–[c]	76	23
Pharmaceutical or drug companies	62	20	73	23
Hospitals	61	18	73	23
Banks	–[c]	–[c]	72	26
Car manufacturers	–[c]	–[c]	69	25
Oil companies	–[c]	–[c]	64	26
Life insurance companies	–[c]	–[c]	63	24
Health insurance companies	44	32	48	47
Managed care companies	34	21	45	42
HMOs	36	25	–[c]	–[c]
Tobacco companies	–[c]	–[c]	32	60

Sources: See below

Note: HMO is health maintenance organization.
[a]Kaiser-Harvard-Princeton Survey Research Associates poll, 1997.
[b]Harris poll, 1998.
[c]Not applicable.

**Exhibit 11.3. Impressions of Managed Care
in a State with Extensive Experience (California)
and the United States, 1997.**

	Percent saying	
	United States	*California*
View of government regulation		
Government needs to protect consumers from being treated unfairly and not getting the care they should from managed care plans	52%	52%
Additional government regulation isn't worth it because it would raise the cost of health insurance too much for everyone	40	35
Rating of the job managed care companies do in serving health care consumers		
Good job	34	27
Bad job	21	19
During the past few years, HMOs and other managed care plans have		
Decreased the quality of health care for people who are sick	51	46
Increased the quality of care	32	31

Source: Kaiser-Harvard-Princeton Survey Research Associates poll, 1997.

Notes: HMO is health maintenance organization. The volunteered responses "mixed," "no effect," and "don't know" are not shown.

If this held true in the case of managed care, we would expect the public to be anxious about the managed care industry in general but not about their own managed care health plan. However, the survey finds that people in "heavy" managed care are more worried than are those with traditional coverage when it comes to the perceived motivations of their health plans. This is true for the four measures used in the study: Americans' perceptions of how likely their plan is to pay for an emergency room visit, how likely it is to pay for most of the cost for care of a serious problem requiring a costly treatment, trust in their plan to do the right thing for their care, and worries that the plan would be more concerned about saving money than about what is the best treatment if they are sick (Exhibit 11.4).[24]

How Important Is Concern About Being Able to Get Care?

Concerns about what happens to people when they are very sick are reflected in what Americans say is most important in choosing a health plan. Although respondents rated each of seven factors on a list as very important in choosing a health plan, when they were forced to choose among them, the number-one factor was how well the health plan takes care of members who are sick (cited by 25 percent), followed closely by how much the patients have to pay (22 percent). Ranked next were whether the plan has a wide range of benefits (17 percent) and whether a person's current doctor is in the plan (15 percent). Further down the list were whether a plan offers a wide choice of doctors (8 percent) and whether one's preferred hospital is in the plan (5 percent). Lowest on the list was whether the plan has passed a review and been accredited (3 percent).[25]

Americans' views are relatively negative about efforts by health plans to limit payment for care that doctors think a patient needs. Many say that they would have a less favorable view of a plan if patients needed to get approval from the plan before they could receive expensive medical treatment (58 percent); if the plan limited payment for certain types of health services when people are sick, to keep costs low (48 percent); and if doctors had to follow certain health plan guidelines on the types of treatments and drugs they can give to patients (44 percent).[26] In addition, 62 percent of Americans said in a previous study that they agreed that health plans should pay for medical treatment even if it costs a million dollars per life.[27] When they learn that some health plans require doctors to follow certain guidelines in treating patients, a majority (56 percent) agree that this is a bad thing because decisions about treatment should be entirely up to the doctor; 39 percent agree that this is a good thing because all patients will benefit from proven techniques.[28]

Exhibit 11.4. Americans' Impressions of How Their Health Plan Will Deal with Them When They Need Help, Currently Insured Persons, by Type of Plan, 1997.

	All Insured	Heavy managed care[a]	Light managed care[a]	Traditional plan[a]
Very likely that your health plan will pay for emergency room visit	64%	56%	63%	78%
Very likely that your health plan will pay for most of the cost if you had a serious problem requiring a costly treatment	55	44	54	69
Trust your health insurance plan to do the right thing for your care just about always	41	30	31	55
Very/somewhat worried that your health plan would be more concerned about saving money than about what is the best treatment for you if you are sick	47	61	51	34

Source: Kaiser-Harvard-Princeton Survey Research Associates poll, 1997.

[a]Under age sixty-five.

Who Benefits from the Cost Savings of Managed Care?

Public concerns about efforts to limit payment are magnified by skepticism about who benefits from the cost savings. Many Americans are uncertain that managed care keeps health care costs down at all (see Exhibit 11.5). A majority (55 percent) believe that during the past few years HMOs and other managed care plans have not made much difference to health care costs; only 28 percent think that they have helped to keep costs down.[29] However, Americans are more optimistic about managed care's ability to contain costs in the future. A slight majority (51 percent) believes that the trend toward more managed care will help to contain health care costs, whereas 42 percent think that it will not help.[30]

In addition, majorities see the money saved by managed care plans as helping health insurance companies to earn more profits (72 percent) and allowing employers to pay less for health insurance (56 percent). Only about half (49 percent) believe that the money saved makes health care more affordable for people like themselves.[31]

Will Report Cards Be the Answer?

Many experts believe that report cards on the performance of managed care plans would help to allay public anxiety about these plans by giving people information they could use to make informed choices. However, public opinion data suggest real limits to the usefulness of this approach.

The public is particularly interested in the experience of sick persons trying to gain access to the care they and their doctors think they need. In contrast, most consumer surveys today report satisfaction levels among all plan members, most of whom are not very sick or burdened with the large medical bills that can be a source of contention with their plan.

In addition, surveys show that a large share of consumers do not rely on objective ratings to make decisions. Health care consumers are much more likely to rely on personal experiences or the recommendation of friends and family members (see Exhibit 11.6). If they had to choose between health plans that cost the same, more Americans would choose a plan recommended by friends and family than one rated much higher in quality by independent experts

Exhibit 11.5. Americans' Views on the Cost Savings from Managed Care, 1997.

	Percent responding
During the past few years HMOs and other managed care plans have[a]	
Not made much difference to health care costs	55%
Helped to keep health care costs down	28
Made costs go up (volunteered response)	12
Don't know	12
The trend toward more managed care will[b]	
Help to contain health care costs	51
Not help	42
Not sure	7
Money saved by HMOs and other managed care plans[a]	
Helps health insurance companies to earn more profits	72[c]
Allows employers to pay less for health insurance	56[c]
Makes health care more affordable for people like you	49[c]

Sources: See below.

[a]Kaiser-Harvard-Princeton Survey Research Associates poll, 1997.
[b]Harris poll, 1997.
[c]Percent responding "yes."

Exhibit 11.6. How Americans Choose Health Plans and Providers, 1996.

	Percent responding
Suppose you had to choose between health plans that cost the same; which would you be more likely to choose?	
One strongly recommended to you by friends and family	52%
One rated much higher in quality by independent experts who evaluate plans	43
Don't know	5
Suppose you had to choose between two surgeons at a hospital; which would you be more likely to choose?	
A surgeon who has treated your family for a long time, but whose ratings aren't as high as those of other surgeons at the hospital	76
A surgeon whose ratings are much higher, but who has not had anyone you know personally as a patient	20
Don't know	4
Suppose you had to choose between two hospitals; which would you be more likely to choose?	
A hospital you and your family have used for many years without any problem	72
A hospital that is rated much higher in quality by experts	25
Don't know	3

Source: Kaiser-Agency for Health Care Policy and Research-Princeton Survey Research Associates poll, 1996.

who evaluate plans. About three in four would choose a surgeon who has treated their family for a long time—even if that surgeon's ratings were not as high—rather than a surgeon whose ratings are much higher but who has not treated anyone the respondent knows personally. Similarly, most would choose a hospital they and their family had used for many years without any problems, rather than a hospital rated much higher in quality by experts.[32]

Research on decisions in other areas of consumer choice has shown a mixed picture. On the one hand, relatively few persons use consumer ratings when making important purchasing decisions. When those who had bought or leased a motor vehicle during the past ten years were asked to think back to the last time they made such a purchase, only one in three (35 percent) said that they turned for information to consumer magazines that test and rate products. As with health plans, the most frequently mentioned source of information was friends and family members (46 percent). In general, only one in five (20 percent) said that they go to an information source such as consumer magazines always or most of the time before making a major purchase.[33]

This tendency to rely on sources of information other than objective measures extends even to the way Americans judge the health of the economy. Asked to choose (from a list of nine possible sources) the two indicators that they think give them the best picture of how the economy is doing, only 32 percent of the public mention news reports on government unemployment and cost-of-living statistics. Nearly as many (28 percent) cite as a key indicator the amount of activity they see in stores. More than half (55 percent) rely on the personal experiences of family, friends, and coworkers.[34]

In addition, four in ten insured Americans (41 percent) report that when they enrolled in their current health plan, they did not have a choice of more than one plan.[35] For this group, report cards will not be directly useful, although their employers might use them as a way of selecting the plan they offer their employees.

Conclusions

We are confronted here with two seemingly contradictory pieces of information. One suggests that Americans are satisfied with their health insurance plans, regardless of whether the plans are traditional fee-for-service or managed care. The other indicates that the public favors regulation of managed care plans, even if it raises costs. How can this seeming inconsistency be resolved?

Findings of these two sentiments derive from different types of inquiry: consumer ratings of health plans and public opinion questions. Consumer ratings measure the average experience of those who use a service, whereas public opinion can often be driven by rare occurrences as well as by people's own experiences and those of their families and friends as day-to-day consumers of health care.

We believe that two important factors are influencing the public backlash against managed care. First, a significant proportion of Americans report problems with managed care plans. Based on five studies on satisfaction with nonfinancial aspects of managed care health plans, results for all enrollees combined showed less satisfaction with managed care plans than with fee-for-service plans.[36] Another study, looking at differences between managed care and fee-for-service plans for persons who are ill, found more complaints about access to specialists, tests, and waiting times by those enrolled in managed care plans.[37]

Second, we believe that the public backlash is also being driven by relatively rare events that seem threatening and dramatic but have been experienced by few consumers personally. A review of polling research in two other service-related areas—airlines and banking—shows that such events (the crash of a ValuJet plane in May 1996 and the savings and loan crisis in the late 1980s) can lead to increased public support for government regulation, even though measures of consumer satisfaction remain stable or even improve.[38]

Prior research shows that an issue is more likely to emerge as part of the public's policy agenda if it involves continuing news coverage and is dramatic in nature.[39] In any given year relatively few Americans are very ill or accumulate very large medical bills, situations that can lead to serious conflicts with their health plans. Because this is the case, we would expect people's negative impressions of managed care to come mostly from sources other than their own direct personal experiences while they were sick—including what they hear or experience through friends and family or what they see or read in the news.[40] Thus, part of Americans' interest in regulation of the managed care industry seems to derive from a concern that regardless of how well their plan performs today, care might not be available or paid for when they are very sick.

Some experts believe that providing report-card ratings of health plans will enable consumers to make the best decisions for their families and negate the need for government regulation. However, report cards will be seen as providing little protection by the large portion of the population who have no experience using this type of rating. As a result, if concerns arise about the threatening behavior of individual health plans, a share of the public is likely to support some degree of regulation rather than depending on report-card ratings as a way of avoiding the consequences of plan decisions. For example, for airline safety, although safety reports and consumer complaints are provided by airlines as a matter of public record, experience suggests that these reports have not quelled the public's desire for some level of government safety regulation. Still, report cards could play a role in the decision making of employers who want to make the best choice of health plans for their employees. This in turn could have an influence on the quality of plans available in the marketplace.

Public concerns about the need for increased regulation of managed care are likely to be with us for the long term. Experience in other industries suggests that Americans have limits on how far they will allow marketplace decisions to put them at individual risk. As with airline safety and banking, public support for regulation is being driven in part by the anxiety the public feels over the occurrence of visible events questioning the behavior of managed care plans, as well as the problems people experience in their own lives. As a result, debate about regulation of the managed care industry is likely to be a permanent fixture on the health care agenda for years to come.

Notes
1. "Health Care in America: Your Money or Your Life," *Economist*, March 1998, pp. 23–26.
2. See, for example, Monroe, A. D. "Consistency Between Public Preferences and National Policy Decisions." *American Journal of Political Science*, January 1979, pp. 3–19; Monroe, A. D. "American Party Platforms and Public Opinion." *American Journal of Political Science*, February 1983, pp. 27–42; Page, B. I., and Shapiro, R. Y. "Effects of

Public Opinion on Policy." *American Political Science Review*, March 1983, pp. 175–190; Shapiro, R. Y., and Jacobs, L. R. "The Relationship Between Public Opinion and Public Policy: A Review." In S. Long (ed.), *Political Behavior Annual*. Boulder, Colo.: Westview, 1989; Wright, G. C., Jr., Erikson, R. S., and McIver, J. P. "Public Opinion and Policy Liberalism in the United States." *American Journal of Political Science*, November 1987, pp. 980–1001; Erikson, R. S., Wright, G. C., Jr., and McIver, J. P. "Political Parties, Public Opinion, and State Policy in the United States." *American Political Science Review*, Sept. 1989, pp. 729–750; Page, B. I., and Shapiro, R. Y. *The Rational Public: Fifty Years of Trends in Americans' Policy Preferences*. Chicago: University of Chicago Press, 1992; Jacobs, L. R., and Shapiro, R. Y. "Public Opinion and the New Social History: Some Lessons for the Study of Public Opinion and Democratic Policy-Making." *Social Science History*, Spring 1989, p. 124; and Jacobs, L. R., and Shapiro, R. Y. "Debunking the Pandering Politician Myth." *Public Perspective*, April–May 1997, pp. 3–5.

3. Hansen, O., Blendon, R. J., Ontmans, J., James, M., Norton, C., Rosenblatt, T. "Lawmakers' Views on the Failure of Health Reform: A Survey of Members of Congress and Staff." *Journal of Health Politics, Policy and Law*, Spring 1996, pp. 137–151. On the decline in public support, see Blendon, R. J., Brodie, M., and Benson, J. "What Happened to Americans' Support for the Clinton Health Plan?" *Health Affairs*, Summer 1995, pp. 7–23.

4. Henry J. Kaiser Family Foundation–Harvard University–Princeton Survey Research Associates poll, Storrs, Conn.: Roper Center for Public Opinion Research, 1997.

5. When interpreting these findings, one should recognize that all surveys are subject to sampling error. Results may differ from what would be obtained if the whole population of adults had been interviewed. The size of this error varies with the number surveyed and the magnitude of difference in the responses to each question. Most national public opinion surveys have sample sizes of about twelve hundred persons, in which the results will, with a 95 percent degree of confidence, have a statistical precision of ±3 percent of what would be obtained if the entire population had been interviewed. The sampling error for five hundred respondents is ±5 percent; for two thousand respondents, ±3 percent. Possible sources of nonsampling error include nonresponse bias, as well as question wording and ordering effects. Nonresponse in telephone surveys produces some known biases in survey-derived estimates because participation tends to vary for different subgroups of the population.

To compensate for these known biases, the sample data are usually weighted in analysis, as they are in the August 1997 Kaiser–Harvard–PSRA survey, using parameters from the most recent available census data. Other techniques, including random-digit dialing, replicate subsamples, callbacks staggered over times of day and days of the week, refusal conversions, and systematic respondent selection within households, are used to ensure that the sample is representative.

6.   In this nonresponse experiment, two surveys were conducted simultaneously asking exactly the same eighty-five questions on a wide range of political and policy issues. The standard survey, using typical polling techniques and interviewing one thousand adults over a five-day period, achieved a 42 percent response rate. The second survey, using a more rigorous methodology over an eight-week period to interview one thousand adults, achieved a 71 percent response rate. The two surveys produced very similar results. Of the eighty-five questions, only five showed statistically significant differences between the two surveys. The differences were sharpest on questions concerning racial issues. Pew Research Center for the People and the Press. *Study of Survey Nonresponse,* Washington: Author, 1998.

7.   Newport, F. "The Pre-Election Polls Performed Well in '96." *Public Perspective,* Dec.–Jan. 1997, pp. 50–51.

8.   Kaiser–Harvard–PSRA poll, August 22, 1997.

9.   KPMG Peat Marwick. *Health Benefits in 1997,* Arlington, Va.: Author, 1997.

10.   ABC News poll, Storrs, Conn.: Roper Center for Public Opinion Research, August 24, 1997; Donelan K., Blendon, R. J., Benson, J. Leitman, R., and Taylor, H. "All Payer, Single Payer, Managed Care, No Payer: Patients' Perspectives in Three Nations." *Health Affairs,* Summer 1996, pp. 254–265; Davis K., Collins, K. S., Schoen, C., Morris, C. "Choice Matters: Enrollees' Views of Their Health Plans." *Health Affairs,* Summer 1995, pp. 99–112; *Los Angeles Times* poll, Storrs, Conn.: Roper Center for Public Opinion Research, June 17, 1995; Minnesota Health Data Institute/Maritz Marketing Research. *You and Your Health Plan: 1995 Statewide Survey of Minnesota Consumers,* Minneapolis: Minnesota Health Data Institute, 1995; Coalition for Medicare Choice. *American Attitudes Toward Managed Care: A Review.* Washington, D.C.: Coalition for Medicare Choice, 1995; and "Regardless of Health Status, HMO and FFS Patients Report Similar Levels of Satisfaction." *GHAA News,* July 26, 1995, pp. 1–3.

11. Kaiser–Harvard–PSRA poll, August 22, 1997.
12. Blendon, R. J., Benson, J. M., Brodie, J., Altman, D. E., Rowland, D., Neuman, P., and James, M. "Voters and Health Care in the 1996 Election." *Journal of the American Medical Association*, April 16, 1997, pp. 1256–1257.
13. Kaiser–Harvard–PSRA poll, August 22, 1997.
14. Princeton Survey Research Associates–Pew Research Center for the People and the Press poll, Storrs, Conn.: Roper Center for Public Opinion Research, February 19, 1998; Wirthlin Worldwide–Patient Access to Responsible Care Alliance poll, Washington, D.C.: Patient Access to Responsible Care Alliance, October 2, 1997; and Henry J. Kaiser Family Foundation–Harvard University–Princeton Survey Research Associates poll, Storrs, Conn.: Roper Center for Public Opinion Research, December 12, 1997.
15. Kaiser–Harvard–PSRA poll, August 22, 1997.
16. Harris poll, New York: Louis Harris and Associates, August 20, 1997.
17. Kaiser–Harvard–PSRA poll, August 22, 1997.
18. Ibid.
19. Ibid.; and Harris poll, New York: Louis Harris and Associates, March 25, 1998.
20. Kaiser–Harvard–PSRA poll, August 22, 1997.
21. Ibid.
22. Blendon, R. J. "The Public's View of the Future of Health Care." *Journal of the American Medical Association*, June 24, 1988, p. 3592.
23. Patterson, K. D., and Magleby, D. B. "The Polls—Poll Trends: Public Support for Congress." *Public Opinion Quarterly*, Winter 1992, pp. 539–551.
24. Kaiser–Harvard–PSRA poll, August 22, 1997.
25. Ibid.
26. Ibid.
27. Blendon, R. J., Benson, J., Donelon, K., Leitman, R., Taylor, H., Koeck, C., Gitterman, D. "Who Has the Best Health Care System? A Second Look." *Health Affairs*, Winter 1995, pp. 220–230.
28. The question read as follows: "As you may know, some health plans require their doctors to follow certain guidelines in treating patients. Some people think this is a good thing because all patients will benefit from proven techniques. Others think it is a bad thing because decisions about treatment should be entirely up to the doctor. Which comes closer to your view?" Henry J. Kaiser Family Foundation–Agency for Health Care Policy and Research–Princeton Survey Research Associates poll, Storrs, Conn.: Roper Center for Public Opinion Research, July 26, 1996.

29. Kaiser–Harvard–PSRA poll, August 22, 1997.

30. Harris poll, August 20, 1997.

31. Kaiser–Harvard–PSRA poll, August 22, 1997.

32. Kaiser–AHCPR–PSRA poll, 1996.

33. Ibid.

34. Blendon, R. J., Hyams, T. S., Benson, J. M. "Bridging the Gap Between the Public's and Economists' Views of the Economy." *Journal of Economic Perspectives,* Summer 1997, pp. 115.

35. Kaiser–Harvard–PSRA poll, August 22, 1997.

36. Miller, R. H., and Luft, H. S. "Does Managed Care Lead to Better or Worse Quality of Care?" *Health Affairs,* Sept.–Oct. 1997, pp. 7–25.

37. Donelan, K., Blendon, R. J., Benson, J., Leitman, R., and Taylor, H. "All Payer."

38. For public opinion on regulation of airlines, see Gallup poll, Storrs, Conn.: Roper Center for Public Opinion Research, August 24, 1987; and CBS News poll, Storrs, Conn.: Roper Center for Public Opinion Research, July 21, 1996. For consumer complaints, see U.S. Bureau of the Census. *Statistical Abstract of the United States: 1997.* Washington, D.C.: Author, 1997, Table 1054. For public opinion on regulation of banks, see *Roper Report 87–7,* Storrs, Conn.: Roper Center for Public Opinion Research, July 18, 1987; and *Los Angeles Times* poll, Storrs, Conn.: Roper Center for Public Opinion Research, April 6, 1991. For consumer ratings of banks, see Gallup–American Society for Quality Control polls, Storrs, Conn.: Roper Center for Public Opinion Research, 1985, 1988, 1991.

39. Downs, A. "Up and Down with Ecology: The Issue-Attention Cycle." *Public Interest,* Fall 1972, pp. 38–50; Rogers, E. M., and Dearing, J. W. "Agenda-Setting Research: Where Has It Been, Where Is It Going?" In D. A. Graber (ed.), *Media Power in Politics,* Washington, D.C.: CQ Press, 1994; and Nelson, B. J. "The Agenda-Setting Function of the Media: Child Abuse." In *Media Power in Politics.*

40. Brodie, M., Brady, L. A., and Altman, D. E. "Media Coverage of Managed Care: Is There a Negative Bias?" *Health Affairs,* Jan.–Feb. 1998, pp. 9–25.

Chapter Twelve

A Foundation Perspective
Core Principles for Regulating Health Care Quality
Karen Davis and David Sandman

For Americans with health insurance, the system they confront today is dramatically different from that of just a few years ago. Coverage of working families has rapidly shifted to managed care. Among employees of firms with two hundred or more workers, 81 percent belonged to a managed care plan in 1997 compared with just 29 percent in 1988.[1] Similarly rapid growth in managed care enrollment has occurred in the Medicaid program; almost half—48 percent—of all Medicaid beneficiaries belonged to a managed care plan by 1997.[2] Some 14 percent of Medicare beneficiaries were enrolled in managed care in that same year, and further growth is expected.[3] At the same time, the number of Americans without any health insurance is also steadily growing.

New Concerns About Quality

As managed care has grown, it has raised new concerns about the quality of health care being delivered. Under a fee-for-service system, people worried that unnecessary diagnostic tests and medical services were being ordered for patients and that the nation's health care costs were out of control. Overutilization of services and inappropriate use of health care resources were viewed as the primary problem. Not surprisingly, managed care's financial incentives have the opposite effect. Now the public and policymakers are concerned that patients are being denied access to medically needed care in efforts to save money. This fear has been supported by changes in the managed care industry itself. Despite evidence that not-for-profit health plans provide better-quality care than for-profit plans, it is investor-owned, for-profit plans that are experiencing the greatest growth.[4] By 1997, 62 percent of all HMO enrollees belonged to for-profit plans.[5]

Expressions of concern can be heard from both patients and physicians. Warning signs about the quality of managed care plans were found in the 1994 Commonwealth Fund Survey of Patient Experiences with Managed Care.[6] This survey of more than 3,347 working adults in Boston, Miami, and Los Angeles found higher levels of patient dissatisfaction and lower ratings for quality of care among those in managed care than those in fee-for-service plans.

Doctors confirm patients' experiences with managed care. The Commonwealth Fund Survey of Physician Experiences with Managed Care, a nationally representative study of seventeen hundred practicing physicians, found that doctors with substantial percentages of managed care patients were more likely to be dissatisfied with their ability to make the right decisions for patients, with the amount of time they can spend with patients, and with the practice of medicine overall.[7]

As such evidence accumulates, it is not surprising that the public and policymakers have become increasingly vocal about the need to assure quality in managed care. In a recent national survey, close to half of all Americans reported that either they personally or someone they knew had a problem with a health plan.[8] In response, Congress is considering numerous proposals to set standards for managed health care. Similarly, more than one thousand proposals affecting managed care were introduced in state legislatures in 1997 and almost two hundred have become law. At least twenty-one states have enacted comprehensive consumer rights bills.

Consumer Bill of Rights and Responsibilities

Against this backdrop, the President's Advisory Commission on Consumer Protection and Quality in the Health Care Industry had a daunting task when it was appointed in March 1997. Its charge was to advise the president on changes occurring in the health care system and to recommend measures to promote and assure quality and protect consumers and workers. The centerpiece of the commission's final report is the Consumer Bill of Rights and Responsibilities (CBRR). Containing more than fifty recommendations, it charts a course for enhancing trust among all players in the health care system, establishing the roles of these participants in assuring quality, and laying a framework for accountability.[9]

Among the provisions contained in the CBRR, those relating to a few themes are especially significant, including the need for adequate insurance coverage, choice, information disclosure, and grievance and appeals mechanisms.

Adequate Coverage

The commission observed that for consumers being insured is the most important quality protection. Decades of health services research has established the incontrovertible truth that health insurance is crucial in assuring adequate access to high quality, affordable care. Work supported by the Commonwealth Fund and others has demonstrated that uninsured patients are at high risk for not receiving primary and preventive care and that when uninsured people do receive care, they often report receiving lower-quality care and are less satisfied than their insured counterparts.[10]

Nevertheless, more than forty-three million Americans are uninsured. Because a quality health care system is one that is accessible to all, the nation must take serious steps to reverse the growth in its uninsured population or far too many Americans will remain untouched by other efforts to promote health care quality.

Choice

For those with insurance, the commission recommended that patients be given a choice among health plans and providers because choice is inextricably linked with quality and satisfaction. The Commonwealth Fund's survey of patients found that individuals who have a choice of plan are much more likely to rate plans high on quality, choice of physicians, access to care, and physician responsiveness to their concerns.[11]

Unfortunately, choice is becoming a luxury that many patients cannot afford. As the health insurance landscape was originally envisioned, patients were to have a choice of multiple managed care plans, as well as traditional fee-for-service coverage. Competition among plans was supposed to assure quality care at a reasonable cost. The current reality is considerably different.

The 1997 Kaiser–Commonwealth National Survey of Health Insurance found that the majority of working Americans do not have a choice of plans provided by their employers. Only 40 percent of workers were offered two or more plans by their own employer.[12] Workers without a choice of plan were more likely to work for a small employer and to have a low income.

The absence of a choice among plans is tied to a lack of choice among providers. In the past, patients with traditional indemnity coverage could obtain care from any physician or hospital they wanted. If they changed insurance coverage—which usually occurred because an employer selected a different carrier—it did not mean they were required to change their physicians. Today, selection of health plan and doctor are linked decisions. Managed care places limits on choice of physician, hospital, and other providers. Among managed care patients who had to change plans, 39 percent also had to change their doctors. Half of those changing their doctors said it was a major or minor problem for them.

The most troubling aspect of lack of choice is its implication for continuity and quality of care. Patients who stay with the same physician for a long period of time are less likely to be hospitalized and more likely to have lower health care costs.[13] Long-term patient-provider relationships are also important in facilitating communication, establishing trust, and promoting compliance with treatment protocols and advice regarding health behaviors.

Information Disclosure

When choices of plans and providers do exist, patients and purchasers cannot properly exercise them in the absence of standardized information on their relative quality and costs. For a competitive market to function properly, data *must* be available to help reliably compare options.

Recent years have witnessed considerable progress in the collection and reporting of quality data.[14] The National Committee for Quality Assurance (NCQA) has made important contributions in this area. For the first time, purchasers are able to make detailed assessments of the quality of care provided by competing plans and to make value-based decisions that balance quality and cost considerations.

The progress made by NCQA in compiling and analyzing the quality of care provided to commercially insured individuals requires expansion to beneficiaries of public programs. Medicare is making strides in this direction by requiring all participating plans to collect and submit Health Plan Employer Data and Information Set (HEDIS) data. Quality monitoring and information disclosure in the Medicaid program, however, have not kept pace with the rate of growth in managed care enrollment.

The information being collected and reported need to encompass the full spectrum of care—including clinical care and patient-centered measures of quality. Both HEDIS and the Consumer Assessment of Health Plans Survey (CAHPS), developed by the Agency for Health Care Policy and Research, are leading sources of information about the actual experiences of patients with their physicians and health plans. Information of this type needs to be collected, audited, analyzed, and publicly reported in ways that are understandable and meaningful to patients. Report cards on health plans are one means of assisting patients to make informed choices.

Grievances and Appeals

When there is no choice of plans, patients are unable to "vote with their feet." As a result, it is especially important to provide fair and effective grievance and appeals mechanisms. Among these protections, the commission was right to recommend the availability of an independent, external review system. The deck is stacked against patients when their sole recourse is to appeal a denial of care or payment to the same plan that issued the initial denial, which has a financial self-interest to affirm an earlier denial.

All patients should be entitled to timely notification of their plans' decisions, expedited consideration of appeals that involve urgently needed care, and resolution of claims by qualified medical personnel who were not involved in the decision that led to the filing of a grievance. Wherever possible, alternatives to litigation for resolving disputes should be encouraged, including the use of consumer ombudsmen programs, which can resolve disputes in a faster and less costly fashion.

Implementation and Enforcement

These qualities—adequate coverage, choice, information, and grievance mechanisms—are among the most important ones recommended by the commission. However, although the commission fulfilled its mandate to identify trends that place quality of care in jeopardy and define ways to protect and promote quality, it was unable to achieve consensus on how such measures should be implemented and enforced. Options range along a spectrum that includes federal and state regulation, market competition, and voluntary actions.

The difficulty in establishing the correct balance between governmental regulations and voluntary private-sector efforts is apparent in the attitude of the public. In a recent national survey, an overwhelming proportion of Americans favored laws that would require plans to disclose more information, establish external appeals procedures, and allow patients with serious medical conditions to see a specialist without getting permission from their primary care doctor to do so.[15] In fact, access to specialists was rated the number-one item that Americans would most like to see enacted in legislation. Interestingly, having the right to sue a health plan for malpractice—one of the most contentious quality provisions currently being debated—was rated as most important by only 8 percent of respondents.

At the same time, support for these types of laws erodes when their potential consequences are also raised. Three in four Americans favor the consumer bill of rights endorsed by the president, but this percentage declines sharply if respondents think it would get the government too involved in health care, increase premium costs, or cause employers to drop coverage for workers. In general, public opinion on who should have the main responsibility for protecting managed care consumers divides between the government, a nongovernmental independent organization, and the managed care industry itself.

President Clinton has already issued an executive order instructing all federal health plans, which cover eighty-five million

Americans, to comply with the CBRR. However, there is still a need to ensure these protections for patients in private health plans. Without comprehensive action at the national level, 122 million Americans could remain deprived of such protections. The guiding principle for any further action should be comprehensiveness; regulating health care on a piecemeal, body part by body part basis is in nobody's best interest and could actually undermine efforts to assure that patients receive high-quality, appropriate care. In the absence of any more sweeping regulation, all plans that participate in Medicare and Medicaid should be required to be accredited and meet minimum quality standards.

Private Sector Leadership

Government efforts alone will not be enough to assure and improve health care quality. Private sector efforts to establish standards, refine quality measurement systems, and make information widely available are essential in meeting and advancing a quality improvement agenda. An alliance between the National Committee for Quality Assurance, the Joint Commission on Accreditation of Healthcare Organizations, and the American Medical Association will coordinate performance measurement activities for the continuum of providers, including physicians, hospitals, and health plans. Collaborations such as this should ease the burden of data collection and allow meaningful comparisons to be made; they deserve the support of the government, the health care industry, and foundations.

Other noteworthy examples of private sector leadership include pioneering health plans such as Kaiser Permanente, Group Health Cooperative of Puget Sound, and HIP. These health insurance plans and cutting-edge employers like GTE have voluntarily implemented sweeping quality assurance mechanisms for their members and employees.

Next Steps Toward Quality

Too often, appointing commissions is a way of avoiding dealing with problems rather than confronting them. This commission deserves applause for its willingness to grapple seriously with some of the thorniest issues involved in health care quality debates. It has provided the nation with a road map for achieving the promise of American medicine and assuring quality health care for all. Yet complex problems are rarely, if ever, amenable to quick and easy solutions. It would be unrealistic to expect that a commission of this type could achieve consensus on some of the most controversial health policy questions of the day.

In particular, further work is required to advance the nation's health care quality agenda. Although managed care has raised new questions and concerns about quality, it has also brought with it new opportunities to hold the system accountable for quality and improve care that were not present in an fragmented fee-for-service system. Next steps should include the following:

Ongoing Monitoring

The commission recommended creating an advisory council for health care quality that would analyze trends in quality and assess the implications of any proposed and enacted legislation. Using MedPac as a model, this advisory council could help ensure that quality considerations, in addition to cost containment issues, drive the emergence of a new health care system.

Improved Data Capacity

Because markets cannot work without information, the nation needs to invest in improved quality measurement and information systems. The commission recommended the creation of a private quality forum that would identify a common set of quality measures, establish rules of the game for the submission of audited quality information by plans, and make comparative information widely available. The forum's top priorities would be to establish a core set of performance measures that are outcome oriented, assist providers to understand and improve their performance, and give consumers the information they need to choose wisely for themselves and their families.

Analysis of Relationship Between Quality and Cost

The greatest impediment to implementing stronger quality protections is the concern that they will increase operating costs and begin a dangerous domino effect, in which premiums will increase, more employers will drop coverage, and the nation's uninsured population will swell as a result. Estimates of the costs involved have ranged from pennies per month to dire predictions that premiums will rise by as much as 23 percent a year, causing millions to lose coverage. Such wide variation is a result of differences in the interpretation of mandates and of assumptions that flow from those interpretations.[16] But most of these estimates have been produced by parties that have a financial interest in the outcome. To sort out myth from reality, independent and credible analyses of the costs of various quality assurance mechanisms are needed. Reliable analyses would help determine if and when cost-quality trade-offs truly exist.

There is little doubt that medical care in the United States ranks among the highest quality care in the world and that choice, information, and fair appeals mechanisms are core ingredients of health care quality. But quality care is often unavailable to Americans who lack health insurance, and changes in the health care system threaten to jeopardize quality even for the insured. The commission has drawn the attention of policymakers and the public to the intertwined issues of quality, access, and affordability. Efforts to control health care spending are crucial, but the drive to save dollars should not be at the expense of patient care. The path to quality health care for all Americans will have many bumps along the way, but it must be pursued with vigor.

Notes

1. KPMG Peat Marwick. *Health Benefits in 1997.* Arlington, Va.: Author, 1997.
2. Health Care Financing Administration. *Medicaid Managed Care Enrollment Report.* Washington, D.C.: Author, 1997.
3. Christensen, S. *Memorandum on Medicare+Choice Provisions in the Balanced Budget Act of 1997.* Washington, D.C.: Congressional Budget Office, 1997.
4. Schoen, C., and Davidson, P. "Image and Reality: Managed Care Experiences by Type of Plan." *Bulletin of the New York Academy of Medicine,* 1996, *73*(2); Kuttner, R. "Must Good HMOs Go Bad?" *The New England Journal of Medicine,* 1998, *338*, 1558–1563; and Greene, J. "Blue Skies or Black Eyes? HEDIS Puts Not-for-Profit Plans on Top." *Hospitals and Health Networks,* 1998, *72*, 26–30.
5. InterStudy. *HMO Industry Report.* St. Paul, Minn.: Author, 1997.

6. Davis, K., Scott Collins, K., Schoen, C., and Morris, C. "Choice Matters: Enrollees' Views of Their Health Plans." *Health Affairs,* Summer 1995, 99–112.

7. Scott Collins, K., Schoen, C., and Sandman, D. R. *The Commonwealth Fund Survey of Physicians' Experiences with Managed Care.* New York: Commonwealth Fund, 1997.

8. Henry J. Kaiser Family Foundation–Harvard University National Survey of Americans' Views on Consumer Protections in Managed Care. Menlo Park, Calif.: Henry J. Kaiser Family Foundation, January 1998.

9. The President's Advisory Commission on Consumer Protection and Quality in the Health Care Industry. "Quality First: Better Health Care for All Americans." Final report to the President of the United States, March 1998.

10. Schoen, C., Lyons, B., Rowland, D., Davis, K., and Puleo, E. "Insurance Matters for Low Income Adults: Results from a Five-State Study." *Health Affairs,* 1997, *16;* and Davis, K. "Uninsured in an Era of Managed Care." *Health Services Research,* 1997, *31.*

11. Davis, K., Scott Collins, K., Schoen, C., and Morris, C. "Choice Matters."

12. Davis, K. "Assuring Quality, Information, and Choice in Managed Care." Testimony before the U.S. House of Representatives, Committee on Commerce, Subcommittee on Health and Environment, Hearing on Managed Care Quality, October 28, 1997.

13. Weiss, L. J., and Blustein, J. "Faithful Patients: The Effects of Long-Term Physician-Patient Relationships on the Costs and Use of Health Care by Older Americans." *American Journal of Public Health,* 1996, *86*(12), 1742–1747.

14. Epstein, A. M. "Rolling Down the Runway: The Challenges Ahead for Quality Report Cards." *Journal of the American Medical Association,* 1998, *279,* 1691–1696.

15. Kaiser Family Foundation–Harvard University National Survey of Americans' Views.

16. Copeland, C. "Issues of Quality and Consumer Rights in the Health Care Market." EBRI Issue Brief no. 196. Washington, D.C.: Employee Benefit Research Institute, 1998.

Chapter Thirteen

The Managed Care Industry
Balancing Market Forces and Regulation
Karen Ignagni

In a market-oriented health care system, regulation is necessarily a balancing act. Its proper role is to promote appropriate accountability and consistency of care without needlessly restricting the freedom to innovate. Whether this balance can be achieved and maintained depends on a number of variables, of which the most important may be the public's perception of the regulatory challenge.

There is a compelling need to look beyond the day's headlines. Reaching the goal of balanced regulatory policymaking requires context. Decisions need to be based on a clear, objective understanding of whether market-based health care reform is, on the whole, working—that is, delivering generally superior care to more Americans at more affordable cost—and if so, whether a relatively heavy regulatory hand is necessary or appropriate to ensure that reform stays on track.

Looking at the Consequences

Context also means recognizing what is at stake when new regulations and restrictions are proposed. For example, increasing the

Rick Smith, vice president, Public Policy and Research, AAHP, and Phil Blando, deputy director, Strategic Planning, AAHP, also contributed to this chapter.

exposure of health plans to lawsuits for damages may have far-reaching consequences for plans and consumers alike. Such regulation could force plans to shift from proactive to defensive care management, in effect authorizing everything instead of systematically reviewing utilization patterns and seeking continually to improve care management protocols and practices. Rather than benefiting consumers, such regulation would make the long-term goal of universal coverage more elusive by adding to the per capita cost of care. Indeed, the threat of malpractice litigation has for many years forced physicians to practice defensively, prescribing tests and treatments regardless of clinical value. With the cost of defensive medicine already estimated to inflate the nation's health care bills by as much as 10 percent annually, the multibillion-dollar price tag associated with defensive medicine raises serious doubts about whether proposals to expose health plans to essentially unlimited liability meet the shorthand test of balanced regulation: promoting accountability without stifling progress.

The key question is whether the state of health care delivery in the United States today warrants major new regulatory initiatives. The discussion needs to be broadly framed by asking, and continually returning to, overarching questions such as these: What are our overall objectives? What problems are we trying to solve? How should we evaluate progress in meeting these goals?

Our overall objectives should include ensuring that comprehensive health care is as broadly available as possible, which requires us to stretch our resources continually by improving the quality of care and measuring its effectiveness. Among the problems we must address is a significant one inherited from the old system: the unacceptably wide range of quality of care—from best in the world to grossly inadequate, from routine overtreatment to chronic undertreatment, from proactive and preventive to reactive and late-stage. The system has served some individuals extremely well but on the whole addressed the needs of large populations unevenly and inadequately. In making a shift to a more public health-oriented model of care, problems of ensuring consistency of care at affordable cost require close attention.

As to the challenge of measuring progress in a market-oriented system that is addressing previously unmet needs, we should rely not on anecdotes but on the best available benchmarking data, and use that data to establish baselines from which to proceed further. Here we are still on relatively new and, for the public, unfamiliar ground. In part because the old system was so fragmented, it could not and did not systematically collect or disseminate performance data. The new system produces better information and is still improving. Unfortunately, however, any evidence of shortcomings tends to be held up against the more subjective standards of the old system, in which consumers knew whether they liked their physician or hospital but did not necessarily know very much about the overall quality of care being provided.

Policymakers interested in balanced regulation cannot afford to be guided by such subjective criteria. They must look to more objective measures to decide whether trends in the organization and delivery of care are positive or negative. The answer will determine whether the nation's approach to regulation should be more or less punitive—that is, whether there should be more governmental micromanagement or more reliance on the system's capacity to demonstrate accountability and continual improvement.

The Regulatory Climate Today

The public view of the regulatory challenge is skewed by the perception that health plans are essentially unregulated. In fact, however, plans operate within a complex, multidimensional regulatory matrix. They compile data on virtually every aspect of their operations—from capitalization to resolution of disputes—and report to a wide range of federal, state, and nongovernmental agencies, including accreditation organizations, multiemployer purchasing groups, and individual employers.

Federal Level

Several federal agencies establish rules and requirements affecting health plans. The Department of Health and Human Services (HHS), acting primarily through the Health Care Financing Administration (HCFA), has a dual role, purchasing health care coverage for Medicare and Medicaid participants and regulating the benefits and services they receive. Under the HMO Act of 1973, HCFA sets standards governing key aspects of health plan design and operations. HCFA also purchases and regulates coverage for Medicare beneficiaries who choose to enroll in health plans. In addition to meeting state licensure and other requirements, a health plan seeking to participate in Medicare must meet a separate set of federal rules and requirements designed to ensure the plan's ability to serve Medicare beneficiaries. HCFA determines whether a plan meets Medicare requirements by reviewing its written application and conducting an on-site visit. Continued compliance is then monitored by means of follow-up visits at the end of a plan's first year of participation and at least every two years thereafter.

Through HCFA, the federal government also establishes requirements for and oversees state Medicaid managed care programs. HCFA reviews each state's plan to determine that its Medicaid managed care program and participating health plans meet numerous federal contractual requirements, and the agency investigates any alleged violation of these requirements.

HCFA is also responsible for promulgating regulations to apply the requirements of the Health Insurance Portability and Accountability Act of 1996 (HIPAA) to "health insurance issuers," a category that encompasses health plans.

The Department of Labor (DoL) has primary responsibility for administering the Employee Retirement Income Security Act (ERISA), including recent amendments made by HIPAA. The DoL's principal regulatory role has been to ensure that individuals with employment-based health care coverage receive adequate notice of their plan's terms and conditions of coverage and that plans deliver promised benefits. Toward this end, ERISA imposes documentation, reporting, and disclosure requirements and preempts state laws (other than laws regulating insurance) that relate to health plans. (For specifics on ERISA and preemption, see Chapter Ten of this volume, by Copeland and Pierron.)

Until the recent changes made by HIPAA, the ERISA statute did not generally regulate the content of employer-based plans. Although ERISA does not directly apply to health insurance issuers, its requirements for employment-based plans influence purchasers' expectations of health plans.

The Office of Personnel Management (OPM) oversees the Federal Employees Health Benefits Program (FEHBP), which provides health coverage to federal employees, retirees, and dependents. It is the nation's largest employer-sponsored health plan. Like HCFA, OPM sets threshold standards to ensure that plans participating in FEHBP have sufficient financial resources, experience, and network capacity.

State Level

State regulators include insurance and health departments as well as labor and personnel departments. Health plans often are regulated by more than one agency in a state, usually the department of insurance (which generally oversees health plans' financial operations) and the department of health (which generally regulates health plans' care delivery systems, including oversight on access and quality of care). Because states also purchase health care for government employees and Medicaid beneficiaries, other state agencies may also be involved in setting and enforcing health plan standards.

The National Association of Insurance Commissioners (NAIC), which drafted a Model HMO Act in 1972 and updates it periodically, assists states in the task of regulating prepaid health plans. Building on precedents set for other types of insurance, the model act requires that plans obtain a state license in order to operate and it conditions licensure on compliance with various requirements. In addition, NAIC has developed numerous model acts and regulations that serve as the basis for state action in a variety of areas including quality assurance, utilization review, and grievances and appeals.

Private Sector

Independent accrediting organizations also set standards for health plans. Increasingly, major employers and other purchasers seek external validation of the plans with which they contract. Accreditation standards, although they do not have the force of law, are influential in shaping key aspects of plan design and operation. Moreover, many state laws explicitly recognize private accreditation, and some require it. And recent changes in federal law have paved the way for HCFA to consider private accreditation of quality assurance programs in determining a plan's compliance with comparable federal standards.

Areas of Regulation

Health plan regulators have addressed numerous aspects of plan operations: quality assurance and utilization review, solvency, benefits, enrollment rules, enrollee information, access to care, provider contracting, premiums and rating practices, grievances and appeals, organizational structure and management, reporting and disclosure, and confidentiality. Because regulatory authority is dispersed among various agencies and organizations, health plans often must comply with multiple standards in each of these areas.

Quality Assurance and Utilization Review

Generally, plans must have quality assurance programs that lay out their activities to monitor quality, assess any quality problems, impose corrective actions, and analyze patterns of care. Also, they may be required to demonstrate involvement of physicians in establishing and reviewing the program and to contract with external organizations to evaluate quality independently.

Solvency

Standards for solvency are intended to ensure that health plans have sufficient resources to provide promised benefits. Most regulators require plans to meet such standards and to update financial data periodically.

Benefits

Federal and state officials have adopted policies requiring health plans to provide specified benefits.

Enrollment

Regulators have established two types of rules regulating enrollment in health plans: those specifying a process (such as open enrollment) and those limiting the conditions under which a plan
may exclude an individual.

Enrollee Information

Virtually all entities that set standards for health plans require
them to provide detailed information to enrollees on various aspects of health plan policies and operations, increasingly in formats that facilitate comparison of plans.

Access to Care

Because many health plans provide benefits primarily through networks of providers, it has become common for regulators to set
standards to assess the network's adequacy—that is, whether there
are enough providers to furnish covered services to an enrolled
population without unreasonable delays. In some cases, other aspects of access—such as member choice of providers and direct access to specialists—are also regulated.

Provider Contracting

Regulators generally impose three types of regulations on health
plan contracts with providers. Some require plans to disclose the
details of their provider contracts in order to monitor compliance.
Others request that contracts include certain substantive provisions. A third type addresses the process that plans use to select the
providers with whom they contract.

Grievances and Appeals

Regulators generally require health plans to have internal grievance
and appeals processes to resolve enrollee complaints. Usually, they
distinguish between the level of review that is required for relatively

minor disputes compared with complaints about determinations that allegedly deny, reduce, or terminate benefits. Some regulators, including HCFA and a number of states, require independent external review of certain determinations resulting in denial of coverage or payment.

Organizational Structure and Management

Regulatory requirements regarding a health plan's organizational structure and management fall into three main categories. Some are intended to assure clear accountability for plan policies by identifiable individuals. Others call for the involvement of individuals with appropriate expertise and experience in specific decision-making areas (for example, physician involvement in development of practice guidelines). Still others exclude from health plan management individuals deemed to have conflicts of interest, or for other specified reasons.

Reporting

Health plans must comply with extensive reporting requirements—particularly in the areas of solvency and quality assurance—and provide reasonable access to plan records to permit verification of reported information. In some cases this information supports activities to verify compliance with applicable standards; in other cases it is used as the basis for consumer information.

Confidentiality

Health plans must comply with applicable state and federal laws intended to protect the confidentiality of information about the health status and treatment of identifiable individuals.

Health Plan Initiatives

With the adoption of an industrywide code of conduct implemented in stages since 1996, the community of health plans has taken a significant and unprecedented step in advancing the regulatory process. Rarely has any industry voluntarily set such performance targets and held itself responsible for meeting them. Members of the American Association of Health Plans (AAHP) participate in developing and refining the code, and all AAHP members—more than one thousand health plans serving more than 160 million Americans—pledge to adhere to its provisions. The code covers a wide range of patient issues, including these:

Information

Health plans will encourage participating physicians to discuss all treatment options with patients and will ensure that every member has access to all information necessary to promote the right care at the right time and in the right setting. This includes information about the plan's structure and provider network, benefits covered and excluded, cost-sharing requirements, and on request, precertification and review procedures and the basis for a specific utilization review decision.

Health plans will also ensure that members can easily obtain up-to-date information about whether a specific prescription drug is included in a formulary or whether a particular physician or practice within the plan's network is accepting new patients; a summary of how participating physicians are compensated; and in the event of a dispute about coverage of experimental treatments and technologies, information providing a basis for determining whether such treatments and technologies should be covered.

Appeals

If a patient disagrees with a health plan's coverage decision or approved course of treatment, the plan will explain the basis for the decision in a timely notice to the patient, accompanied by an easily understood description of the patient's appeal rights and the time frames for an appeal. The plan will seek to resolve the appeal as rapidly as warranted by the patient's situation and will provide an expedited appeals process for situations in which the normal time frame could jeopardize a patient's life or health.

Confidentiality

Health plans are pledged to protect the confidentiality of each patient's records and will implement appropriate safeguards to do so. Patient-identifiable information will not be disclosed without the patient's consent except under clearly specified circumstances (for example, when necessary to provide needed care, perform essential plan functions such as quality assurance and administration of claims, support research or public health purposes, or comply with a law or court order).

Choice of Family Physicians

Plans will offer members a choice among primary care physicians participating in their network and available to accept new patients, and members will be free to change primary care physicians.

Access to Specialty Care

Plans will offer timely and appropriate access to specialty care available within the plan's network.

Transition from One Provider to Another

Plans will facilitate the transfer of care from one provider to another, including from a nonnetwork to a network provider and when a practitioner treating a patient leaves a network.

Access to Emergency Care

Plans will cover emergency room screening and stabilization for conditions that reasonably appear to constitute an emergency.

Quality Assessment and Improvement Programs

Programs to monitor patient care in order to identify opportunities for improvement should be physician-directed, and participating physicians should be involved in the design and implementation of such programs.

Practice Guidelines

Plans' practice guidelines will be based on current scientific and medical evidence, designed to involve participating physicians in their development and review, updated regularly, and open to physician-requested modification based on the presentation of relevant evidence.

Utilization Management

Plans' utilization management programs will be based on current scientific and medical evidence, directed by an experienced physician, and involve participating physicians in reviewing utilization management criteria. Treating physicians should have the opportunity to provide clinical information supporting a rationale for a specific course of treatment prior to a utilization review determination, and health plans will provide a physician-directed exceptions process for cases in which a participating physician believes that a utilization management decision does not adequately take into account the unique characteristics of the patient.

Prescription Drug Formularies

Plans will involve participating physicians in developing, reviewing, and updating formularies. Selective formularies will include an exceptions process for cases in which a patient or participating physician wishes to present science-based medical evidence to support coverage for a prescription drug not routinely included in the formulary.

At AAHP's request, an independent survey was conducted in June 1998 by Peter D. Hart Research Associates to determine the status of health plans' compliance with the code. They found that 95 percent of AAHP member plans complied with at least six of the seven principles in effect, two-thirds were in compliance in all seven areas, and all of the plans not in compliance were in the process of making necessary changes in policies and practices to ensure full compliance within twelve months.

The code of conduct addresses three primary issues of overriding concern to consumers, policymakers, and regulators: the right to know, assured access to the right care at the right time and in the right setting, and the right to fair and equitable administrative processes, including the right of appeal. The code by itself does not, of course, obviate the need for other forms of regulation. But it does reflect the commitment of health plans to meet high and consistent performance targets—which, in turn, reflects the maturing of the industry. The existence of the code and the demonstrable seriousness of the health plans in honoring it underscore the appropriateness of developing a regulatory system that reinforces rather than inhibits the ongoing quality and service initiatives of health plans.

Quality and Service: What the Research Shows

Given the array of regulatory tools already in place, a significant challenge for policymakers is to decide whether others are needed. That requires determining whether the glass is half-empty or half-full—that is, whether the transition taking place in health care is more to the detriment of patients than to their benefit. Proponents of micromanagement of health plans argue the former. Research, however, supports the view that the transition from unmanaged, uncoordinated care—the failed fee-for-service system—to comprehensive coverage and coordinated, evidence-based care has been and continues to be beneficial for patients and for the nation.

A 1997 analysis by Robert H. Miller and Harold S. Luft, two highly respected health care researchers, of quality-of-care studies published between late 1993 and early 1997 showed that according to most measures health plans were delivering care comparable or superior to that provided by the fee-for-service system. These findings were consistent with their 1994 analysis of studies issued between 1980 and 1994, which showed that in fourteen of seventeen indicators of quality care, health plans' care equaled or exceeded that provided in other settings.[1]

During the 1990s, as enrollment in network-based health plans increased dramatically, at least seventeen new peer-reviewed, government, or accreditation agency studies have reinforced Miller and Luft's conclusion that the quality of care provided to health plan patients is as good as or superior to that given to patients in fee-for-service arrangements. As the Centers for Disease Control and Prevention has noted, the comprehensive and coordinated nature of services provided by health plans "offers a medical home to those whose care has traditionally been episodic and fragmented"—a description that fits the medical histories of millions of Americans. Health plan patients have been shown to be more likely to receive appropriate treatment (including early detection) for a range of conditions including various kinds of cancer, heart disease, diabetes and hypertension, rheumatoid arthritis, back pain, and appendicitis. Health plans have also demonstrated their ability to provide superior prenatal care in complex pregnancy cases and to help patients manage a range of chronic illnesses from asthma to osteoporosis.[2]

The following examples illustrate some of the ways in which patients enrolled in health plans are likely to receive better care than those covered by fee-for-service arrangements:

- A person with diabetes is more than three times as likely to have a crucial diagnostic eye exam.
- A person who has suffered a heart attack is nearly 2.5 times as likely to be given beta blockers to prevent subsequent attacks.
- A person who smokes is nearly two times as likely to be counseled to quit smoking.
- A woman is nearly 1.5 times as likely to be screened for breast cancer and 1.4 times as likely to be screened for cervical cancer.
- Women with complicated pregnancies are more likely to receive thorough, coordinated prenatal care.
- Medicare patients are more likely to have cancer diagnosed early.
- Patients treated in intensive care units have lower levels of mortality.

And on the downside, fee-for-service patients who develop appendicitis are 20 percent more likely to suffer a ruptured appendix than those in a health plan.[3]

Similarly, in a number of areas relevant to pending regulatory proposals, research shows that health plans are responsive to consumers' expectations:

Physician-Patient Communication

A 1997 General Accounting Office (GAO) study found no evidence that health plans use so-called gag clauses. Not one of the 1,150 physician contracts with 529 health plans examined by GAO had clauses that specifically restricted physicians from discussing all appropriate medical options with patients.[4]

Health Status of Enrollees

Despite claims that health plans disproportionately enroll healthy people, numerous studies show that managed care plans and indemnity plans enroll similar proportions of people in poor health. A 1998 Congressional Research Service (CRS) report noted that average health status, as measured by the percentage of patients with chronic health problems, differs very little between the two groups. Among patients interviewed in 1994, the percentage reporting having a medical condition of any kind was the same—37 percent—for both health plan and indemnity patients. And the difference among patients reporting one or more chronic medical conditions was statistically insignificant: 30.7 percent for indemnity patients versus 29.9 percent for health plan enrollees.[5]

In addition, compared with indemnity contracts, health plans enroll a higher proportion of lower-income individuals—who generally are believed to be in poorer health than higher-income individuals—in part because they cannot afford the high out-of-pocket costs of indemnity plans. A 1997 National Research Corporation survey of 165,000 households found that 40 percent of insured individuals under age sixty-five in families with annual incomes below $25,000 were enrolled in health plans. Only 18.6 percent of individuals in such families were in fee-for-service arrangements.[6]

Physician Recommendations and Utilization Review

Health plans and physicians are generally in agreement about care recommendations. A recent study of more than two thousand physicians caring for patients in health plans found that in eight categories of care the final coverage denial rate for physician recommendations was, at most, 3 percent, and generally lower. Most physicians reported no coverage denials for any recommendations. Moreover, physicians were found to be spending more time with their patients than they did a few years ago and were using just 3 percent of their time on insurance paperwork.[7]

Hospital Length of Stay

Length-of-stay patterns for indemnity and health plan patients are similar. In general, effective and appropriate care often means less time in the hospital than was thought necessary several years ago. This is true regardless of the type of coverage. For example, an AAHP analysis of Medicare data shows a 21 percent decline in average lengths of stay for all diagnoses among fee-for-service Medicare patients between 1990 and 1995.[8]

Moreover, lengths of stay for health plan enrollees coincides with physicians' recommendations. An AAHP analysis found that 95 percent of both health plan and indemnity hospital admissions had a length of stay that either fell within or exceeded the high end of the range recommended by surgeons surveyed by the American College of Surgeons (ACS) regarding ACS-identified procedures. The other 5 percent fell below the recommended length-of-stay range for both health plan and indemnity enrollees.[9]

In addition, although health plans use practice guidelines to promote continual care improvement, these guidelines do not dictate treatment. A recent AAHP comparison of actual lengths of stay in health plans with the Milliman & Robertson (M&R) Optimal Recovery Guidelines shows that 62 percent of all health plan admissions (compared with 67 percent of indemnity admissions) for selected diagnosis-related groups (DRGs) had a length of stay that was longer than recommended in the M&R guidelines.[10]

Mastectomy Care

Much-publicized criticism of health plans for requiring outpatient mastectomies has been proven to be misplaced. New York Department of Health data show, for example, that 72 of the 124 outpatient mastectomies performed in New York in 1995—58 percent—were performed on patients in traditional Medicare; 2 of them—1.6 percent—were performed on women in Medicare health plans; and 15 of them—13 percent—involved patients in commercial health plans. An AAHP-commissioned study of 1993–1994 commercial market data found that, overall, differences in outpatient mastectomy rates among health plans and indemnity plans were not statistically different. More important than a comparison of outpatient mastectomy rates alone, however, is that women enrolled in health plans are more likely to receive the mammograms that make it more likely that breast cancer will be detected at a relatively early stage.[11]

Patient Satisfaction

Many surveys report high levels of consumer satisfaction with health plans. In 1998, a comprehensive review of surveys on public attitudes toward managed care found "little evidence of widespread or serious dissatisfaction with health care arrangements among those who have [health plan] coverage." The same review also revealed that large majorities of those enrolled in health plans would recommend their plan to others.[12] These findings hold true both for enrollees who are generally healthy and for those who, because of poorer health, have more extensive experience with health care services.[13]

Unintended Consequences

As this brief overview shows, health plans have demonstrated their capacity both to provide quality care to millions of Americans *and* to respond to consumers' concerns about how that care is organized and delivered. It follows that policymakers should proceed with caution in adopting new regulatory initiatives that could have the unintended consequence of making this kind of care less accessible and affordable.

Cost

At AAHP's request, KPMG Peat Marwick's Barents Group recently analyzed and attempted to quantify the impact of four specific legislative and regulatory initiatives, developing models to estimate their effect on health plan premiums and the impact of premium increases on businesses, households, and government. The four initiatives in question would: increase the exposure of health plans to malpractice liability; deny health plans the freedom to make policy and practice determinations based on utilization reviews; prohibit plans from playing any role in determining the medical necessity of coverage and treatment recommendations; and require plans to accept any willing provider into their networks as long as the provider meets certain qualifications and is willing to abide by plan policies.

The potential adverse effects associated with increasing health plan liability alone are staggering. Barents estimates there would be a premium increase of 2.7 to 8.6 percent. If employers absorbed all of the increased cost and reduced wages to offset it, the wage loss per covered household from 1999 to 2003 is estimated to be from $475 to $1,512. Alternatively, if cost increases were shared by employers and employees, from 1999 to 2003 these increases are projected to

- Increase total employment-based health care spending by $38.7 billion to $123.1 billion for private firms, households, and government
- Increase costs by $109 to $346 per covered household
- Decrease employment by 75,200 to 239,500 people
- Decrease the number of insured individuals by 54,300 to 1,787,800 (1999 only).[14]

Because regulation may add to the cost of care, it is important that it add value as well. Regulation that provides guidance to health plans and other providers and encourages them to achieve quality-improvement performance targets meets this test. Regulation that primarily encumbers them and forces them to function defensively does not. It is worth keeping in mind that in the abstract consumers generally respond affirmatively when asked if they want more health care regulation, but when asked if they are willing to have the cost of their care increase as a result they are much less positive. In considering the pros and cons of various approaches to legislation, legislators need to be mindful that in the long run consumers are unlikely to support the addition of new regulatory surcharges—in effect, new taxes—to the overall cost of health care.

Pitfalls

Among the other pitfalls to be avoided in designing a regulatory model appropriate to a market-oriented health care system are these:

Solving Market Problems in the Legislative Arena

Legislative micromanagement of health care processes and practices has generally proven to be undesirable and unworkable. It has resulted, for example, in arbitrary mandates that may conflict with current best practices, discourage innovation, and drive up costs without adding value. As a general rule, the legislative arena is an appropriate forum in which to debate public policy goals and set broad performance and regulatory criteria; it is less suited to the task of addressing the constantly evolving spectrum of health care processes and practices.

Turning Back the Clock

One of the risks of overreliance on regulation is that it narrows the opportunities for health plans and other providers to make the most effective use of their own quality-assurance systems. When care managers and administrators have their hands too tightly bound by regulation—lacking the freedom to implement practice guidelines, utilization review procedures, and other quality improvement tools—the clock is effectively turned back to the point where no one can be held broadly accountable for the quality of care delivered to defined covered populations. This was the case before the evolution of managed care, a situation that produced, among other things, enormous inconsistencies in care and runaway costs that had the effect of pricing quality health care out of the reach of millions of working Americans and their families.

Assuming That Everything Needs to Be Done by Government

In the ongoing debate about how best to regulate health care there is inevitable tension between the traditional government-centered regulatory approach and a model better suited to a market-oriented delivery system. With that model still evolving, it is understandable that the impetus to rely on the traditional approach remains strong. But this tends to result in thinking within the narrow horizons of conventional wisdom. It limits opportunities to explore alternative ways of assigning regulatory roles to private or quasi-governmental entities such as those presently involved in accreditation and quality oversight.

Goals for a Regulatory System

The ideal regulatory model should operate at the balance point between public and private and between general guidance and micromanagement, setting performance targets and providing a means of ensuring they are met. The next challenge, then, is to outline broad goals for a market-sensitive regulatory system, goals that allow the evolution of health care to proceed while simultaneously protecting consumers against remaining system deficiencies and providing criteria against which proposals can be measured and tested.

An important step in shaping and refining goals is to identify the challenges that the stakeholders in the nation's health care system must meet. Through its Policy Advisory Council, its Committee on Quality Health Care, and in other settings, AAHP has been working to identify these challenges and articulate a vision for quality improvement. Among the questions that health plans believe should be addressed are these:

- What does our nation want our health care system to achieve? What level of resources is the nation willing to commit to achieve these goals?
- What are the principal quality-related issues in our health care system? How do we structure all aspects of the system—including health plans, hospitals, and practitioners—to improve quality systematically?
- What needs to be done to promote the concept of evidence-based care, that is, care that demonstrably improves outcomes and overall health?
- What effect has the employment-based health benefits structure had on the delivery of health care services and on quality?

- Health plans are currently regulated at multiple levels. Is this the optimum design? How well do current and proposed regulations promote quality and affordability?
- What is the optimum role for private sector activities such as accreditation?
- Should we be developing new models of regulation that move beyond the transaction- and process-oriented models of the past?
- Within the regulatory context, what must be done to preserve and promote innovation in health care coverage and health care services?

Of course, these are complex and difficult questions. That is why they need to be continually addressed, not just by health plans but also by consumers, employers, the media, and lawmakers in an ongoing discussion that moves the debate beyond rhetoric. It is reasonable to expect that out of such a discussion a consensus will emerge about the broad goals that a model market-oriented regulatory system should be pursuing, which are likely to include the following:

Affordability

If we accept the premise that every proposal has a cost and that one of our highest priorities as a nation is to do everything possible to bring care within the reach of all, it then becomes imperative to measure the costs as well as benefits of any proposal.

Quality

One of the core tenets of care management is that quality can be continually improved by promoting consistency of care and measuring outcomes. Health plans, along with all providers, should be accountable to a regulatory structure that facilitates advances in information technologies leading to better care measurement.

Coordination of Care

In a nation with an aging population and other medically vulnerable groups, there is a strong need for proactive maintenance of health and management of complex and chronic illnesses. Abundant opportunities exist to develop effective new collaborations among care practitioners—between health plans and multidisciplinary physician practices, for example, and between health plans and academic medical centers. This is part of the evolution of health care to meet the needs of the next century; regulation should be designed to encourage rather than restrain such innovation.

Consumer Trust and Patient Satisfaction

Regulation can play a major role in determining whether consumers generally trust the health care system and whether patient satisfaction is consistently high and rising. The more complex the regulatory environment, the more it becomes an arena exclusively for expert adversaries, leaving consumers on the sidelines. A goal, therefore, should be to keep regulation as simple and streamlined as possible. This is consistent with the continuing need to help consumers become comfortable with care management and aware of its advantages in meeting both individual and societal needs.

Fair and Equitable Administrative Policies

In a market-oriented health care system there are powerful incentives for health plans to respond to consumer concerns and to address procedural shortcomings as well as any major failures of care or flaws in the design and administration of services. The regulatory environment needs to allow room for health plans to make such midcourse corrections unencumbered by unduly punitive provisions.

Uniformity

There is a strong case to be made for considering any regulatory approach in light of whether it promotes consistency regardless of where, when, or how health care services are delivered or received. Inconsistencies from state to state, from state to federal, or from governmental to nongovernmental regulation should be avoided. This argues for moving toward a system in which entities with broad authority work closely with the health care community to develop and implement reasonably uniform performance targets.

Equity

In a market-oriented society it is important that regulatory initiatives neither deliberately nor inadvertently distort the market by providing differing standards for various approaches to health care and for different providers to meet. Whatever the issue—from credentialing to the guarantee of an effective appeals process to exposure to litigation—rules should be applied equitably across the board. To put it another way, regulators should not regulate by *product* but by *function*. Rather than singling out managed care for scrutiny, the objective should be to evaluate all providers of care under the same spotlight.

Performance Standards

The regulatory structure should be configured (and, as necessary, reconfigured) to increase emphasis on the guidance of plans and other providers by establishing clear, consistent performance standards that all providers are expected to meet.

Benchmarking Purposes

Because health care is a work in progress with quality improvement a constant objective, the regulatory framework should foster progress by offering a means of measuring performance over time. Its objective should be to demonstrate that the populations served by *any* provider arrangement are receiving care and services that meet or exceed agreed-upon performance benchmarks that are pegged to uniform indicators of health status, affordability, consumer satisfaction, and other relevant measures.

A Public-Private Partnership

In broad outline, the ideal regulatory model of tomorrow promotes continual quality improvement by setting performance targets for health plans and other providers to meet. It plays a key role in the development and deployment of increasingly sophisticated and consistent data to measure progress and inform consumers. It provides efficient mechanisms to resolve conflicts between providers and consumers. It promotes consistency of licensing and performance requirements nationwide. And it recognizes the importance of initiatives within the health care community to maximize the traditional advantages of the competitive marketplace in fostering innovation and superior service.

A coherent vision of the appropriate role of regulation in a market-oriented health care system necessarily takes time to develop. This poses a particular challenge for the legislative process, which is geared to act in response to the demands of constituents and within the time frames of legislative sessions. The process does not readily lend itself to careful study, which is an essential step in designing a regulatory system that can meet the needs and expectations of consumers without setting back the progress that has already been made in creating our uniquely accountable, adaptable, and affordable health care system.

Ideally, the regulatory system of the future will be a genuine public-private partnership. The role of government may be augmented or partly superseded by the evolution of independent organizations charged with broad responsibility for setting performance criteria, overseeing quality-improvement initiatives, and reporting to consumers and policymakers. This approach offers much promise as a means of streamlining the existing system.

One of the key tests of any regulatory design will be whether it mitigates or increases the administrative overhead of the nation's health care system. Given the inescapable cost pressures that the system faces in the future—from an aging population, large demographic cohorts with special needs, and high-tech medicine, among others—there is increasing urgency to address administrative costs.

Finally, the unmet needs of the nation must always be kept in mind. If regulation mainly represents an increasing cost burden, or a way to protect the status quo or turn back the clock, it will have the effect of postponing the day when coverage can be extended to the forty-three million among us who are uninsured and the day when all Americans can count on having access to the right care, at the right time, and in the right setting.

The health care revolution, with its emphasis on preventive care, early intervention, coordination of care, continual quality improvement, and affordability, has moved that day closer than it ever was under the old system. Above all, the role of regulation in a market-oriented health care system should be to help keep the evolution of patient-centered health care moving forward.

Notes

1. Miller, R. H., and Luft, H. S. "Does Managed Care Lead to Better or Worse Quality of Care?" *Health Affairs,* Sept.–Oct. 1997, pp. 7–25; Miller, R. H., and Luft, H. S. "Managed Care Plan Performance Since 1980." *Journal of the American Medical Association,* 1994, *271*(19), 1512–1519.

2. American Association of Health Plans. *Quality of Care* (research brief). Washington, D.C.: Author, 1998.

3. Information on diabetes, beta blockers, smoking, cancer screening from the National Committee for Quality Assurance, *The State of Managed Care Quality,* 1997; on appendicitis and prenatal, *The New England Journal of Medicine,* 1994; on Medicare, *American Journal of Public Health,* 1994; on ICUs, *JAMA,* 1996.

4. General Accounting Office. *Explicit Gag Clauses Not Found in HMO Contracts, But Physician Concerns Remain.* Washington, D.C.: Author, 1997

5. Congressional Research Service. "Health Insurance and Medical Care: Physician Services Under Managed Care." *CRS Report for Congress,* Report #98–352EPW. March 30, 1998; National Center for Health Statistics. *Health Interview Survey.* Hyattsville, Md.: Author, 1994.

6. National Research Corporation. *Healthcare Market Guide VI.* Lincoln, Neb.: Author, 1996.

7. Remler, D., and others. "What Do Managed Care Plans Do to Affect Care?" *Inquiry,* 1997, *34,* 196–204; and "How Doctors Spend Their Working Hours." *Medical Economics,* November 24, 1997.

8. American Association of Health Plans. *An Analysis of Inpatient Hospital Length of Stays for Selected Diagnosis Related Group.* Washington, D.C.: Author, 1997.

9. Ibid.

10. Ibid.

11. New York State Department of Health, Bureau of Quality Management and Outcome Research. *1995 Outpatient Mastectomy Data.* New York: Author, 1996; American Association of Health Plans. *The Regulation of Health Plans: A Report from the American Association of Health Plans.* Washington, D.C.: Author, 1998.

12. Bowman, K. *Health Care Attitudes Today.* Washington, D.C.: American Enterprise Institute, 1998.

13. Ladd, E. C. Op-Ed Piece. *The New York Times,* July 23, 1998.

14. Barents Group. *Characteristics of Health Plan Choices Available to Employees Through Employer-Based Health Benefits.* Arlington, Va.: KPMG Peat Marwick, 1996.

Chapter Fourteen

Regulation from a Consumer's Perspective

Ronald F. Pollack

In 1995, nearly three out of four Americans with health insurance coverage provided by their employers received their health care through managed care plans: health maintenance organizations (HMOs), preferred provider organizations, and point-of-service plans. This is a dramatic change from a decade earlier, when fewer than three out of ten people were enrolled in such plans.[1] The rapid rise of managed care was spurred by the dramatic escalation in health care spending in the late 1980s and early 1990s. As health care budgets grew dramatically, many consumers were encouraged—or required—to sign up for managed care through the employer or government programs (Medicaid and Medicare) that paid a large part of the bill for their care.

Managed care was seen as a necessary component of the drive to bring health costs under control. The traditional fee-for-service health care system—in which patients first sought care, then asked their insurance plans to pay for it—was believed to have offered perverse incentives that drove up spending. Consumers could see any doctor, whether generalist or specialist, as often as they wanted: the choice was theirs. Doctors and hospitals were rewarded for providing more services, regardless of their value or necessity. Managed care turned this system on its head. Incentives that encouraged providers to see patients frequently and to test and treat them aggressively were replaced by incentives that encouraged the delay or denial of care.

On paper, managed care seems like a sensible way to hold down health care costs *and* maintain or even strengthen quality of care. Managed care can promote primary and preventive care, and it can ensure proper care coordination. It can also reduce the use of unnecessary, even harmful, treatments and procedures. By developing a more accountable system of care, managed care also has the potential to enable good science to play a more central role in determining the efficacy of a course of treatment.

Half a century ago, the seeds of managed care were planted when Henry J. Kaiser and others fought to establish a new system of financing and delivering health care: prepaid health plans. The pioneers of managed care believed that this new system would revolutionize health care. Members paid a fixed amount each month to cover all the costs of providing their care; the prepaid plans built clinics and hired doctors to staff them. Besides controlling costs, the prepaid plans managed and coordinated patients' care and emphasized preventive care, which often was not covered by health insurance.

But managed care as we know it today is very different from the health delivery system envisioned by HMO pioneers fifty years ago. Many HMOs today do more to manage health care risks and distribute those risks to others than to manage care. Moreover, the managed care pioneers who spawned the earliest HMOs did so mainly through nonprofit organizations; by contrast, today's managed care industry is dominated by insurance and HMO corporations whose primary mission is to generate net revenues for their shareholders. The combination of forces at work in managed care today—built-in incentives to control costs by delaying or denying care and pressure to generate profits—has created serious problems for health care consumers. Too often, health care decisions are no longer made by physicians and other trusted health professionals; instead, those decisions are made or heavily influenced by individuals who never see affected patients and may have had no medical training.

In order for managed care to realize its potential for providing high-quality care, the federal government must regulate the marketplace, ensuring basic protections for health care consumers. This regulatory oversight should *not* dictate how to provide clinical treatment and should not be directed at designing benefit pack-ages. *But it should establish reasonable procedural protections to ensure that health plan enrollees actually receive, on a timely basis, the services promised to them in their benefit packages.* That is what a patients' bill of rights is designed to achieve.

Patients' rights legislation encompasses a series of different procedural rights, including these:

- The right for a patient to go to an emergency room and have the managed care plan pay for the resulting care, if that patient reasonably believes he or she is experiencing an emergency
- The right for a patient to appeal denials of care through a process that is external to, and independent of, the health plan
- An established procedure that enables a doctor to prescribe for a patient, and for that patient to receive, specific prescription drugs that are not on a health plan's drug formulary
- The right for a patient to receive health care from an out-of-network provider and have that care paid for by the HMO when the health plan's network of providers is inadequate
- Prohibitions against plans' use of so-called gag rules—rules that prevent or inhibit physicians and health providers from fully disclosing treatment options to patients or from advocating on behalf of their patients
- The right for a person with a serious illness or disability to use a specialist as a primary care provider
- The right for a seriously ill person to receive standing referrals to health specialists so that he or she does not need to visit a primary care physician each and every time a specialist consultation is needed
- The right for a seriously ill patient or pregnant woman to continue receiving health care for a specified period of time from a physician who has been dropped from the health plan's network of providers
- Prohibitions on plans' reliance on inappropriate financial incentives to deny or reduce necessary health care
- Established protections that prevent health plans from prohibiting participation in clinical trials

Why We Need Federal Regulation

There are several reasons why reasonable federal regulatory protections are needed. First, federal legislation is needed because the protections that exist today constitute a veritable jumble that is unpredictable, undecipherable, and extraordinarily uneven. There are enormous differences in the protections that are afforded to people based on the happenstance of their state of residence. People who live in Michigan may be guaranteed treatment in a medical emergency but are not assured direct access to women's health providers; in Tennessee, the reverse is true.[2] Even worse, vast differences in patients' rights exist even for people living in the same state, depending on the source of their health coverage. Different rules apply to Medicare beneficiaries, to those who buy insurance on their own, to those who receive coverage through an employer who buys insurance, to those who receive coverage through an employer who self-insures, and to people in the Medicaid program.[3]

Although a significant number of states have enacted strong consumer protection laws, these laws do not apply to a large number of their residents. Some 51 million Americans are in self-insured employer health plans that are exempt from most state laws under the federal Employee Retirement Income Security Act of 1974 (ERISA), and approximately 123 million people are precluded by ERISA from securing state remedies to compensate for wrongful denials of care.[4] Instead, they dwell in a regulatory never-never land, where they have weak or nonexistent patient protections. A federal patients' bill of rights, therefore, would establish a regulatory floor for everyone, thereby providing predictability and greater clarity of rights and responsibilities for all.

Second, there is no realistic alternative to a federal patients' bill of rights to promote patient protections. In theory, the health care marketplace could provide such an alternative. Some economic theorists argue that patient protections and quality of care will be promoted as people choose to leave bad plans and enroll in good plans. Under this theoretical construct, good health plans would be rewarded by increased enrollment and bad plans would be disciplined as enrollees "vote with their feet" and leave the plan. In fact, however, a large portion of the American public has no opportunity to make such a choice. This is especially true for people who receive health coverage through their employers, which is the most common way for people to receive health coverage in our nation today. A 1997 Kaiser–Commonwealth national survey of health insurance found that the majority of working Americans do not have a choice of plans provided by their employers. Thus, most consumers cannot influence health care quality because they do not have the opportunity to vote with their feet.

Even when consumers do have a choice of plans, it appears that choice may not be enough to ensure quality care. This is illustrated by a 1997 report issued by Families USA entitled *Comparing Medicare HMOs: Do They Keep Their Members?* This publication reported the results of a Families USA study examining the rates at which Medicare enrollees voluntarily quit, or "disenrolled" from, HMOs. The study covered every HMO that served more than a thousand Medicare beneficiaries throughout 1996. The study found a wide disparity in the rate at which enrollees voluntarily left their plans during the course of the year, ranging from a low of 2 percent to a high of 81 percent.[5]

The study found a disturbing trend in Florida and Texas, two states that had high disenrollment rates and enough HMOs to offer Medicare beneficiaries a meaningful choice of plans. In Texas, five plans had disenrollment rates in excess of 20 percent. In these plans, more than one in five enrollees voluntarily left during the year. Yet every one of those five plans—notwithstanding their incredibly high disenrollment rates—had a higher total enrollment at the end of the year than at the beginning of the year. Every one of those plans had a higher market share at the end of the year than at the beginning of the year. In Florida, out of fourteen plans with disenrollment rates in excess of 20 percent, nine plans had a higher enrollment at the end of the year than at the beginning of the year.

Clearly, each and every one of those plans was more successful at drawing people in than at satisfying and retaining enrollees. Even though Medicare beneficiaries were voting with their feet by disenrolling in droves from those plans, an even larger number of people were signing up. Presumably, the new enrollees knew little about the large number of people who voluntarily quit those plans. Although disenrollment rates per se are not absolute proof of poor-quality service, it is clear that the market's mechanism for expressing mass dissatisfaction did not appear to be hurting those plans' bottom lines.

Last, the American public wants and needs consumer protections. A recent study by the Kaiser Family Foundation and Harvard University's School of Public Health found that the majority of Americans believe managed care plans make it harder for sick people to see medical specialists. In addition, over half of those surveyed said that managed care has hurt the quality of care for people who are sick. And in one of the most alarming findings, most consumers (55 percent) said they were at least "somewhat worried" that if they became sick their "health plan would be more concerned about saving money than about what is the best medical treatment."[6]

Reasonable regulatory oversight through a patients' bill of rights would help to restore the confidence that the public has lost in our changing health care system. It would also help restore the faith that patients have traditionally had in their physicians, a faith that is weakened when people wonder whether their physicians will be loyal to their patients or to the plans that hire them.

The Cost of Regulation

Reasonable patient protection legislation is cost-effective. All of the studies prepared by independent analysts—those analysts who are neither proponents nor opponents of patients' rights legislation—have found that the cost of a patients' bill of rights is extraordinarily low. Only analyses supported by the insurance and HMO industries, which have spent many millions of dollars to defeat patients' rights legislation, contradict these findings.

For example, the Henry J. Kaiser Family Foundation estimated that major provisions of the Consumer Bill of Rights and Responsibilities endorsed by President Clinton would increase the annual premium for a typical HMO by 0.61 percent, adding approximately $31 per person per year to the cost of the average family insurance policy.[7] The President's Advisory Commission on Consumer Protection and Quality in the Health Care Industry found that the costs of an independent right of review of health service denials would only cost between $0.003 and $0.07 per person per month.[8] And the Congressional Budget Office estimated that the Patients'

Bill of Rights, the most comprehensive bill pending in the 105th Congress, would raise premiums by only 4 percent.[9]

As low as these costs are, they overstate the net effect of patients' rights legislation on consumers' pocketbooks. There are two reasons for this. First, none of the estimates factor in the costs to consumers of securing care outside their HMOs—and paying out-of-pocket for that care—when the care is improperly denied by their HMOs. If patients' rights protections are put in place, consumers will save money when their plans pay for care that is currently being denied. Second, some of the key provisions in patients' rights legislation are designed to reduce costs, and those savings are not reflected in cost estimates. For example, patients' rights legislation would provide a woman with the right to visit her obstetrician and gynecologist without first going to, and receiving a referral from, a primary care physician. Enabling a woman to get the care she needs through one doctor's visit rather than two would undoubtedly save money. Similarly, by enabling seriously ill patients to receive standing referrals to the specialists treating them, patients' rights protections would also obviate unnecessary visits to primary care physicians, thereby saving money.

Legal Recourse to Remedy Wrongful Denials of Care

One of the most contentious issues in the patient protection debate is whether patients should have legal recourse to meaningful remedies when they are harmed by a wrongful denial of care. The issue arises from the restrictions established under the federal ERISA statute.

Under ERISA, two important obstacles were placed in the path of aggrieved consumers. First, state laws establishing the right of patients to sue an insurance company or HMO that improperly denies care do not apply to those who have employer-provided coverage governed by ERISA. This limitation applies to virtually all (approximately 123 million) people who receive health coverage from an employer, except for state government workers. Second, although ERISA creates a right to sue in federal courts, it severely limits the remedies that patients can receive. Neither compensatory nor punitive damages are available in federal courts under ERISA.

The only remedy allowed for a patient who proves that an HMO wrongfully denied care is the ultimate provision of the wrongfully withheld service or a payment for the cost of that service. In many cases, this is an illusory remedy because it comes too late to be of any help.

The absurdity of these limitations is illustrated by the tragic case of Frank Wurzbacher.[10] Wurzbacher had prostate cancer and was receiving periodic injections of leupron at no cost. When his employer switched health plan administrators, the new administrator informed him that he would have to pay $180 per injection, an amount he could not afford. Wurzbacher complained that this unaffordable payment must be a mistake, especially because the scope of his coverage had not been changed. The plan administrator, however, rebuffed him. Seeking advice from his physician, Wurzbacher learned that his only alternative was to be castrated, and the health plan agreed to pay for his castration. On the day he returned from the hospital after his castration operation, a letter awaited him from the health plan indicating that they made a mistake about the $180 copayment requirement. Now when Wurzbacher seeks recourse, the only remedy he can secure from federal courts is the right to receive these obviously useless injections for free, a remedy that is a cruel joke.

When ERISA was enacted nearly a quarter of a century ago, such an injustice could not have been foreseen by policymakers. In the mid-1970s, almost all health care was provided in a fee-for-service context. In that context, disputes between patients and insurance companies virtually always focused on denials of payments for health services that had already been provided. Thus, the right to sue in federal court for the cost of such service was reasonably designed to provide full relief to a complainant.

This, however, is not true in a managed care context. Today, legal disputes focus not just on the payment for services but, far more significantly, on the actual provision of those services. Hence, during the lengthy time often consumed by litigation, the complainant is likely to be harmed to a considerably greater extent because crucial health care is being withheld. Thus, although the ERISA statute may have made abundant sense when it was enacted, today it is outdated, producing tragic, unintended consequences.

Originally intended to protect employees in pension and health plans, ERISA has become a protective shield for managed care plans. This lack of meaningful remedies invites abuse. Regardless of a managed care company's indifference, callousness, willfulness, or negligence in refusing to authorize medically necessary treatment, the worst that can happen is that it will have to pay for the services originally denied. As a result, a managed care company has every financial incentive to deny or delay care because it will never incur a liability greater than the value of the service being denied. *The ERISA statute, therefore, takes away any meaningful deterrent against inappropriate health service denial decisions by managed care companies.*

The injustices resulting from the ERISA statute's limitations have drawn strong criticism from federal judges. Although these judges faithfully implemented the restrictive remedial features of ERISA, a significant number have accompanied their decisions with stinging rebukes of the unjust results. In one case that resulted in the death of a managed care enrollee, the court found that the health plan's and utilization reviewer's conduct, although "extraordinarily troubling," were less "disturbing" than "the failure of Congress to amend a statute that, due to the changing realities of the modern health care system, has gone conspicuously awry from its original intent."[11] In yet another case, the court concluded:

> The result ERISA compels us to reach means that the [plaintiffs] have no remedy, state or federal, for what may have been a serious mistake. . . . While we are confident that the result we have reached is faithful to Congress's intent neither to allow state-law causes of action that relate to employee benefit plans nor to provide beneficiaries in the [plaintiffs'] position with a remedy under ERISA, the world of employee benefit plans has hardly remained static since 1974. Fundamental changes such as the widespread institution of utilization review would seem to warrant a reevaluation of ERISA so that it can continue to serve its noble purpose of safeguarding the interests of employees.[12]

Other federal judges have similarly admonished the Congress to amend the ERISA statute, a most unusual step for members of the judiciary to take.[13] There are two ways in which ERISA may be adapted to the changes in the health care system. Congress can either authorize the states to establish legal remedies for improper denials of health care or it can establish a uniform system of remedies in federal court that compensates patients for the harms caused by their HMOs. The latter alternative can be accompanied, if Congress so decides, with reasonable limitations on court awards, including limitations relating to punitive damages, guidelines for jury awards, or caps on such awards. But if Congress fails to amend the ERISA statute, consumers will continue to suffer from health plans' lack of accountability for harm caused by their wrongful denials of care.

Making Protections Work

With a number of patient protection laws already on the books in most states, and as Congress considers managed care legislation in the year ahead, there is an overwhelming need for consumers to be better equipped to pursue their health care choices, rights, and responsibilities. To make consumer protections work and help consumers understand and navigate our increasingly complex health care system, it is important that consumer assistance—or ombudsman—programs be established. Consumers need help in figuring out how to choose health plans if they have more than one alternative available to them. They need to know where to take their complaints, questions, and grievances. Should they go to the state insurance commissioner, an employer benefits relations administrator, the Department of Labor's regional office, the Health Care Financing Administration, the state Medicaid agency, or some other source? They may need help with administrative reviews of their complaints, either in internal HMO reviews of benefit denials or in independent, external reviews. Any and all such help can be provided through a consumer assistance program.

Such assistance would help to demystify managed care and our bewilderingly fragmented health care system. It would empower individuals to navigate the health care system and become thoughtful participants in health care choices. It also would help to resolve problems at earlier, less formal stages, and obviate the need for more contentious proceedings, such as litigation.

Consumer assistance programs should provide the following types of services:

- They should help consumers make choices about health plans by providing information and answering potential enrollees' relevant questions.
- They should help those who have enrolled understand their rights and responsibilities within their plans.
- They should set up toll-free phone numbers to respond to questions and potential problems.
- They should assist enrollees with their nonlitigious appeals, both those handled internally by health plans and external administrative appeals.
- They should make referrals, as appropriate, to health plan administrators, employers, and regulators.
- They should keep accurate records of, and report on, the help provided to consumers so that everyone has good data and information about consumer inquiries and concerns.

To work well, these consumer assistance programs must be nonprofit, nongovernmental organizations that are independent of plans, providers, regulators, and payers. However, because these programs can only work if they have a reasonable resource base, they should be supported with public funds—preferably a block grant to states that would issue requests for proposals from qualified nonprofit organizations.

There is significant precedent for such consumer assistance programs. For approximately two decades, ombudsman programs have operated effectively on behalf of families of nursing home residents. The Institute of Medicine, in a thoughtful analysis released in 1995, found that these ombudsman programs have played an important role in improving quality of care in nursing homes around the country.[14] Similarly, we have seen fledgling programs provide such assistance to some Medicare and Medicaid beneficiaries. And most recently, the Center for Health Care Rights has established an ombudsman program for people in the Sacramento area, a program currently supported with funding from three California philanthropies.

As this concept is developed, a number of issues undoubtedly will need to be addressed. First, none of the ombudsman funding should be used for policymaking advocacy but instead should be used exclusively to provide direct services to consumers. Second, the creation of publicly supported consumer assistance programs should complement, not supplant, already existing services—such as those currently provided by some employers and public agencies. And third, a balance needs to be drawn so that consumer assistance programs, on the one hand, serve all consumers, no matter the source of the health coverage, and on the other hand, have the capability and specialized expertise to serve people with significantly divergent needs.

Conclusion

The revolution in health care has been unsettling for the American public. As more and more people experience denials of care or learn about such denials from friends, relatives, and the news media, the public becomes increasingly apprehensive. Consumers who have lost the right to choose their physicians or health plans experience or hear about improper denials of care and are bewildered and don't know what they can do to protect their families.

Consumers need a set of uniform national protections that are guaranteed to them as purchasers of insurance. Such protections are affordable and would add little to the cost of providing care. They would provide predictability and uniformity by establishing a floor of national standards applicable to everyone. They would restore public confidence in the health care system. Finally, they would enable managed care to realize its potential for simultaneously controlling health care costs while providing high-quality care to all consumers.

Notes

1. The President's Advisory Commission on Consumer Protection and Quality in the Health Care Industry. "Quality First: Better Health Care for All Americans." Final report to the President of the United States, March 1998.

2. Families USA Foundation. *HMO Consumers at Risk: States to the Rescue.* Washington, D.C.: Author, 1996; Families USA Foundation. *Hit and Miss: State Managed Care Laws.* Washington, D.C.: Author, 1998.

3. Families USA Foundation. *Hit & Miss.*
4. Ibid.
5. Families USA Foundation. *Comparing Medicare HMOs: Do They Keep Their Members?* Washington, D.C.: Author, 1997.
6. Henry J. Kaiser Family Foundation–Harvard University National Survey of Americans' Views on Managed Care. Menlo Park, Calif.: Henry J. Kaiser Family Foundation, November 5, 1997.
7. Coopers & Lybrand. *Estimated Cost of Selected Consumer Protection Proposals: A Cost Analysis of the President's Advisory Commission's Consumer Bill of Rights and Responsibilities and the Patient Access to Responsible Care Act (PARCA).* Menlo Park, Calif.: Henry J. Kaiser Family Foundation, April 1998.
8. Dobson, A., Steinberg, C., and Finley, D. *Consumer Bill of Rights and Responsibilities Costs and Benefits: Information Disclosure and External Appeals.* Report submitted by The Lewin Group to the Presidential Commission on Consumer Protection and Quality in the Health Care Industry, November 1997.
9. Congressional Budget Office. *Cost Estimate: H.R. 3605/S. 1890, Patients' Bill of Rights Act of 1998.* Washington, D.C.: Author, July 16, 1998.
10. *Wurzbacher v. Prudential Insurance Co. of America,* Civil Action No. 96–97 (E.D. Ky. 1998).
11. *Andrews-Clarke v. Travelers Insurance Co.,* 984 F. Supp. 49 (D. Mass. 1997).
12. *Corcoran v. United HealthCare, Inc.,* 965 F. 2d 1321, 1338 (5th Cir. 1992).
13. Pear, R. "Hands Tied, Judges Rue Law That Limits H.M.O. Liability." *The New York Times,* July 11, 1998, p. A-1.
14. Harris-Wehling, J., Feasley, J. C., and Estes, C. L. (eds.). *Real People, Real Problems: An Evaluation of the Long-Term Care Ombudsman Programs of the Older Americans Act.* Washington, D.C.: Institute of Medicine, 1995.

Chapter Fifteen

Regulation from an Insurance Industry Perspective

Bill Gradison

Any discussion of health plan regulation can be informed by a brief review of how the health care marketplace has changed—and continues to change—in response to the demands of consumers. In fact, over the past ten to fifteen years, health insurance and health plans have evolved in response to what consumers wanted, and the result has been no less than a revolution in how health care is financed and delivered.

Employers who purchase health plans, and the employees and dependents enrolled in the plans, are the two primary groups of consumers to dominate today's health care marketplace. It is the combined interests of these consumers that have transformed the health care system. As a recent KPMG Peat Marwick study shows, a majority of health plan executives believe that consumers influence the policy, strategy, operations, even the investment decisions of their organizations. And 90 percent said that their plans expanded the number and type of services they offer based on consumer preferences.[1] The conclusions of this survey are also reflected in the recent history of change in the health care marketplace.

A Brief History of Managed Care

More than a decade ago, businesses said: "Health insurance is too expensive." And it was. Purchasing health benefits was moving beyond the reach of many firms. While policy analysts and legislators debated the pros and cons of various "fixes," the marketplace responded with broad-based innovation aimed at containing costs while enhancing quality. Managed care played a critical role: HMOs gained in popularity, and indemnity plans adopted managed care techniques to eliminate unnecessary and inappropriate services. As the market share of HMOs grew and as managed care techniques such as utilization review and case management became prevalent, health care inflation started to slow down and employers saw their premium increases begin to level off.

But some consumers wanted more options than those offered by the HMOs of the period, without paying the price of traditional fee for service. In reality, what consumers wanted out of the health care system seemed almost impossible to achieve. They wanted a greater variety of plans from which to choose, better choice of physicians, more direct access to specialists, and the ability to go "out of network"—all without paying a high price tag.

Yet with surprising ease and speed, the market obliged. In less than a decade, preferred provider organizations (PPOs) and point-of-service (POS) plans emerged, and hybrids—combinations of two or more managed care systems—became commonplace. In essence, as cost-containment pressures mounted and competition increased, insurers adjusted their systems to make them more attractive.

Increasingly, workers covered by employer-sponsored benefit plans are offered a choice of two or more health plans.[2] And 74 percent of health plans offer a point-of-service option, up from roughly 20 percent four years ago.[3] PPOs have become the dominant form of employer-based coverage, and 92 percent of eligible employees in employer-sponsored plans are offered an option for selecting nonnetwork physicians.[4]

Direct access to specialists—particularly among women seeking access to ob/gyns—is also easier. As shown in a Commonwealth Fund study, whereas in 1985 women enrolled in HMOs were "substantially more likely to see a generalist, women in HMOs in 1995 are much more likely to obtain care from specialists."[5] Managed care, then, has not only contributed to curbing health care premium inflation, which is now in line with the overall inflation rate (down from two or three times the CPI of five to six years ago),[6] but has proven to be flexible—yielding an array of options for health care consumers. No wonder, then, that most Americans are satisfied with their health plans.

Satisfaction and Quality

Despite the media bias against health plans displayed in the recent barrage of negative press, most insured Americans have always rated their own health plans favorably.[7] More significantly, most Americans are happy with the quality of care they receive.[8] A recent survey of research on managed care plan performance indicated favorable quality of care results for HMOs.[9] And in a review of fifteen studies, the authors noted that "evidence of significantly better quality covers a wide spectrum of enrollees."[10]

Other data, such as those collected by state insurance departments, corroborate these findings. The New York State Insurance Department, for example, seems to experience ten times more complaints against physicians than against HMOs (and complaints against plans often are not upheld by the department).[11] More specific surveys that look at particular plans also report favorable data. The federal government's Office of Personnel Management asked federal employees nationwide what they thought of a popular private plan with a PPO component.[12] The results were impressive:

Eighty-seven percent of those surveyed are satisfied, very satisfied, or extremely satisfied with this option.

Eighty-nine percent are satisfied with coverage.

Ninety-seven percent are satisfied with access to care.

Eighty-eight percent are satisfied with choice of physicians.

Eighty-seven percent are satisfied with their ability to get an appointment when sick.

Ninety-five percent are satisfied with the quality of care received.

Ninety-seven percent thought their providers were competent and thorough.

Ninety-five percent were satisfied with their health plan.

In light of these data, it is not surprising that a new national survey of health plan satisfaction found that 83 percent of people in employer-sponsored health plans say they will not switch their health plans at the next opportunity.[13] And that percentage is consistent along all product lines—fee for service, HMO, PPO, and others.

The Cost of Regulation

Despite the vigor and inventiveness of the health care industry, and the many new goods and services it has brought to the marketplace, the urge to regulate it remains strong among legislators and certain interest groups. But health insurance is already heavily regulated, as is discussed in detail by Karen Ignagni in Chapter Thirteen.

At the state level, elected and appointed insurance commissioners administer myriad rules on how insurers are to do business. Although some of the regulations on the books embody important consumer protections, others—like a multiplicity of mandated benefits—are both superfluous and costly. Likewise, the federal government is increasing its involvement: the Health Insurance Portability and Accountability Act of 1996 (HIPAA) established a major federal role in the regulation of private group and individual coverage, and the Balanced Budget Act of 1997 will strongly affect insurers who will be enrolling Medicare beneficiaries under Medicare+Choice. In addition, Congress is considering proposals that would increase federal oversight of managed care plans; legislative activity in this area is occurring on both sides of the aisle.

But there are trade-offs involved in the legislative proposals under consideration. Virtually every proposal on the table would require administrative outlays and other expensive systems. Thus, regulation tends to increase costs, drive up premiums, reduce marketplace innovation, and decrease choice. In the long run, this almost certainly translates into fewer employers offering coverage, greater cost-sharing by employees, and fewer workers having the financial resources to enroll in their employer's plan. Well-intentioned actions by government adopted ostensibly on behalf of consumers have in this way often harmed the very people they were meant to help. And it is important to note that the Government Accounting Office reports that millions of Americans are already unable to enroll in health plans offered by employers because they have difficulty paying their share.[14]

Regulation is a double-edged sword. Although it may seem to protect consumers, its hidden effects may be harmful. Consider one of the front-burner issues before Congress today: whether to legislate national regulatory standards for all health insurers and plans in the form of a patients' bill of rights. Although well-intentioned, such federalized consumer protection standards would be highly duplicative. In addition to existing state and federal laws and regulations, many private accreditation initiatives protect the interests of consumers.

But perhaps more important is the voluntary commitment made by health plans to enhance quality and satisfy customers, employers and insureds alike. A satisfied customer doesn't change plans (and keeps paying premiums). So it makes sense that plans and insurers focus on quality enhancement because, by so doing, they gain the greatest possible competitive advantage when it comes to retaining current customers and attracting new ones.

In spite of this, the federal legislative challenge that emerged has gained momentum. As 1998 was an election year, this is not surprising. Few issues are more personal than health care, or more central to the concerns of consumers. Unfortunately, health care is also an issue that lends itself to overblown rhetoric, if not outright falsehoods. And one of the most conspicuous falsehoods heard in this debate is that more stringent regulation—meaning more government intervention—is always better for the public. This simply is not the case with regard to the dynamic, consumer-oriented, customer-driven health insurance marketplace. Passing laws that leave fewer people with coverage, and those covered paying higher premiums, will serve the interests of no one, and do far more harm than good.

Certainly, health insurers and health plans do not claim to be perfect. But in a constant quest to improve, the market offers some things that no legislated mandate can: more choice rather than less, and real-time responsiveness to changing circumstances. Most of all, today's system shows a sensitivity to cost and coverage issues, offering plans that are inherently flexible and suit different kinds of consumers. Unneeded regulation should not be afforded an opportunity to interfere with the trend over the last fifteen years to accommodate the needs and desires of consumers and create better ways to serve policyholders and patients.

Notes

1. KPMG Peat Marwick. *New Voices: Consumerism in Health Care.* Evanston, Ill.: Northwestern University's Institute for Health Services Research, 1998.
2. Barents Group. "Health Care Choices." Report commissioned by American Association of Health Plans, December 1997.
3. Health Care Advisory Board. "The Impact of Managed Care on the Health Care Industry." Washington, D.C.: Author, 1997.
4. Barents Group. "Health Care Choices."
5. Weisman, C. S. "Women in Managed Care and Measuring Quality of Care for Women." Paper presented at the Commonwealth Fund Commission on Women's Health Symposium: Access, Leverage and Quality in Women's Health: Are the Issues Changing? Washington, D.C., January 27–28, 1998.
6. U.S. Bureau of Labor Statistics. *Consumer Price Index, All Urban Consumers, Annual Average 1988–1998.* Washington, D.C.: Author, n.d..
7. Health Insurance Association of America. *Monitoring Attitudes of the Public.* Washington, D.C.: Author, 1989–1995.
8. KPMG Peat Marwick. "New Voices."
9. Miller, R. H., and Luft, H. S. "Does Managed Care Lead to Better or Worse Quality of Care?" *Health Affairs,* 1997, 16(5).
10. Ibid.
11. State of New York Insurance Department. *Health Insurance Complaint Ratios—All Companies.* New York: Author, 1997.
12. U.S. Office of Personnel Management. *Guide to Federal Employees Health Benefits Plans for Federal Civilian Employees.* Washington, D.C.: Author, 1997.
13. National Research Corporation. *NRC Healthcare Market Guide.* (7th ed.). Lincoln, Neb.: Author, 1997.
14. U.S. General Accounting Office. *Private Health Insurance—Continued Erosion of Coverage Linked to Cost Pressures.* Washington, D.C.: Author, 1997.

Chapter Sixteen

Regulation Misses the Big Issue—The Uninsured

Larry S. Gage

The debate over health industry regulation reminds me of an old "Peanuts" cartoon. Lucy is bent over examining an object on the sidewalk. "This is a rare butterfly from Brazil," she informs Linus. "You don't see many of them in this part of the world."

"That's a potato chip," Linus points out.

"Hmmm, you're right," says Lucy, now looking more closely. "I wonder how this potato chip got here from Brazil?"

From the vantage point of America's safety-net hospitals and health systems, the debate over regulation of managed care is rather like Lucy's effort to find meaning in a Brazilian potato chip. Although some observers see virtue (largely defined as the lowest possible price) in a free and unfettered marketplace, others argue that health care defies normal economic principles and must be regulated as an essential human good. But the purists on both sides seem to be discussing the health system of a country with which I am unfamiliar.

A Heavy Burden?

For example, the American Association of Health Plans developed an exquisitely labyrinthine chart purporting to illustrate the many

The author is indebted to Lynne Fagnoni, chief financial officer, and Jennifer Tolbert, analyst, of the National Association of Public Hospitals and Health Systems, for their assistance in preparing this chapter.

ways in which health plans are already "overregulated." A comparison can be made instantly to Senator Arlen Specter's famous 1994 chart "describing" the Clinton health plan; it too appeared complicated and exotic to the average viewer. Senator Specter's graphic configuration included each office or agency of every health program funded or touched in any way by the federal government—whether it was already in place or would be eliminated, consolidated, or created by the Clinton plan. It included the Veterans Administration, Champus, Medicare, Medicaid, Indian Health Service, the FDA, many PHS programs, and so on. Although in hindsight the Clinton plan was somewhat misguided (and certainly bungled in the selling), the reason why the plan, like the chart, was so complex was because it tried to address every aspect of the nation's trillion-dollar health system.

Similarly, most of the elements in the American Association of Health Plans (AAHP) chart refer to requirements a health plan generally must meet simply to get paid by (or otherwise do business with) various components of the health system. In fact, much of this "regulation" is purely voluntary. No one requires health plans to engage in the industry's voluntary accreditation process, or participate in the Medicare or Medicaid programs. But if they do, they must meet the pertinent requirements—a cost of doing business that is generally no greater for health plans than for any other component of the health system.

In fact, an argument can be made that the regulatory "burden" on health plans is far less than that on hospitals and other providers. Providers not only have to cope with the complex (and often different) bureaucracies imposed on them by health plans and other public and private payers but also must respond to many other requirements. These include a full range of fraud and abuse laws, as well as the various rules and responsibilities that address access for the poor and uninsured (including Medicaid and Medicare participation requirements, COBRA antidumping laws, and Hill-Burton).

What is perhaps most striking about AAHP's description of the regulatory burden is what is missing: any reference to or requirement that managed care plans participate in financing or providing care to the uninsured and underinsured. Nor is any such requirement found in even the most comprehensive managed care "consumer protection" bills that are likely to be reconsidered by the Congress in 1999. The "patient bill of rights" proposals are just that: protection for those who already have insurance coverage against real or perceived market-driven abuses of managed care.

The Most Important Shortcoming

Indeed, the biggest problem with the debate over health plan regulation is that it largely misses the most important shortcoming of our nation's health system: the utter failure of so-called competitive health care to meet the short-term needs (or solve the long-term dilemma) of the rapidly growing number of uninsured Americans. Yet unless we address this dilemma—with an appropriate level of participation and responsibility of health plans generally and managed care in particular—we might as well be talking about a foreign country. As long as the managed care industry can continue to ignore the uninsured and underinsured, and absent any other coherent plan to address the needs of these populations, no amount of either regulation or free market capitalism should give any comfort to consumers that their health care is adequate.

In actuality, the dilemma of the uninsured overshadows other regulatory issues. It affects our health system generally (and health plans and safety-net providers in particular) as well as the role and responsibility of health plans in sharing the burden.

Prosperity and the Uninsured

The U.S. health insurance system is a combination of employer-sponsored insurance (serving 64 percent of nonelderly Americans) and government-sponsored health insurance (through Medicaid and state and local indigent care programs where 13 percent of nonelderly Americans receive coverage).[1] A small percentage of individuals (7.5 percent) purchase insurance on their own.[2] This leaves the uninsured Americans, whose numbers are projected to increase to almost forty-five million by 2002.[3]

Since our most recent failure in the early 1990s to enact universal health coverage, the numbers of uninsured and underinsured have continued to grow. This growth, combined with cost-containment pressures by Medicare, Medicaid, and private insurers, has placed an escalating burden on public and private safety-net hospitals and health systems that serve as an essential backstop in the nation's health system.

It is ironic that such pressures on the safety net are increasing at a time of unprecedented economic prosperity in America. Unemployment is at a twenty-eight-year low. The federal budget was balanced last year for the first time in decades. And many states are seeing larger budget surpluses than at any time in recent memory. Why do we face this paradox of an extraordinarily robust economy and increasing problems in coverage and access to care? There are several likely reasons, including these:

- Many of the new jobs being created are in small businesses or service industries that do not provide adequate insurance coverage.
- Many lower-income workers, especially younger individuals, faced with rising costs, are giving up coverage or refusing to accept optional personal or dependent coverage.
- Welfare and immigration reforms have led to reduced eligibility for Medicaid and other programs among some low-income and vulnerable populations.
- In most states a large proportion of those eligible for Medicaid and other programs are simply never enrolled, or at least not until they fall seriously ill.
- Incremental reforms—such as the 1995 Kennedy-Kassebaum legislation and the 1997 Child Health Insurance Program (CHIP)—have been slow to bear fruit and will likely end up helping far fewer uninsured individuals than originally anticipated.

Meanwhile, legislative constraints and budget reductions adopted throughout the 1990s, culminating in the Balanced Budget Act of 1997, have affected many of the traditional sources of funding for safety-net health systems (such as Medicare and Medicaid disproportionate share hospital or DSH payments, and cost-based reimbursement) for Federally Qualified Health Centers (FQHCs).

The Uninsured and the Underinsured

We have seen a shift in the cost of health insurance from the employer to the employee, with fewer workers opting for coverage as a result. In fact, U.S. Department of Labor (DoL) data show that the percent of workers employed in medium and large firms with coverage fully financed by their employers went from 74 percent in 1980 to just 37 percent in 1993.[4] A study by The Lewin Group revealed that over three-quarters of the decline in employer-sponsored coverage between 1989 and 1996 was the result of the growth in the employee share of premiums.[5]

Furthermore, employers are dropping dependent coverage, or employees are refusing to pay for dependent coverage because the cost sharing is too high. DoL data show that dependent coverage fully financed by the employer was available to 54 percent of full-time workers in 1980, compared with 21 percent in 1993.[6]

The nature and scope of the underinsured population are fundamental to this discussion because inadequate insurance coverage or coverage limits for chronic illnesses (including limits on mental health and substance abuse or lifetime caps) can affect individuals' ability to cover fully the costs of their care in the event of catastrophic sickness or chronic conditions.

The term *underinsured* may be defined in several ways, but the most commonly used definition refers to individuals whose medical expenses would exceed 10 percent of their income if they faced a catastrophic illness. Using this definition, almost 19 percent of the population under sixty-five years old was underinsured in 1994, representing twenty-nine million individuals, as compared with 12.6 percent or twenty million people in 1977.[7] The income group with the greatest likelihood of being underinsured is individuals below 125 percent of poverty (61.6 percent), with the second greatest risk for individuals between 125 and 200 percent of poverty (31.7 percent).[8]

Another study reveals that almost 20 percent of Americans have problems paying medical bills, and of those, three-quarters have private insurance.[9]

The Erosion of Cost Shifting

During most of the 1980s and early 1990s, private payers increasingly reimbursed more than the cost of care, whereas governmental payers like Medicaid and Medicare reimbursed less than the cost of care (with the exception of 1985 and 1986, when Medicare payment-to-cost ratios were positive).[10] In fact, the Congressional Budget Office estimated that by 1989, private payers offset 55 percent of unreimbursed costs (shortfalls on governmental payers and uncompensated care), whereas other nonpatient sources offset 30 percent of unreimbursed costs, and state and local subsidies offset 10 percent.[11] Thus, a significant and growing share of uncompensated care was reimbursed by hospitals' overcharging privately insured patients.

Between 1992 and 1994, however, that trend began to reverse, as the ratio of private payments to costs fell for the first time from a high of 1.31 in 1992 to 1.24 in 1994.[12] Employers were no longer willing to accept increases in premiums that far exceeded inflation, applying price pressure on care providers and introducing price competition into the marketplace. Simultaneously, the widespread implementation of managed care to control costs and introduce predictability in pricing resulted in cost containment and creation of further excess capacity.

These factors resulted in intense competition among hospitals for patients with private sources of payment. An Employee Benefit Research Institute (EBRI) issue brief noted that "cost shifting appears to have died, killed off by new forms of insurance, price competition among hospitals, and greater cost consciousness in health care."[13] Thus, the private sector commitment to financing uncompensated care is shrinking in the current turbulent health care environment.

Telling Snapshots

Anecdotes help illuminate the impact of the erosion of cost-shifting and rise of competition.

- A recent *Washington Post* story bore the misleading headline: "Maryland Hospitals Strain Under Rate System." In fact, the state's hospitals are not straining because payment rates are too low—but rather because they are too high. Under Maryland's unique rate review system, hospitals are permitted to incorporate the uncompensated cost of serving the uninsured into their rates for all payers (except Medicare). As a result, private employers, insurers, and managed care plans are all described as diverting their patients to Washington, D.C., hospitals, which are free to offer discounts with no such humanitarian constraints.

• The effects of managed care on providers were highlighted in a recent *AHA News* article. It cited a New York State comptroller report that predicted a loss of over $100 million for the New York City Health and Hospitals Corporation (HHC) over the next four years because of lower Medicaid rates resulting from the shift to managed care.

• States have used managed care to contain costs in their Medicaid programs and in some instances have attempted to expand coverage to the uninsured with a portion of the savings, which should reduce the level of uncompensated care. In contrast, intense competition for patients brought on by managed care has jeopardized an important financing mechanism for uncompensated care. Competition has forced hospitals to seek out any patient who is insured—even those who are publicly insured.

What these stories tell us is that neither state Medicaid plans nor private employers and insurers will likely participate in funding care for the uninsured unless someone forces them to do so. And meanwhile, ever-hungrier providers show no remorse about turning on one another, happily accepting patients diverted away from institutions whose higher costs reflect their willingness to provide more uncompensated care.

Impact on Safety-Net Providers

As we have seen, the number of uninsured and underinsured Americans continues to increase. Although the burden of uncompensated care for the hospital industry has remained relatively constant over the last decade (when measured as a percent of expenses), underlying trends indicate that it is becoming more concentrated among a few safety-net hospitals. These are shouldering an increasing responsibility for care to the uninsured and underinsured, even while they are experiencing changes in the financing of this care that could undermine their ability to meet their safety-net mission in the future.

The American Hospital Association reported that hospitals across the country provided a total of $18 billion in uncompensated care in 1996.[14] As a percent of total expenses, uncompensated costs averaged 6.1 percent for all hospitals in that year.[15] However, this average belies important differences among types of hospitals. In 1994, uncompensated care as a percent of total costs ranged from 4.0 percent in proprietary and nondisproportionate share hospitals to 17.6 percent in public major teaching institutions.[16] Among members of the National Association of Public Hospitals & Health Systems (NAPH), uncompensated care as a percent of total expenses averaged 26 percent in 1996.

In a profile of uncompensated care, Mann and others analyzed 1994 data that revealed the disproportionate burden of uncompensated care among provider types. They found that urban public hospitals provided over 35 percent of all uncompensated care in that year, even though they represented only 15 percent of all hospital expenses; this was the only group by ownership whose burden of uncompensated care was disproportionate.[17] The aggregate expenses of the members of the National Association of Public Hospitals represented only 7 percent of hospital expenses nationally, although these institutions provided nearly 24 percent of uncompensated care.

In addition, the data showed that teaching institutions disproportionately offered uncompensated care. Major public teaching hospitals provided 26 percent of uncompensated care in 1994 but only represented 9 percent of total hospital expenses; minor public teaching hospitals provided 21 percent of all uncompensated care with just 2 percent of hospital expenses.[18] Another study, by Reuter and Gaskin, revealed that only 125 academic health centers (or 7 percent of hospitals in their market) provided 37 percent of all uncompensated care in their markets.[19]

Similarly, according to Mann and others, hospitals with high Medicaid patient loads disproportionately provided uncompensated care; those in the highest third in terms of Medicaid volume contributed 56 percent of all uncompensated care but only represented 38 percent of all hospital expenses.[20]

This concentration of uncompensated care in hospitals with large Medicaid shares has significant implications for the financing of uncompensated care. As competition for Medicaid patients increases among providers, hospitals contributing a lot of uncompensated care risk losing an important source of financing in terms of Medicaid and the DSH payments that are attached to Medicaid revenues.

Sources for Financing Uncompensated Care

Hospitals rely on a number of sources to finance the uncompensated care they provide, as NAPH survey data on revenues and costs at urban safety-net hospitals demonstrates. Using NAPH data from 1989 to 1996, researchers calculated the ratio of revenues to costs for patient care revenue and cost sources, including Medicare, Medicaid, commercial insurers, self-pay and uncompensated care, and other payers. The ratios were also calculated for nonoperating revenue and sources such as philanthropic donations and interest expenses.

These findings illustrate the erosion of cost shifting (and thus the diminished role of health plans) as a source of financing care for the uninsured. As with all hospitals, the surveyed institutions shifted the costs of care for the uninsured to commercial payers wherever possible. However, their ability to transfer these costs has declined since peaking in 1993; the surveyed hospitals gained only 6 percent on revenues from commercial payers in 1996 compared with 14 percent in 1993. Interestingly, even at the peak safety-net providers were unable to manage the 30 to 50 percent margins on commercial payers achieved by hospitals with larger commercial patient proportions.

Managed care has further eroded safety-net providers' base of Medicaid patients in the 1990s, jeopardizing this important financing mechanism for uncompensated care. Most of the patients lost by high uncompensated care providers are lower-cost Medicaid clients, such as obstetrics patients. Between 1989 and 1994, public teaching hospitals' share of Medicaid deliveries dropped from 25 percent of the market to 12 percent, a decline of over 50 percent (even though their proportion of Medicaid deliveries was still triple their representation in the market).[21] The same hospitals experienced a slight increase in their share of self-pay deliveries (from 15 percent to 19 percent) during this period. Most of the market share of Medicaid deliveries went to nonteaching, nonprofit hospitals, whose proportion of Medicaid deliveries rose from 27 percent to 37 percent.

Attempts at and Barriers to Health Plan Involvement

Taken together, these pressures on our health system—extreme emphasis on price, erosion of cost-shifting opportunities, the increase in Medicare and Medicaid managed care, and the ability of most health plans to escape any responsibility for the uninsured— are formidable. They will likely accelerate the day when major safety-net systems collapse unless ways can be found to harness the resources of the entire health system, including health plans, in support of the uninsured. But although there have been efforts to impose additional obligations on health plans to address these needs, significant barriers remain.

The Health Insurance Portability and Accountability Act

The Health Insurance Portability and Accountability Act of 1996 (HIPAA) was intended to reform insurance practices including denial of coverage to individuals with preexisting conditions and to reduce employee "job-lock"—that is, fear of changing jobs because of the possibility of being denied coverage or of waiting periods. It guaranteed issue and portability to individuals moving from one group insurance plan to another or from a group plan to an individual one. There would, in theory, be no waiting periods or preexisting condition exclusions as long as the individual maintained coverage with no gaps.

Primarily, the act protected individuals who already had insurance, rather than expanding coverage to uninsured people. Even that limited goal has proved elusive, however. A recent Government Accounting Office report on HIPAA implementation revealed the difficulties of these types of insurance reforms when they are not accompanied by rate regulation. The report showed that some insurers are charging from 140 percent to 600 percent over standard rates, essentially treating HIPAA eligibles as if they were high-risk purchasers.[22] Thus, although insurance companies must offer plans to individuals, they are likely to charge unaffordable premium rates.

Further, a survey by Kaiser and the Commonwealth Fund determined that only 3 percent of the uninsured lacked coverage for health reasons.[23] Thus, although HIPAA sought to address concerns about loss of insurance for those who have coverage, it is not likely to assist the uninsured in any material way.

Employee Retirement Income Security Act

Another important barrier has been the Employee Retirement Income Security Act (ERISA), passed in 1974, which exempts companies that self-insure from state health insurance laws. It also prevents states from imposing employer mandates or other insurance reforms on self-insured plans, and from taxing or assessing surcharges on these plans for the purpose of financing uncompensated care pools. Thus, states are limited in their ability to require all components of their health care systems to contribute to reform efforts by imposing charges or taxes on health plans. In order to implement meaningful programs and policies to cover the uninsured, ERISA would need to be amended. Hawaii, which is the only state to possess statutory exemption from the act's requirements, comes the closest to providing universal health coverage. (For more discussion of ERISA, see Chapters Nine and Ten.)

Clinton Plan

In 1998, there were proposals at the federal level to continue expanding coverage to other populations. President Clinton submitted a plan to permit individuals from fifty-five to sixty-four years old to buy into the Medicare program. The plan has three parts: (1) allowing individuals ages sixty-two to sixty-five to buy into Medicare by paying two different premiums before and after age sixty-five to offset the cost fully over their lifetimes; (2) allowing workers ages fifty-five to sixty-one to buy into Medicare if they lose employer-sponsored health insurance at a premium that fully finances the cost of the premium; (3) and giving retirees age fifty-five and over, whose health benefits have been terminated, the chance to buy COBRA coverage until they are sixty-five years old.

Although this fifty-five- to sixty-four-year-old age group is the least likely to be uninsured (13 percent),[24] it is one of the poorest and sickest of all uninsured groups and the most unlikely to be employed or have an employed spouse.[25] People in this group have greater difficulty purchasing private insurance coverage at affordable rates because of age and preexisting conditions. Research by the Center for Studying Health System Change estimates that individuals would have to spend 20 to 25 percent of their income on premiums under the president's plan, which makes the proposal unaffordable to many of the uninsured in this age group.[26] The administration estimates that only 15 percent of the uninsured population between ages fifty-five and sixty-four would be able to take advantage of the program.

Other Proposals

Several other proposals have been discussed in the 105th Congress, including accelerating the timetable for allowing individuals to deduct health care expenses from income taxes; requiring an individual mandate to have health insurance coverage; establishing an employer mandate for health insurance coverage for firms over a certain size; providing a new range of tax credits to encourage individuals to buy health insurance; and creating a program like the Federal Employees Health Benefit Plan (FEHBP) to permit employers to purchase into a "health mart" to offer plans to their employees at affordable rates. It is unclear which, if any, of these proposals will get serious consideration.

Two Types of Reforms

If as we have seen the health care safety net is unraveling in good times, what will happen if the healthy economy sours? If unemployment increases? If inflation and high interest rates return, and the stock market crashes?

If we are to be truly prepared for such an eventuality, we need to address these issues now. Recognizing that a single approach to universal health coverage is unlikely to win passage, we must nevertheless adopt a national policy agenda that includes a broad enough range of specific reforms to provide hope that the problem will not continue to grow worse and that the gaps can begin to be closed. To begin with, we must recognize that our current system has two major parts: a public and private insurance component, consisting of private insurers, HMOs, and public entitlement programs like Medicare and Medicaid; and an institutional component, consisting of a certain amount of "free care" provided by a broad range of hospitals and other providers but with an important foundation of a relatively small number of government-funded health centers and public and nonprofit hospitals and health systems.

All policymakers need to understand that the institutional component of our nation's health safety net is every bit as important as the insurance system in meeting the needs of the uninsured and underinsured. It is time to contemplate a broader sharing of this burden, including a more appropriate and explicit role for private health plans.

Too often, America's institutional health safety net has received short shrift in national debates about budget balancing and health care reform. As a result, the safety net has been more often targeted for budget cuts than for necessary strengthening, whereas most health plans have improved their ability to evade any responsibility for the uninsured. This can no longer be the case. We must now consider a full range of reforms and proposals on both sides of this equation. Initiatives can be categorized into two types: insurance and coverage reforms, and institutional safety-net reforms.

Insurance and Coverage Reforms

First and foremost, it is essential that we reinstate the ultimate goal of achieving universal health coverage, even if we remain unlikely to achieve it in the short run. Other recommendations include these:

- Expand appropriate coverage under existing programs or create new ones (such as SCHIP) for certain homogeneous and easy-to-identify populations (for example, children or fifty-five-to sixty-four-year-old retirees).
- Create a coordinated nationwide outreach program, directed by the federal government (and preferably organized under the leadership of a prominent American), to achieve higher enrollment levels among individuals and families already eligible for public or private coverage.

- Pay careful attention to state-based reform programs that have been operated for several years under federal waivers to determine what works and what does not and to identify the needs and gaps in those programs.
- Give states much broader latitude to experiment with mandates and other innovations in the area of private insurance, through a combination of waivers and a relaxation of ERISA restrictions.

Finally, we need to address the accessibility issue for smaller employers and individuals by establishing a congressionally chartered "national health plan," with the goal of making new and affordable insurance products available, on a voluntary basis, to anyone who may wish to take advantage of them. Although this proposal is similar to the health mart concept now being advocated by some members of Congress, I propose carrying it a step further by creating a semiprivate corporate structure, modeled on such highly successful federal organizations as the Federal National Mortgage Association (Fannie Mae). Such a national health plan could function both as a FEHBP or CalPERS type of purchasing cooperative as well as an innovator of new products.

Institutional Safety-Net Reforms

In the short term, we must halt the erosion of funding for—and in fact strengthen—programs that directly support safety-net institutions, including Medicare and Medicaid DSH payments and direct subsidies for community, migrant, and rural health centers. Program enhancement efforts should focus on institutions and systems that serve the highest proportion of the uninsured and underinsured, and they should be broadened where necessary to include outpatient as well as inpatient care.

The imperative for change, particularly for institutional subsidies, is real. Incremental coverage expansions that would greatly affect the number of uninsured, particularly the populations most often treated by safety-net providers, are not likely to be realized in the near future. As institutional subsidies are cut back, safety-net providers are increasingly failing to meet the realities of current health care delivery. Yet these subsidies are a lifeline for the organizations struggling to provide care to the indigent. Because we will continue to rely on these providers, as a society, we must finance them rationally. How should this be done?

In particular, Medicare disproportionate share hospital payments (like medical education payments) must be carved out of Medicare managed care premiums. To balance the success of many health plans and employers in reducing cost shifting, the formula for determining DSH eligibility should be tightened to focus more on providers caring for the uninsured. And because safety-net institutions often suffer from reduced access to capital and technical assistance, we need to provide support to improve their systems and infrastructure—including areas such as information system and integrated delivery system development, and bricks and mortar to rebuild or reengineer structures.

Indigent Care Trust Fund

In the longer term, we need tap Medicare and Medicaid DSH and other funding sources to create a national indigent care trust fund to provide a steady source of support for the highest-volume providers of care to the uninsured and underinsured. This trust fund should have a single qualifying criterion and payment methodology. If properly directed to health care providers based on their provision of uncompensated care, the total amount of financing for the fund probably would be less than is spent in the various existing programs, freeing up funds for coverage expansion. At the same time, such a trust fund could serve as a vehicle for the participation by health plans in meeting the needs of the uninsured, perhaps through a small national premium tax dedicated to the fund.

In any case, nonsafety-net institutions and health plans must continue to be encouraged—or if necessary, required—to share the burden of serving the uninsured and underinsured. This can be done through a combination of incentives and a strengthening of legal requirements, such as the COBRA antidumping laws and managed care benefit coverage and emergency room payment requirements.

Finally, federal, state, and local programs aimed at particularly vulnerable populations should continue to be funded and strengthened, and incentives provided directly to safety-net institutions themselves to develop innovative new programs to provide access to needed services.

Maximizing individual health insurance coverage must continue to be our nation's primary goal for enfranchising the uninsured, giving them an opportunity for improved quality of care resulting from choice. In a health system with more than forty-five million people who are uninsured, we do not have the luxury of limiting our policy debate to the desirability of legislating patient protections (and otherwise imposing new regulations) on health plans for insured individuals. Unless and until universal coverage becomes politically fashionable again, it is far more important to consider how best to "regulate" the broadest possible participation of all elements of our health system in providing and financing this burden.

Notes

1. Winterbottom, C., Liska, D. W., and Obermaier, K. M. *State Level Databook on Health Care Access and Financing.* The Urban Institute, 1995, p. 18.
2. Ibid.
3. Sheils, J. F., and Alecxih, L.M.B. *Recent Trends in Employer Health Insurance Coverage and Benefits.* Unpublished study. The Lewin Group, p. 4.
4. Fronstin, P. *Sources of Health Insurance and Characteristics of the Uninsured.* Employee Benefit Research Institute, Nov. 1997, p. 22.
5. "Millions More Workers Will Be Priced Out of Insurance, Study Predicts." *American Hospital Association News,* February 23, 1998, as cited in The Lewin Group estimates (1998).
6. Fronstin, P. *Sources of Health Insurance,* p. 22.
7. Short, P. F., and Banthin, J. S. "New Estimates of the Underinsured Younger Than 65 Years." *Journal of the American Medical Association,* 1995, *274*(16), 1305–1306.
8. Ibid., p. 1306.
9. Blendon, R. J., and others. "Paying Medical Bills in the United States: Why Health Insurance Isn't Enough." *Journal of the American Medical Association,* 1994, *271*(12), 950.

10.   Congressional Budget Office. *Responses to Uncompensated Care and Public-Program Controls on Spending: Do Hospitals "Cost Shift?"* Washington, D.C.: Author, 1993; and Altman, S. H., and Guterman, S. "The Hidden U.S. Healthcare Safety Net: Will It Survive?" In S. H. Altman, U. E. Reinhardt, and A. E. Shields (eds.), *The Future of the U.S. Healthcare System: Who Will Care for the Poor and Uninsured?* Chicago: Health Administration Press, 1998, p. 174.

11.   Congressional Budget Office. *Responses to Uncompensated Care,* p. 35.

12.   Prospective Payment Assessment Commission. *Report and Recommendations to the Congress.* Washington, D.C.: Author, March 1, 1997, 18–19.

13.   Morrissey, M. A. *Hospital Cost Shifting, A Continuing Debate.* Washington, D.C.: Employee Benefit Research Institute, 1996, p. 12.

14.   American Hospital Association. *Uncompensated Hospital Care Cost Fact Sheet.* Chicago: Author, 1998, p. 3.

15.   Ibid.

16.   Altman, S. H., and Guterman, S. "The Hidden U.S. Healthcare Safety Net." p. 179.

17.   Mann, J. M., and others. "A Profile of Uncompensated Hospital Care, 1983–1995." *Health Affairs,* July–Aug. 1997, p. 228.

18.   Ibid.

19.   Reuter, J., and Gaskin, D. J. "The Role of Academic Health Centers and Teaching Hospitals in Providing Care for the Poor." In S. Altman, U. E. Reinhardt, and A. E. Shields (eds.), *The Future of the U.S. Healthcare System: Who Will Care for the Poor and Uninsured?* Chicago: Health Administration Press, 1998, p. 155.

20.   Mann, J. M., and others. "A Profile of Uncompensated Hospital Care, 1983–1995," p. 228.

21.   Data provided by the Association of American Medical Colleges from the AHCPR Nationwide Inpatient Sample.

22.   U.S. General Accounting Office. *Health Insurance Standards: New Federal Law Creates Challenges for Consumers, Insurers, Regulators.* Report to the Chairman, Committee on Labor & Human Resources, U.S. Senate. Washington, D.C.: Author, 1998, p. 8.

23.   Davis, K., and others. "Health Insurance: The Size and Scope of the Problem." *Inquiry,* 1995, *32,* p. 197.

24.   Fronstin, P. *Sources of Health Insurance,* p. 19.

25.   Cunningham, P. *Issue Brief on Next Steps in Incremental Health Insurance Expansions: Who Is Most Deserving?* Washington, D.C.: Center for Studying Health System Change, 1998, p. 2.

26.   Ibid., 3.

Managed Care Regulation in Practice

In this final section, we focus on the practical side of instituting regulatory reform. First we consider how a regulatory apparatus might be structured, then we review the structure that was recommended in California. Finally, we examine the cost of proposed managed care regulations and consider why there has been such a large variation among the different researchers who have estimated the costs.

In the first chapter, Phil Nudelman provides an overview of different models that could be employed in setting and enforcing standards. Observing the rapid change that has occurred in health markets and the proliferation of regulatory measures to deal with those changes, Nudelman recognizes the need for both consistent and enforceable standards. Indeed, he speaks of a "flexible regulation model for national enforceable standards." The challenge, as he sees it, is to ensure adequate protection of consumers without impeding the ability to innovate and improve quality, while at the same time being mindful of the cost. He considers a range of options balancing the responsibility of creating standards among public, quasi-public, and private bodies, with the responsibility of enforcement divided among the states, the federal government, and voluntary accreditation.

Sara Singer and Alain Enthoven report on the California Health Care Improvement Task Force. This task force was created by the governor of California in 1997 and issued a comprehensive report that included seventy-seven multipart recommendations. Similar to many of the previous authors, Singer and Enthoven describe an effort to balance market forces, industry self-regulation, and government regulation. Three areas in which government intervention is needed, they assert, are ensuring consumer protection, making markets work well, and subsidizing public goods. The California experience could provide a road map for other states that are considering regulatory reform.

The final chapter concerns the cost of health care regulation. In the fall of 1997, the President's Advisory Commission on Consumer Protection and Quality in the Health Care Industry asked the Lewin Group to assess the cost of a patients' bill of rights. Allen Dobson and Caroline Steinberg report on that effort and explain the difficulty of comparing widely varying cost estimates. They identify the differences in assumptions and interpretations employed by different estimators and highlight the importance of more precise language in the drafting of legislation. As policymakers consider regulatory reform in the future, accurate and independent estimates of the cost of regulation will be critical to the decision-making process.

Chapter Seventeen

Creating Standards

A Practical Approach

Phil Nudelman

America's medical care system is a work in progress. Historically, it has been characterized by little information about what worked and what did not, uninformed consumers, the delivery of much inappropriate care, and a lack of preventive care. But the system has undergone dramatic change in just a decade, driven in part by efforts to improve delivery systems and in response to rapid growth of costs. Change was needed to ensure that average people could continue to afford quality medical care and that government health care programs would not collapse.

With the growth of managed care, Americans have begun to experience the benefits of coordinated care. By integrating the financing and delivery of care, health plans are bringing together on the patient's behalf the frequently uncoordinated activities of a whole set of caregivers. Wellness and prevention have become priorities. There is recognition that higher quality can also mean reduced costs, and a questioning of the assumption that more care is always better. These changes have resulted in the provision of quality affordable care, the development of best practices, and the dissemination of unprecedented amounts of information to consumers.

Concerns Associated with Change

However, such significant change inevitably is associated with public concern and anxiety. Managed care imposes a new approach on health care delivery that is mystical to many and laden with new terminology. Accordingly, health plans have a responsibility to communicate better with consumers.

Concerns about declining consumer trust and confidence in managed care have led to an unprecedented push for greater regulation of health plans at both the state and federal levels. A patchwork of inconsistent and duplicative health plan standards has resulted. Many stand ready to build on this unsteady foundation in order to satisfy political goals, but such an approach does not further the goal of quality health care. Instead, it threatens to divert more resources from patient care to the implementation of duplicative and often-unnecessary regulations.

Fortunately, health care policymakers, in conjunction with consumers, employers, other purchasers, health care professionals, providers, and plans, have opened a dialogue to reevaluate the appropriate role of government in health care and determine the best course of action to address consumer concerns. These discussions consider the following questions:

- What is the relationship between regulation and quality?
- What standards are appropriate for federal adoption?
- What standards are more appropriate for state or voluntary adoption?
- What is the right balance between regulation and the promotion of an innovative, market-based system?
- How can we best promote competition in a regulated environment?
- Will added regulation improve the health status of Americans?
- Will added regulation improve consumer confidence in health care?

Consumer Satisfaction with Managed Care

It is useful to consider the context for the debate about health care regulation. Reviewing the recent evolution of managed care is key to establishing a perspective on consumer concerns.

Managed care enrollment growth has been dramatic. In 1996, 77 percent of active employees were enrolled in managed care organizations (including PPOs, POSs, HMOs), up from 52 percent in 1993[1]. Among retirees, 52 percent under age sixty-five were enrolled in managed care in 1996 as were 29 percent of retirees age sixty-five or older.[2] The rapid growth in enrollment can be attributed to the value HMOs provide for the premium, which includes accountability, comprehensive benefits, coordination of care, an emphasis on health promotion, and of course, lower costs. In 1996, employers with ten or more employees paid 15 percent less per active employee for HMO coverage than for traditional indemnity insurance.[3]

According to the American Association of Health Plans' (AAHP) annual national survey, virtually all HMOs covered unlimited hospital services—more than 65 percent of HMOs without any cost-sharing requirements such as copayments, coinsurance, or deductibles. With nominal copayment, HMOs also covered an unlimited number of primary care visits and preventive care such as well-baby care, prenatal care, well-child care, and childhood immunizations. In contrast, traditional indemnity coverage most often required enrollees to pay an average deductible of $538 per family and 20 percent of the cost of care. In addition, indemnity coverage usually has not covered preventive care.[4]

In general, consumers are satisfied with their managed care plans.[5] According to a National Research Corporation survey, members of HMOs, PPOs, and fee-for-service plans report similar satisfaction levels with their health plans whether they are in good-to-excellent or poor-to-fair health. For example, of respondents under age sixty-five who said they were in either poor or fair health, 79 percent of HMO members, 75 percent of PPO members, and 78 percent of fee-for-service members were satisfied.[6]

However, despite the overall satisfaction of most health plan enrollees with their care, too many consumers report experiencing problems with their health plans. In a survey taken by the 1997 Managed Health Care Improvement Task Force, appointed by Governor Pete Wilson and the California legislature, 42 percent of Californians had a "problem" with their health insurance last year.[7] At the same time 76 percent reported they were satisfied with their health plan.

Some people believe that many surveys are susceptible to misinterpretation by those who wish to attack managed care. Alain Enthoven, chair of the California Managed Health Care Improvement Task Force, has challenged journalists and politicians interpreting surveys on satisfaction with managed care to ask themselves the following questions: Were the "problems" serious? What is a reasonable standard of comparison? Was the problem created by the health plan or the doctor? Would the patient's complaint have been judged meritorious by an impartial panel of medical experts?[8]

Health Plans Address Anxieties

The rise in managed care enrollment has forced consumers to respond rapidly to a new system of care with its unfamiliar terminology: PCP, formulary, triage nurse, consulting nurse, benefits managers. The resulting confusion and anxiety sometimes erode patient confidence and create doubts. Unsure how to access care and lacking clarity on covered benefits, patients may perceive that choice of providers is constrained and question the incentives for the decisions providers make.

Some health plans have shown leadership by responding to consumer concerns in a variety of ways. Many have increased their investment in customer service by assigning a personal customer service agent to each enrollee or by introducing an ombudsman program. Others have developed point-of-service or preferred provider products.

Health plans also have taken a variety of actions to enhance consumer trust. Some have endorsed and committed to implement the Consumer Bill of Rights and Responsibilities (CBRR) developed by the President's Advisory Commission on Consumer Protection and Quality in the Health Care Industry. One employer, GTE, requested all of its health plan providers to implement the Bill of Rights on a voluntary basis. Kaiser Permanente, Group Health Cooperative of Puget Sound, and HIP Health Insurance Plans in partnership with Families USA and AARP developed and endorsed their own very similar Principles for Consumer Protection. In addition, the American Association of Health Plans developed the Putting Patients First program. All these initiatives advocate specific policies that promote high-quality care in a manner that meets the needs of individual patients.

Despite the efforts by health plans to be responsive to patient concerns, an environment fanned by the media, provider organizations, and politicians has been established in some quarters and resulted in a barrage of legislation at the state level. More than 182 state laws on managed care were passed in 1997, an increase from the 100 passed in 1996. At least nineteen states enacted comprehensive managed care laws in 1997.[9]

In addition, there have been efforts to review the impact of managed care in a more general sense and develop new frameworks for consumer protection. The California Managed Health Care Improvement Task Force—which is the subject of Chapter Eighteen—adopted more than sixty recommendations for both private-sector and regulatory solutions, including one that would create a new state entity for regulation of managed health care.

Differing Approaches to Regulation

A discussion of a variety of means for regulating managed care follows. Some of these methods are currently being employed, others are available for expanded roles for future models.

Expanded Federal Role

The federal government's role has been primarily as a major purchaser of health care. The Health Care Financing Administration developed and implemented many regulations for plans participating as federally qualified HMOs and for those participating in Medicare and Medicaid. The Office of Personnel Management and the Department of Defense likewise regulate health plans that participate in the Federal Employees Health Benefits Program (FEHBP) and Tricare, respectively.

In a recent State of the Union address, President Clinton called on Congress to enact standards for health plans to ensure that individuals have the right to know their medical options, the ability to choose the doctor they want, the access they need for emergency care, and the right of confidentiality. And in February 1998, he issued an executive memorandum requiring all health plans that participate in government contracts with the Health Care Financing Administration (HCFA) for Medicare and Medicaid, or the Office of Personnel Management (OPM) for FEHBP, or the Department of Defense (DoD) for Tricare, to comply substantially with the CBRR. As a public purchaser, the government can continue to use its current authority or request through the Congress expanded authority to regulate health plans that participate in government programs.

Recently, the role of the federal government in regulating plans has expanded. Congress has taken steps to address specific issues of national concern, including recent legislation on health insurance portability and accountability (COBRA and HIPAA), maternity length of stay, and mental health parity. These new laws address features of health plans that have traditionally been within the purview of the states. For example, the Health Insurance Portability and Accountability Act (HIPAA) provides for guaranteed issue, guaranteed renewability, portability of coverage, and health care market reforms—in specific situations.

Despite concerns about Congress legislating how medical care is provided and about duplicating state oversight responsibilities, a national approach could have important benefits. First, because national standards could reach all plans and consumers, they could serve to streamline regulation and provide greater consistency of protection for plans, consumers, and employers. Currently, such protections differ depending on geographic location, political jurisdiction, and type of plan. There are extensive compliance costs for plans that operate in multiple states and participate in federal programs and therefore must meet overlapping and redundant requirements.

State, Voluntary, and Public-Private Entities

Regulation of health plans has traditionally been a state function. Usually, both a state department of health and department of insurance play roles in ensuring that plans meet certain marketing, benefit, quality assurance, and financial standards. States vary in the extent to which they regulate plans. Although the National Association of Insurance Commissioners has developed model HMO acts, these have not been consistently adopted by states. A limitation of state regulation is that it applies only to state-regulated plans. Such regulation is preempted for self-insured plans offered by employers in accordance with provisions in the Employee Retirement Income Security Act of 1974 (ERISA).[10]

The private sector, led by employers and government purchasers, increasingly is encouraging standard setting for plans. More and more plans are voluntarily pursuing accreditation by independent entities such as NCQA and JCAHO to meet the needs of purchasers and to demonstrate quality to consumers. Standards set by such accrediting organizations will affect many plans, but some will not seek voluntary accreditation. Purchasers too have begun to set specific performance standards for plans, linking payments to the plans' ability to meet them.

National Regulatory Options

Several proposals for new health plan standards have been introduced in Congress recently. The Patient Access to Responsible Care Act (H.R. 1415, S. 644) proposes new standards in areas such as access, emergency care, choice, nondiscrimination, appeals, and remedies. Although this bill has a large number of cosponsors, it has engendered substantial opposition because of its potential adverse impact on the cost of health coverage.

The challenge for Congress as it considers possible legislation is how to ensure adequate protection for consumers while minimizing increases in costs. A decision to adopt additional federal legislative standards for health plans will have broad implications for the health care system and the nation. The approach must take into account health plans' need for flexibility in order to fulfill their role in achieving a higher-quality, more affordable health care system. Congress should not adopt standards in the name of consumer protection that impose unnecessary burdens on the health care system and impede the ability of health plans to innovate and improve quality. Further, Congress must consider the roles of states and accreditation entities in developing and enforcing standards and determine whether states should be preempted from further regulation in areas that have been addressed at the federal level.

Congress should give consideration to the following basic options for national standard setting:

- Set detailed standards, or delegate some of the details to federal agencies, such as HHS.

- Identify subject areas for standards and charter an independent entity to develop and make recommendations. Models include the National Academy of Science's Institute of Medicine (IOM) or the Financial Accounting Standards Board (FASB). Congress could have stand-by authority if the entity failed to meet its responsibilities.

Options for enforcing standards and encouraging compliance include the following:

- A federal agency or agencies could review and certify compliance and enforce standards among plans.
- State-regulated plans could be enforced through existing state regulatory authorities (a model adopted to implement HIPAA standards). Federal agencies such as Medicare, OPM, or the Department of Labor could have responsibility for enforcement of federal programs and self-insured plans to the extent that the standards are applicable to these plans. Congress could have stand-by authority to enforce standards if states failed to meet this responsibility.
- Congress could establish standards for voluntary compliance and denote complying plans as "federally recognized." Voluntary compliance could be encouraged with incentives, such as exemptions from conflicting regulation for federally recognized plans. A federally approved private accrediting organization, or state and federal agencies, could certify compliance. Plans receiving such certification would be deemed to meet federal standards.

Implementation and Need for Flexibility

There are trade-offs in each of these models and there are proponents and opponents of each approach. Evaluation of the models could include consideration of whether they:

- Ensure that standards are appropriately set, with input from key stakeholders
- Foster consumer trust
- Ensure accountability for health plans

- Streamline regulation of plans to promote greater consistency, lower costs, and efficient regulation
- Allow for continued flexibility and innovation in care delivery
- Promote cost-effective implementation, including reliance on existing state and private-sector expertise
- Promote incentives to comply rather than mandates to comply
- Improve or reduce access for the uninsured
- Enhance the environment for continuous quality improvement and innovation in the delivery of care and health outcomes

Approaches to Implementation

Given the nature of potential standards and the policy goals to be achieved, there may not be a one-size-fits-all approach to standard setting. It is likely that each standard should be handled differently depending on several factors:

- Importance of achieving national uniformity and consistency in consumer protection across jurisdictions and plans
- Importance of achieving efficiency and nonduplication in regulation of plans and systems
- Extent to which existing regulatory entities, such as those at the state level, are already performing oversight functions
- Degree of complexity of a standard, including the likelihood that it will continue to evolve and be refined, and the degree of expertise required to develop the standard
- Need to insulate standard setting from political influences

To contribute to the ongoing dialogue, and to allow for different points of view, the following paragraphs offer some themes for consideration in implementing a flexible regulatory model to achieve national enforceable standards.

Review of Proposed Standards

An independent entity could be established to consider potential national standards. It could determine whether a national standard is needed, analyze the potential costs and effects on health plans, and make recommendations about the appropriate development and enforcement mechanisms.

Core National Standards

For the small number of important issues that require enforceable, consistent national standards, Congress could explicitly define them (such as the "prudent layperson" standard for emergency care). For topics that are complex, likely to evolve, and require specific expertise to set standards (such as performance measurement), development could be delegated to an independent body similar to an IOM or FASB entity.

Enforcement would be through the states for state-regulated plans, through the Department of Labor (if self-insured plans are subject to the standards), and through the HCFA for Medicare and Medicaid, OPM for FEHBP, and DoD for Tricare.

A subset of these standards (such as performance measurement) could be enforced by a single federal agency to ensure consistent and uniform application of complex standards. Plans could voluntarily seek accreditation through federally approved accrediting organizations. If accredited, they would be deemed to meet the core standards. Conflicting state regulation in these areas would be preempted.

Incentives to Comply with National Standards

Congress could identify subject areas for voluntary standards and could either set the standards or delegate this task to chartered independent entities. If adopted by federal programs such as Medicare or FEHBP, the standards would become conditions of participation for plans that contract with these entities. State and federal entities could certify compliance with these voluntary standards or a federally approved accrediting organization could do so. Plans adopting the standards would be exempted from conflicting state standards in the same subject areas.

Regardless of what actions, if any, are taken—and whether they are private or public, voluntary or regulatory—they must be geared toward continuous quality improvement on behalf of all patients.

As debate continues about various options, the overall guiding aim for the work of all stakeholders should be to continuously reduce the impact and burden of illness, injury, and disability and to improve the health and functional status of the people of the United States.

As we enter a new era in health care—one in which performance measurement and outcomes research will be critical to providing high-quality, evidence-based care regardless of ability to pay—health plans are rising to meet new challenges. By continuing to explore the important questions of consumer protection and health plan standards, health plans in partnership with consumers, providers, and purchasers are at the forefront of efforts to ensure that all Americans have access to accountable, affordable, patient-centered care.

Notes

1. Foster Higgins National Survey of Employer-Sponsored Health Plans, 1997, p. 9.
2. Ibid., p. 41 (tables).
3. Foster Higgins National Survey of Employer-Sponsored Health Plans, 1996.
4. American Association of Health Plans, 1996 national survey.
5. California Managed Health Care Improvement Task Force Survey.
6. National Research Corporation. *Healthcare Market Guide VI.* Lincoln, Neb.: Author, 1996.
7. California Managed Health Care Improvement Task Force Survey.
8. Enthoven, A., chair of the California Managed Health Care Improvement Task Force, in letter to California Governor Pete Wilson, president pro tempore, speaker, and members of the California legislature, January 6, 1998.
9. "Are HMOs the Right Prescription?" *U.S. News and World Report,* October 13, 1997, p. 63.
10. KPMG Peat Marwick. *Health Benefits in 1996.* Arlington, Va.: Author, 1997, p. 4.

Chapter Eighteen

California's Struggle with Regulation

Sara J. Singer and Alain C. Enthoven

Government regulation is one of several tools for making the health care system function effectively to ensure high-quality, cost-effective care. Market forces that include purchaser and competitor initiatives—driven by consumer preferences based on information and appropriate incentives—also regulate health care, as does the industry itself through self-regulation. Just as government should not be the only regulator of the health care industry, complete reliance on the free market for the distribution of health care is also inappropriate. Health care is far too complex for such an approach, and furthermore, for the needy to do without health care is morally unacceptable. To enable the market to achieve a tolerable result requires significant government regulation.

In California, regulation by government, the market, and the industry are all at work. In April 1997, then-governor Pete Wilson instructed members of the California Managed Health Care Improvement Task Force that their mission was to improve the state's largely market-driven and managed care-based health care system.

The authors' work on this chapter and on the California Managed Health Care Improvement Task Force was supported by a grant from the California Health-Care Foundation. We would like to gratefully acknowledge Maureen O'Haren, executive vice president, Legislative Affairs, California Association of Health Plans, for her assistance in the description of current California law.

To do so, the task force recommended the use of all available tools for improvement—each where it is most effective—to achieve an optimal balance among them.

As this chapter discusses in some detail, the result was seventy-seven multipart recommendations directed at state and federal government, industry, and the market. Building on a substantial base of existing public and private regulation, the recommendations were aimed at enhancing the balance among these regulatory forces.

Success of Market Forces

Although our society supports government intervention and litigation where necessary, in general we look to the market, made up of responsible purchasers and competing sellers, to allocate resources efficiently. We associate competition with quality improvement, customer service, cost reduction, and desirable innovation.

In California, cost reduction has been the most evident success of market forces in health care so far. Since 1992, premiums for large purchasers and purchasing groups in the state have been constant as a result of competition and the shift to managed care. For example, the 1997 California Public Employees Retirement System (CalPERS) premiums were about the same in dollars as they were in 1992 for essentially the same standard benefit package, and when adjusted for inflation they were down about 13 percent. If 1987 to 1992 trends had continued to 1997, CalPERS premiums would now be more than twice what they are, at a cost to employees or taxpayers of $1.5 billion per year, or $4,300 per employee. Most other large California employment groups have experienced similar savings. Of course, continued savings are not assured, and many are predicting that premiums will again increase.[1,2] Kaiser Permanente announced premium increases of up to 11 percent for 1999.[3]

Large buyers and purchasing groups, both public and private, are able to use their substantial expertise and negotiating power to deal effectively with some of the important concerns in our health care system. Certainly, government is a major purchaser of health care coverage and should use its ability to influence the market. In 1995, government paid for 46 percent of health care services in the United States, so its purchasing power, as well as its obligation to beneficiaries and taxpayers, is great. About 3.65 million Californians are enrolled in Medicare, of whom some 40 percent were members of HMOs in 1994.[4] About 5 million are in Medi-Cal, of whom 23 percent were in HMOs in 1995.[5] In addition, the state created the Health Insurance Plan of California (HIPC) to improve the market for small employment groups in the private sector, and Healthy Families, which offers choices through a purchasing group, with federal support, to cover children of low-income families.

Well-organized, large purchasers have significant tools to make the market work better for consumers—tools that they have used only to a limited degree so far. The list includes the following:

- Creating equitable rules within which health plans must compete
- Expanding multiple choice of plan at the individual level
- Providing an incentive for employees to seek and for health plans to offer value
- Demanding new products and product innovations
- Obtaining and publishing quality-related information that consumers can use to make better decisions and clinical providers can use to improve their medical results
- Risk-adjusting premiums so that plans and providers have financial incentives to enroll and develop expertise in caring for even the most sick among us, reducing risk-skimming behavior

The California Managed Health Care Improvement Task Force made a number of recommendations to purchasers and competitors to encourage them to make the market function more efficiently. First, the task force recommended that more employers voluntarily offer individual choice of health plans. Such choice is important both because it makes plans compete at the individual level and because it minimizes the number of people who cannot get to the doctors they prefer. The latter problem is less troubling because most people who are offered only one plan are offered a plan with a nonnetwork component that allows members to seek care from nonnetwork providers at some additional expense.[6] However, this appears to be less true in California, where employers offering only one plan are more than twice as likely to offer a closed-network HMO.[7] When the task force surveyed Californians, it found that 25 percent of consumers in California who knew the number of choices they were offered directly (and indirectly through their spouses) reported that they had only one plan option.[8]

To ensure that individuals can access the doctors they prefer, the task force recommended that stakeholders convene to examine ways of increasing choice of providers on a cost-neutral basis. The task force also considered requiring employers to offer individual choice. However, to compel choices at the state level would require changing the federal preemption of state law under the Employee Retirement Income Security Act of 1974 (ERISA). In addition, task force members were legitimately concerned that as long as employer-sponsored insurance remains voluntary, compelling individual choice may reduce the willingness of employers, especially small ones, to offer coverage.

To provide an incentive for employees to seek and health plans to offer value, the task force recommended that stakeholders collaborate to design standard reference packages against which plans could be required to compare their products to facilitate consumer understanding. And it encouraged employers' to include health benefits as a separate line item on employees' pay stubs to increase their awareness of the proportion of compensation represented by health benefits.

There is a great deal of work ongoing to develop useful quality information in the private sector. In California, the Pacific Business Group on Health (PBGH) is leading an effort involving plans, providers, and purchasers to develop standardized eligibility, enrollment, and encounter data. To foster such efforts and the publication of quality-related data, the task force recommended that the California state government coordinate its information-collection efforts with the private sector.

To minimize incentives for risk selection, the task force also recommended that large public and private purchasers work toward risk adjustment of premiums and, when feasible, payments to providers. This would build on the example of the HIPC, which implemented premium risk adjustment in 1996, and ideally would involve a large enough share of the health plans' members to affect their practices.

Industry Self-Regulation

In California and elsewhere, the HMO industry needs public confidence. On its own initiative or in response to problems identified by employers, consumers, and regulators, the industry ought to develop improved standards for consumer protection. There is a history of such self-regulation, for example, in the securities industry and in the accounting profession; the Financial Accounting Standards Board is a private, profession-sponsored organization whose findings are usually ratified by the Securities and Exchange Commission.

The health care industry has taken some initiative to self-regulate, and these efforts may help create new standards for industry practice.[9] However, until the health insurance market makes progress toward risk adjustment of premiums, the industry's incentive to self-regulate will, in part, be influenced by the competitive necessity to engage in some degree of skimming the healthy and avoiding the sick.

The task force directed a number of its recommendations to industry participants, including the following:

- Transition away from prior authorization and concurrent review by making greater use of provider precredentialing, practice guidelines, clinical pathways, retrospective review, and outcomes-based data in utilization monitoring.
- Assess compensation arrangements to identify best and poor practices and influence industry practice and to recommend any necessary changes in regulatory oversight.
- Develop consistent mandatory standards for dispute resolution processes across health plans so patients who complain will receive full explanations for decisions no matter which plan they join and access to an expert, independent third-party review in cases related to questions of medical necessity, appropriateness, and experimental treatment.

In several areas, task force recommendations call for new legislation. These are all issues that the industry could and should address on its own but for which legislation may be necessary in the absence of industry response to consumer and purchaser demands.

For example, to ensure that patients who are undergoing treatment are not forced to change physicians suddenly, the task force recommended that in cases of involuntary plan changes health plans and medical groups should be required to provide continuity with health care practitioners through a course of treatment, up to a maximum of ninety days, or safe transfer of the patient. Similarly, it recommended that plans should be required to ensure continued receipt of a drug removed from a formulary, as long as the doctor continues to prescribe it, for an ongoing condition, so no patient will be forced to change drugs. The task force also proposed a requirement to assure patients standing referrals to specialists for chronic conditions or for a complete course of treatment. Finally, it recommended that plans be required to do much more to involve consumers in plan governance and design of their practices.

In each of these areas, the industry could go further than the task force recommendations to satisfy consumer demand and ensure the good health of their enrollees. For example, in an effort to provide continuity of care following termination of the provider contract, the task force recommended a mandated ninety-day window for patients undergoing treatment. In comparison, CalPERS requested that participating health plans establish contracts with medical groups and independent practice associations to provide eighteen months of continuity for enrollees in the event of contract termination. Compliance so far with their request has been minimal.[10]

Why Markets Fail

Although health insurance markets in California and other states work better today than they did several years ago, particularly for large employers and purchasing groups, and although implementation of the task force recommendations are likely to cause further improvement, markets are still prone to failure. Even large purchasers have not been able to get the kinds of cost reductions and quality and service performance increases they believe are possible.

Free markets inevitably fail, for example, to generate sufficient quantities of public goods. Special characteristics of health care and health insurance also cause the market to fail, including the following:

- The incentive effects of health insurance undermine cost-consciousness (moral hazard).
- Uninsurance is a result of unaffordability, unavailability, and free-riding by those who forego coverage and take advantage of the safety net. For example, a healthy young adult with low expected medical expenditures might choose not to purchase insurance because the combination of moral hazard, pooling with people with higher expected medical expenditures, mandated benefits, administrative costs, and profit make his premiums far exceed his likely medical expenses.
- Information is very expensive and asymmetrical (doctors know important information patients do not have and vice versa).
- Definitions in medical insurance contracts are complex and often lacking.
- Enforced standards are lacking.
- Competition is lacking among delivery systems when multiple health plans contract with nearly identical provider networks.
- Wide variation in medical risks (which creates incentives for insurers to avoid people who are likely to need costly medical care) makes pooling difficult.

Finally, in the California market and elsewhere, two important reasons why purchasers and health plans are not better serving covered employees are lack of relevant information to evaluate quality for providers, purchasers, payers, and consumers, and lack of choice for many consumers who are not covered through large employers or pools.

Because health care has a special moral status, market failures that leave people without necessary care are unacceptable—and therefore reliance on the market and industry alone is insufficient. In a sense, universal access to necessary health care is a public good. Collective action at some level is needed to make the market work with tolerable efficiency and to make access and coverage widespread. However, when seeking an appropriate regulatory balance, it is important to keep in mind that even if collective action could fix all existing market failures, some people would still be dissatisfied with the outcome, especially because of limitations of medical technology. This would be true in any system. In addition, there will continue to be normal human error. Also, expectations will continue to be extremely high as long as insurance shields its beneficiaries from paying personally for what they demand.

Government Role in Consumer Protection

Government intervention is required in several areas because purchasers, competitors, and the industry cannot or do not satisfy desired goals. Some of the essential roles of government include consumer protection, helping the market work well, and subsidizing public goods. In California, significant regulation in these areas already exists, and the task force called for substantially more.

One of the most fundamental tasks of government is to create the conditions for markets to serve consumers effectively. Well-conceived rules can help markets work better and increase satisfaction all around. For example, the rule that permits airlines to overbook and then auction vouchers to induce volunteers to take later flights creates a "win-win" situation.

Health insurance contracts are extremely complex and hard to understand. Terminology is imprecise, and it is impossible to provide for every eventuality. So special arrangements are needed to ensure that patients are treated fairly. In the area of health and safety, consumers need special government protection because when they get sick they are unable to "shop" for themselves as they would for other goods in the marketplace. Advocacy groups for the poor and disenfranchised are natural allies in the government's efforts to protect health care consumers; regulators should view them as such.

Substantial Existing Regulation

Government has been active in defining and securing patients' rights under health care coverage contracts. The California legislature has instituted regulation of health care coverage through two major bodies of law, which are enforced by two governmental departments. The Insurance Code provides a regulatory framework for indemnity insurers and preferred provider organizations and is enforced by the Department of Insurance (DoI). The Knox-Keene Health Care Service Plan Act of 1975, a portion of the Health and Safety Code, governs health care service plans and is enforced by the Department of Corporations (DoC). These two bodies of law, which contain many similar provisions, provide consumer protections through financial standards, contractual requirements, quality assurance programs, required grievance and appeals processes, oversight of soliciting and marketing practices, and mandatory basic benefits.

In particular, the Knox-Keene Act contains numerous, specific, consumer protection requirements. For example, it requires health plans to file extensive documentation on their proposed delivery systems prior to licensure as well as quarterly and annually thereafter to ensure that they can provide sufficient quality assurance, recourse through grievance and appeals processes, continuity of care, and access to providers. Plans also undergo regular financial audits and may be placed under closer examination if their financial reports indicate danger of insolvency.

The Knox-Keene Act also contains extensive requirements in the areas of consumer protection relating to patient care. It requires all health plans to have grievance and appeals processes that allow enrollees to submit disputes to the plan and receive a timely response, including expedited review of grievances involving serious conditions. The act also allows enrollees to seek assistance from the DoC if they are unsatisfied with the health plan's response. When a plan denies coverage for care, it must disclose to patients and providers the criteria or clinical basis for the decision upon request. The act also contains an outside, independent review process for terminally ill patients who have been denied coverage for experimental treatments. Finally, the act prohibits unethical marketing and solicitation practices, such as using statements in advertising that are false, deceptive, or misleading. All advertising and marketing materials must be submitted to the DoC for review prior to use.

Improving the Dispute-Resolution Process

Adding to such existing regulation, the task force made a series of recommendations to expand consumer protections by improving the dispute-resolution process. They address nonurgent and urgent timing requirements, periods of limitation, communication of processes and examples of appeals, the ability of consumers to appear in person at grievance hearings, full and complete explanations of grievance and appeals decisions, common standards for collecting information about complaints by health plans, periodic public reports of complaints made to both health plans and the state regulatory agency, and a single phone number for consumers to reach all state health regulatory agencies.

Further, the task force recommended that consumers receive a bill of rights and responsibilities on enrollment, as well as adequate information upon a denial or grievance incident, about next steps, explanations, and opportunity for a qualified, plan-paid second opinion. Also, it advocated that health plans be required to establish arbitration standards that provide for expeditious resolution, including rapid selection or default appointment of neutral arbitrators and a written opinion to accompany an award (excluding confidential information) made available to the public upon request, and that prohibit a plan that has engaged in willful misconduct from requiring a party to continue in arbitration.

The task force considered but declined to support a recommendation to expand tort liability of HMOs contributing to medical decisions—a recommendation that would have required both state law and a federal amendment to ERISA to be effective. The measure narrowly failed after task force members voted to strike out reference to current California malpractice award limits intended to avoid creating incentives for costly lawsuits. Opponents of an expansion of the tort system objected because it would be a costly and counterproductive way of dealing with medical injuries, which are common in any system.[11] In fact, fear of tort liability is a major impediment to quality improvement in medicine and a destructive force attacking the doctor-patient relationship, which must be based on trust. The threat of malpractice induces "defensive medicine" that raises costs without benefiting patients.[12] Unlimited tort liability may also induce "defensive utilization management," causing health expenditures to soar again with very destructive consequences, including pricing coverage out of reach for even more families of moderate means. Finally, the tort system is a poor method for compensating the injured. (Most of the malpractice premium dollar goes to lawyers and insurance companies to pay the cost of litigation—about 30 percent each—and only about 40 percent goes to patients. The Harvard study on medical malpractice found sixteen times as many patients were injured as received compensation.)

Requirements for Insurance Contracts

The complexity of health insurance contracts necessitates special rules to ensure there is a meeting of minds between buyers and sellers and that what is being sold is what is being delivered. Such rules and processes should lead to the reasonable expectations of reasonable persons being met.

The Knox-Keene Act and its underlying regulations, which govern HMOs in California, sets comprehensive standards for the contracts between health plans and consumers. All contracts between plans and enrollees, plans and employers, and plans and providers must be filed with the DoC for review and approval, and must meet a statutory "fair and reasonable" requirement. Some requirements are spelled out specifically. For example, health plans must cover all medically necessary basic health care services as defined by law, including emergency care in accordance with a "prudent layperson" standard. In addition, statutory mandates apply to specific services—such as preventive care for children and reconstructive surgery and prosthetics for mastectomy patients—which are not subject to negotiation and must be provided in any benefit package. In addition, numerous mandates require plans to offer to employers the opportunity to purchase coverage for services such as acupuncture and infertility procedures. The act sets out specific disclosure requirements pertaining to these benefit mandates, as well as other disclosures regarding exclusions, limitations and co-payments, and physician payment arrangements.

The Knox-Keene Act also protects consumers in ways that help expand access to coverage. It prohibits the use of genetic information in underwriting so individuals with genetic predispositions to certain diseases cannot be denied coverage simply because of that predisposition. And the act prohibits plans from denying coverage or services to individuals for any of a long litany of health status, demographic, and socioeconomic characteristics.

The task force recommendations would add to the existing list of contract requirements by allowing women direct access to their reproductive health care providers in a manner that permits and encourages coordination and integration of services. Coordination of care is a very important component of this recommendation, which intends that primary care physicians and obstetrician-gynecologists be partners or agree to work together to inform the patient about which problems should be taken to which doctor, and to share records.

Further, the task force recommended that plans be required to disclose significant additional information, including a standard product description to facilitate direct comparison of plans by consumers, up-to-date and specific information on provider access, information on referral patterns to specialty centers, and plans' or medical groups' written treatment guidelines or authorization criteria. Health plans would also be required to disclose the scope and general methods and incentives paid to contracting provider groups, and health plans, provider groups, and health practitioners would be required to disclose the specific methods of compensation they paid or received upon request.

Quality Standards and Innovation

Regulators and large purchasers, the task force believes, should generally focus on managed care deliverables rather than the delivery process, in order to preserve maximum opportunity for efficiency-improving innovation. However, broad standards of operation are not inappropriate. Legislation that attempts to address care delivery specifically inevitably fails to account for technological innovation and process improvement, freezing into place current practice.

The Knox-Keene Act requires that every health plan have in place a quality assurance program that is designed to review continuously the quality of care provided, review problems and complaints, and design corrective action plans that prevent problems health planwide. In addition, plans undergo a medical audit every three years to determine whether they are meeting the requirements of the law regarding quality assurance as well as access to care, continuity of care, and provision of benefits. These audits include examinations of patient records and documents from quality assurance committee meetings to ensure that problems have been corrected in a systematic way.

The Knox-Keene Act also prohibits any contractual requirements that would inhibit a provider from discussing treatment options with his or her patient and also prohibits incentive arrangements that would induce the delay, denial, or reduction of medically necessary and appropriate care. State law prohibits any termination or disciplinary action against a provider for advocating appropriate health care on behalf of a patient. The Knox-Keene Act and its underlying regulations also require that medical decision making be separated from fiscal and administrative functions so that these functions do not hinder the medical decision-making process. When a claim is denied for clinical reasons and appealed, for example, it must be reviewed by a licensed professional with competency in the clinical area in question. Individuals who are hired to review claims may not be compensated on the basis of the number of claims denied or the dollar amount of the claims involved. These provisions of the act are designed to ban inappropriate financial incentives that may lead to inappropriate denials.

The task force added to this long list of quality standards by recommending that so-called nuclear capitation be prohibited. There was relative consensus that capitation of one physician for the substantial cost of referrals for that physician's patients would create too intense an incentive to be safe.[13] In addition, where incentives for individuals or small medical groups are tied to the substantial cost of referrals and where small groups are capitated for the substantial cost of referrals, these compensation arrangements should be more carefully scrutinized. Plans would be required to ensure the use of stop-loss, sufficient reserves, or other verifiable mechanisms for protecting against losses due to adverse selection for practitioners at "substantial financial risk." However, the more powerful recommendations regarding physician compensation are likely to be those related to disclosure. These are intended not only to give consumers peace of mind because they can request information about any physician's specific compensation methods but also to eliminate less desirable compensation arrangements through greater public visibility.

Government Role in Making the Market Work Well

In a system that is based on voluntary insurance, with a large proportion made up of individuals and small groups, government action is needed to require or encourage the healthy to subsidize the sick. Three main ways in which this is done in our society are public programs supported by taxes such as Medicare and Medicaid; employment-based health insurance (motivated by incentives in the exclusion of employer-paid health insurance from taxable incomes of employees); and state laws limiting the variation in small group premiums.

Pooling Risks

If everyone could obtain coverage through a large employer or purchasing group that organized and managed a choice of health coverage options for group members, the market would be likely to provide a satisfactory result. However, much of the population works for small employers, works part-time, is self-employed or unemployed, and therefore does not have access to purchasing groups. Because small groups of healthy people, like individuals, prefer not to subsidize the costs of small groups that include sick or high-risk individuals, it is difficult to pool small groups on a purely voluntary basis. Although there are more people in purchasing groups in California than in other states, purchasing groups are not currently growing and forming rapidly enough to provide access for everyone in the foreseeable future.

State and private entities have attempted to form purchasing groups, but so far they have experienced limited growth. In 1993, California passed legislation creating a purchasing pool for small businesses—the HIPC. The same legislation set a narrow range around a health insurer's average premium within which it may price its premiums in the small group market. And it required guaranteed issue and renewal and allowed for the creation of two standardized benefit packages so that small employers and their employees could better compare each plan. This legislation solved some of the difficulties small employers were facing in obtaining affordable coverage. In 1996, the California lawmakers passed legislation that created a statutory framework for the creation of purchasing pools. In addition, to induce the formation and expansion of purchasing groups, the task force recommended an expansion of existing small group reforms to the fifty-one-to-one-hundred-employee market.

Enabling Comparative Information

Government action is likely to be needed to secure the timely production of accurate quality-related data and health plan performance results that consumers and purchasers need to make well-informed decisions. California's health plans and medical groups have cooperated voluntarily in the collection and reporting of the Health Plan Employer Data and Information Set (HEDIS) and other information without government intervention; still, data needed for risk-adjusted medical outcomes studies by hospitals, health plans, and providers in California are lagging behind other states.

Currently in California, collection of information from hospitals and other health facilities requires that individual data elements be specified in law. To facilitate the government's role in the collection of data for comparison of medical outcomes for particular conditions, the task force recommended enabling the relevant state agency to require specific reporting elements *without* legislation, upon the advice of an advisory group. The task force also suggested that the public and private sectors coordinate information collection efforts.

Preventing Entry Barriers

It is important to be sure that government does not inadvertently create artificial barriers to market entry by new health plans. For instance, the time and cost for Department of Corporations approval of a new Knox-Keene license have been reported to be very substantial, and its requirement for contiguous expansion makes growth more difficult for new health plans. Such requirements lead some to seek less onerous regulation under the Department of Insurance because ultimately consumers pay for entry barriers through fewer choices and higher costs.

The task force made several recommendations for streamlining specific aspects of existing government regulation. Most significant were proposals to eliminate audit redundancy by giving medical groups the option to submit to one periodic solvency audit and one quality audit conducted by authorized auditors, rather than one for each plan as currently required. This will save time and money for everyone involved.

Subsidizing Public Goods

Public goods are goods that benefit everyone and from which no one can be excluded. Public goods, like national defense, would be underproduced in a purely private market. In health care, government has a central role in subsidizing the public goods of education, research, care for the poor and uninsured, public health initiatives such as epidemic control, and information (for example, hospital reporting to support risk-adjusted measures of outcome) that are not adequately provided for in the private market.

Large government subsidies for health care services flow to individuals through Medicaid and Medicare. In California, the state provides Medi-Cal coverage to 5.4 million recipients. In addition, the state provides subsidies for health care by sponsoring programs such as the Major Risk Medical Insurance Program, Access for Infants and Mothers Program, and as of 1997, Healthy Families.

The task force determined that engaging in significant deliberations regarding the problems posed by the large and growing numbers of uninsured in California was out of the scope of its mandate. However, members did agree that the number of uninsured Californians is an issue that needs to be addressed and that managed care has implications for the current systems that care for the uninsured. They also strongly encouraged the governor, the legislature, and private-sector groups to address the issue of the large number of uninsured Californians.

Inappropriate Role for Government

As the government knows little of the complexities of medical organization it should, in general, not mandate its details. Government should not attempt to micromanage medical care through legislation, such as by prescribing lengths of hospital stay or appropriateness of outpatient surgery, unless practices clearly threaten health and safety. When governments do get into these areas, they are likely to do several things: create vested interests that resist change, make unsound medical judgments, lose sight of costs, unfairly impose some people's preferences on others, protect providers rather than patients, and cause employers to retreat to self-funded plans protected from state regulation by ERISA. These are good reasons for government to stay out of regulation of the details.

Any evaluation of proposed consumer protections should include the following criteria. First, one should be reasonably sure the problem or abuse actually exists in practice and is not merely hypothetical or an aberration. Second, because workers and taxpayers and not health plans will ultimately bear the costs, the benefits of the proposed protection should outweigh the costs. Third, one should be sure that what is being proposed is consumer protection and not provider protection masquerading as consumer protection. And fourth, if the market is likely to solve the problem in a reasonable period of time, it should be left to do so.

The state of California has enacted its share of laws that would not pass an evaluation based on these criteria. In 1997, then-governor Wilson added one law to this list when he signed a bill to conform California law to federal law that prohibits health plans from restricting coverage for normal vaginal delivery to less than forty-eight hours.[14]

In some cases, there may be good reason for violating these guidelines. In the current highly charged, negative environment in which HMOs operate in California, the task force, for example, thought it appropriate to prohibit "nuclear capitation" without any evidence to support the existence of such practices. Similarly, California and other states imposed laws banning "gag clauses." Later, the U.S. General Accounting Office published a study finding no such gag clauses in HMO contracts.[15] One could argue that, without evidence, such laws are unnecessary. However, by prohibiting such clearly undesirable practices, alarm about them can be diffused, and discussion can be redirected to more productive topics.

Implementation of legislation, through regulation, can also be appropriate or inappropriate to the task. Regulators often have significant power and flexibility over an industry and its participants. So far in California, the Department of Corporations has regulated the HMO industry. This was appropriate when HMOs were few but has become increasingly less so as the industry has grown to the largest in the state, now covering well over half of all Californians. The regulatory structure it imposes was primarily designed in 1975 when the original Knox-Keene Act was passed, and the industry has evolved significantly since then. Given the size, the complexity, and the degree of public interest in managed care, the task force recommended the creation of a new regulatory agency, one devoted specifically to managed care organizations, whose leadership would have the expertise and vision necessary for effective regulation.

As we have seen, government need not and should not attempt to regulate the health care industry alone. Neither should a completely free market be left to distribute health care; because of market failures, it cannot do so in a morally acceptable way. But the market, made up of purchasers and competitors, the industry, and government together can structure an appropriate set of incentives that will create accessible, quality health care for consumers.

Notes

1. Pear, R. "Business Coalition to Fight Legislation Protecting Patients' Rights." *The New York Times,* January 21, 1998, p. A18.
2. Freudenheim, M. "Progress on Health Costs, But Nagging Woes Persist." *The New York Times,* January 5, 1998, p. D10.
3. Sinton, P., and Russell, S. "Kaiser Raising Rates Up to 11 Percent." *San Francisco Chronicle,* March 31, 1998, p. D1.
4. "Medicare and Medicaid Statistical Supplement" (Table 21). *Health Care Financing Review,* 1997, pp. 56–58.
5. California Department of Health Services, Managed Care Division, 1997.
6. According to a study by the Barents Group, 86 percent of workers who are offered one plan only are offered a plan with a nonnetwork component. Barents Group. "Health Care Choices." Report commissioned by American Association of Health Plans, December 1997.
7. California Managed Health Care Improvement Task Force. "Expanding Consumer Choice: Background Paper." Sacramento, Calif.: Author, 1998. Data for 1996 were provided by KPMG Peat Marwick, Tysons Corner, Va., 1997.
8. California Managed Health Care Improvement Task Force. "Public Perceptions and Experiences with Managed Care: Background Paper." Sacramento, Calif.: Author, 1998.

9.   See for example, Patients First, sponsored by the American Associ-
     ation of Health Plans (1997), and Principles for Consumer Protec-
     tion, proposed by a cooperative group consisting of the American
     Association of Retired Persons, Families USA, and several nonprofit
     HMOs (1997).
10. California Managed Health Care Improvement Task Force. "Physi-
     cian-Patient Relationship: Background Paper." Sacramento, Calif.:
     Author, 1998.
11. Harvard Medical Practice Study to the State of New York. *Patients,
     Doctors, and Lawyers: Medical Injury, Malpractice Litigation, and Patient
     Compensation in New York,* 1990. This study examined hospital care
     in New York in 1984 (when managed care was minimal there) and
     estimated that in that year there were 98,609 cases of unintended
     injuries caused by medical management. Of these, 27,179 cases were
     due to negligence. The deaths of 14 percent of the injured patients,
     or 13,805, were at least in part a result of their adverse event, and
     about 2,500 cases of permanent total disability resulted from med-
     ical injury.
12. Kessler, D., and McClellan, M. "Do Doctors Practice Defensive Med-
     icine?" *Quarterly Journal of Economics,* May 1996, pp. 353–390. This
     study analyzed "the effects of malpractice liability reforms using data
     on all elderly Medicare beneficiaries treated for serious heart dis-
     ease in 1984, 1987, and 1990. [They found] that malpractice reforms
     that directly reduce provider liability pressure lead to reductions of
     5 to 9 percent in medical expenditures without substantial effects
     on mortality or medical complications."
13. California Managed Health Care Improvement Task Force. "Finan-
     cial Incentives for Providers in Managed Care Plans: Background
     Paper." Sacramento, Calif.: Author, 1998.
14. A.B. 38, Figueroa, Newborns' and Mothers' Health Act of 1997, now
     part of the California Health and Safety Code, section 1367.62, and
     the California Insurance Code, section 10123.87.
15. U.S. General Accounting Office. *Managed Care: Explicit Gag Clauses
     Not Found in HMO Contracts, But Physician Concerns Remain.* HEHS
     publication no. 97–175. Washington, D.C.: Author, 1997. The study
     found that out of 529 HMOs none used contract clauses that specif-
     ically restricted physicians from discussing all appropriate medical
     options with their patients.

Chapter Nineteen

The Cost of Regulation
How the Estimates Vary
Allen Dobson and Caroline Steinberg

Much of the impetus for President Clinton's health care reform initiative derived from national attention on costs spiraling out of control and resultant fears about security of coverage. Today, with the strong economy mitigating concerns about loss of coverage, it is not surprising that national attention has turned away from coverage and systemic health care reform toward issues of quality and access.

Although managed care has largely been credited with temporarily bringing health care inflation under control, the processes of managing care are in conflict with a culture used to unlimited freedom of choice among providers and an inviolate physician-patient relationship. In the quest for lower costs and increased profits, some managed care organizations are perceived as having gone too far in limiting access and utilization. This perception is reinforced by anecdotal reports of the most egregious incidents of denial of care and coverage, which have become a mainstay of news coverage in both the national and the local press. As a result, managed care plans have become a lightning rod for criticism.

In response to highly publicized issues and concerns, both the executive and legislative branches of the federal government have developed proposals, and a majority of states have passed legislation on one or more issues of consumer protection. In March 1997, President Clinton established the President's Advisory Commission on Consumer Protection and Quality in the Health Care

Industry. This group, broadly representative of providers, insurers, employers, and consumers, drafted a Consumer Bill of Rights and Responsibilities (CBRR), which was enthusiastically endorsed by the president and subsequently applied to federal programs. Other bills have been introduced in Congress, each containing a different set of consumer protections. The Patient Access to Responsible Care Act (PARCA) and the Patients' Bill of Rights Act of 1998 (PBRA) both offer many of the protections outlined in the CBRR.

The Debate About Costs

In the fall of 1997 the President's Advisory Commission asked The Lewin Group to determine the costs and benefits of information disclosure and external appeals as they pertain to CBRR. Our findings were highly controversial because studies conducted by other groups produced results that on face value were twenty to forty times greater than ours. The 1998 Princeton conference made clear the utility of an analysis of cost estimates both to inform policymakers on this issue and, more generally, to understand cost-building methodology. How can cost estimates presumably reflecting the same set of policies vary so dramatically? Such differences are highly confusing to the press, to legislators, and to others attempting to keep abreast of the debate.

The issue of consumer protection cost estimates is hotly debated. Consumer and provider groups are largely in favor of consumer protections and argue that if sensibly implemented, resulting costs would be minimal. Business and insurance groups, however, claim that consumer protections, if legislated, would result in a significant increase in the cost of insurance. This cost increase, they assert, would cause employers to drop coverage and thereby result in greater numbers of uninsured. Groups on both sides of the issue cite studies of the cost impact of various consumer protections that support their diverse views. In turn, they link the cost increases to employment levels and the number of uninsured.

The purpose of this discussion is to compare the cost estimates of four analyses that address aspects of the Consumer Bill of Rights, PARCA, and the Patients' Bill of Rights Act, and to comment on a fifth report that looks at the impact of cost increases. Our primary purpose is not to vindicate our analyses but rather to demonstrate how varying assumptions can produce widely differing cost estimates. In an era where cost estimating has a profound effect on the policy process, a look inside what may be called the cost estimators' black box could be revealing and helpful to policymakers attempting to determine the true costs of consumer protection. The specific analyses included in our investigation are outlined in Table 19.1. They yielded radically different results.

The Lewin Group and Coopers & Lybrand analyses are fairly close in their estimates of individual protections. Coopers & Lybrand used The Lewin Group analysis as a starting point, and the differences in assumptions are clearly articulated. But the Milliman & Robertson and Coopers & Lybrand analyses of the same protections can vary by as much as a factor of ten. The overall "best" numbers reported for PARCA in these latter two reports vary by a factor of thirty. The Congressional Budget Office cost estimate of PBRA includes far more protections than the other analyses, yet it yields a cost impact lower than the Milliman & Robertson analysis.

Sources of Variation

The reasons why these analyses yield such different results can be grouped into six categories: choice of consumer protections included in the analyses; entities included in the analysis of impact; interpretation of the language used in PARCA, CBRR, and PBRA; assumptions about the extent to which a certain provision is (or will soon be) common practice; time frame for implementation; and data sources and included costs. Each subject is discussed in the following paragraphs.

Consumer Protections Included

As noted in Table 19.1, the analyses focus on radically different sets of protections. The Lewin Group examines only two aspects of the CBRR: information disclosure and external appeals. Coopers & Lybrand's analysis looks at a broader range of protections and differentiates between how the same protection is described in the CBRR and PARCA. Milliman & Robertson consider only selected PARCA protections but also look at the indirect effects of the protections

Table 19.1. Cost Analyses of the CBRR and PARCA.

Organization That Conducted the Analysis	Organization That Funded the Analysis	Consumer Protections Analyzed
The Lewin Group	The President's Advisory Commission on Consumer Protection and Quality in the Health Care Industry	• Information disclosure • External appeals
Coopers & Lybrand	The Henry J. Kaiser Family Foundation	• Information disclosure • Mandatory point of service • Access to emergency care • Direct access to specialists • External appeals • Changes in plan liability for medical decisions • Impact of potential changes to ERISA
Milliman & Robertson	Self	• Access to emergency and urgent care • Direct access to specialists • No inducement to reduce services • Elimination of limits on certain benefits • Mandatory point of service • "Administrative requirements" (not clear which protections are included in this category)
The Congressional Budget Office	N/A	• Protections included in the Patients' Bill of Rights Act of 1998
Barents Group	The American Association of Health Plans	• Looks at the impact of premium increases on the rates of employment and uninsurance

as a whole. For example, they evaluate the impact of "adverse selection against rate increases" on the theory that PARCA will increase rates and "result in lapsation of healthy insureds and/or groups resulting in the need for an additional rate increase."[1] The Milliman & Robertson analysis also looks at the composite effect of PARCA on "administrative requirements" for HMOs, although it is unclear whether these include information disclosure. The Congressional Budget Office analysis addresses thirty protections included in the PBRA. Finally, the Barents Group study begins with a range of assumptions about what patient protections might do to premiums but does not analyze any of the provisions or provide a basis for the range of cost increases used. This study primarily looks at the impact that a range of premium increases would have on employment and on the numbers of uninsured.

Most of the variation between the Coopers & Lybrand and Milliman & Robertson studies can be explained by considering which provisions were analyzed. Although each analysis presents a composite effect, some of the biggest-ticket items in the Milliman & Robertson study are not costed at all in the Coopers & Lybrand analysis (see Table 19.2).

The Congressional Budget Office study looks at the most comprehensive array of protections but yields a total cost that is significantly less than even the lowest Milliman & Robertson estimate (see Table 19.3).

Entities Included

Each study differs as to which entities are included in the analysis of impact. Whereas the CBRR would be applied to all types of plans (HMOs, PPOs, and indemnity, for example), the Coopers & Lybrand analysis only estimates costs as they relate to HMO plans. The Lewin Group estimates the cost of the information disclosure requirements for all types of plans, as well as for hospitals and physicians. It does not, however, include other types of providers, such as mental health and long-term care facilities or nonphysician providers such as chiropractors or naturopaths. The Milliman & Robertson report includes premium increases for the "non-Medicaid, non-Medicare insured population."[2] It provides an average cost increase across all types of plans and then a range of

Table 19.2. Cost Estimates: Coopers & Lybrand, Milliman & Robertson, The Lewin Group.

Consumer Bill of Rights and Responsibilities

C&L[1,2]			M&R[3]			The Lewin Group[4]		
	Best	Low	High	Best	Low	High	Best	Low	High
Information disclosure	0.40%	0.37%	0.67%				0.40%	0.28%	0.53%
Prudent layperson Standard	0.11%	0.11%	0.29%						
Direct access to specialist	0.02%	0.02%	0.08%						
External appeals	0.08%	0.02%	0.13%				0.016%	0.001%	0.03%
Total	0.61%	0.52%	1.17%						

Patient Access to Responsible Care Act

	C&L[1,2]			M&R[3]			The Lewin Group[4]		
	Best	Low	High	Best	Low	High	Best	Low	High
Information disclosure	0.08%	0.06%	0.18%						
Prudent layperson Standard	0.11%	0.11%	0.29%	0.50%					
Direct access to specialist	0.02%	0.02%	0.04%	0.20%					
No inducement to reduce services				9.50%	2.00%	17.00%			
External appeals	0.08%	0.02%	0.13%						
Mandatory POS	0.48%	0.32%		0.30%	0.30%				
Equivalent benefits[5]			5.73%	5.50%	0.00%	11.00%			
Administration				2.00%	1.00%	3.00%			
Elimination of limits on certain benefits				5.50%	1.00%	10.00%			
Adverse selection				4.50%	4.50%				
Plan liability	0.25%								
Total	0.77%	0.53%	6.37%	23.00%	7.00%	39.00%			

[1] "Estimated Costs of Selected Consumer Protection Proposals: A Cost Analysis of the President's Advisory Commissions's Consumer Bill of Rights and Responsibilities and the Patient Access to Responsible Care Act (PARCA)," prepared for the Kaiser Family Foundation by Coopers & Lybrand, April 1998.

[2] "Impact of Potential Changes to ERISA," prepared for the Kaiser Family Foundation by Coopers & Lybrand, June 1998.

[3] "Actuarial Analysis of the Patient Access to Responsible Care Act (PARCA)," Milliman Robertson, November 7, 1997.

[4] Consumer Bill of Rights and Responsibilities Costs and Benefits: Information Disclosure and External Appeals," prepared by The Lewin Group for the President's Advisory Commission on Consumer Protection and Quality in the Health Care Industry, November 18, 1997.

[5] Potential adjustment to mandatory POS if plans are required to use the same copayments and deductibles for in and out of network use.

Table 19.3. Cost Estimates: Congressional
Budget Office. (In percent)

Provision	Percent Increase in Premiums
Section 101—Access to Emergency Care	0.2
Section 102—Offering of Choice of Coverage Options	0.1
Section 103—Choice of Providers	a
Section 104(a)—Obstetrical and Gynecological Care	0.1
Section 104(b)—Specialty Care	a
Section 105—Continuity of Care	0.2
Section 106—Coverage for Clinical Trials	0.4
Section 107—Access to Needed Prescription Drugs	b
Section 108—Adequacy of Provider Network	0.1
Section 109—Nondiscrimination in Delivery of Services	b
Section 111—Internal Quality Assurance Program	0.2
Section 112—Collection of Standardized Data	0.3
Section 113—Process for Selection of Providers	b
Section 114—Drug Utilization Program	b
Section 115—Standards for Utilization Review Activities	b
Section 116—Health Care Quality Advisory Board	0
Section 121—Patient Information	b
Section 122—Protection of Patient Confidentiality	b
Section 123—Health Insurance Ombudsmen	0
Section 131—Establishment of Grievance Process	0.3
Section 132—Internal Appeals of Adverse Determinations	c
Section 133—External Appeals of Adverse Determinations	c
Section 141—Prohibition of Interference	b
Section 142—Prohibition of Improper Incentive Arrangements	b
Section 143—Participation of Health Care Professionals	0.1

Note: Congressional Budget Office Cost Estimate, H.R. 3605/S. 1890, Patients' Bill of Rights Act of 1998, as modified by the sponsors, p. 3.

what different individuals might experience based on their plan type. The Congressional Budget Office study estimates premium increases for "all nonfederal employer-sponsored plans, including plans that would face no increase in costs."[3]

The choice of entities included affects both the cost number calculated and the percentage increase arrived at. In general, the impact of consumer protection legislation depends on the current practices of the insuring entities included in the analysis. For example, "direct access to specialist" will have no impact on indemnity plans because they already allow direct access. More restrictive plans could experience significant change. Analysts looking at this feature only as it relates to HMOs will see a much larger percent increase in premiums than if they average the impact across all types of plans.

Interpretation of the Language in PARCA, CBRR, and PBRA

CBRR, PARCA, and PBRA are open to interpretation. Without clear regulations that define, for example, "symptoms that would reasonably suggest to a prudent layperson an emergency medical condition" or "special health care needs and chronic conditions," it is hard to say that the interpretation of one group or another is unreasonable. For example, Coopers & Lybrand assumes that the direct access to specialist provision in PARCA would apply only in selected situations; the Milliman & Robertson analysis assumes the provision would ban "gatekeeper" systems altogether.

Another debatable aspect of PARCA is the degree to which a certain provision indirectly results in a mandated benefit. For example, the Milliman & Robertson study assumes that plans that do not cover emergency room visits at all would be forced to do so under PARCA. But Coopers & Lybrand assumes that only a certain portion of emergency room visits currently denied would not be covered. The PBRA stipulates that the provision related to emergency services applies only to plans that cover emergency services. The Congressional Budget Office analysis of the prudent layperson standard of PBRA is within the range estimated by the Coopers & Lybrand analysis of PARCA.

The Milliman & Robertson analysis assumes that section 2773(c) of PARCA (provider nondiscrimination) would require plans to cover services of professionals not routinely offered (chiropractic and acupuncture, for example) and to disallow limits on the number of visits to such providers. The other analyses do not provide cost estimates for this provision of PARCA.

It is not surprising that different interest groups often assume interpretations that support their case for or against the proposals. This strategy supports greater clarification of the legislation (presumably to the benefit of the interest group) before it is passed on to the regulators. For example, although some might consider it extreme to interpret the intent of the direct access to specialist provision as allowing unfettered access rather than removing unreasonable barriers, it is possible that regulators or the courts might do so, unless legislation is very carefully worded. Milliman & Robertson even note in their report that some of the most expensive (according to their analysis) features of PARCA "depend heavily on interpretation."[4]

Assumptions About Common Practice

Each study's assumptions about the extent to which provisions of the bill are (or will soon become) standards of practice have a strong impact on cost estimates. Both Coopers & Lybrand and The Lewin Group explicitly account for the existing information that plans and providers already supply based on state regulations, purchaser demands, or accreditation standards. The Congressional Budget Office does not. The Coopers & Lybrand analysis also assumes that other protocols are becoming common practice—such as standing orders for specialty referrals and a prudent layperson standard for approving emergency room visits. The Congressional Budget Office study takes into account existing state laws regarding access to ob/gyns, gag clauses, and some other provisions. Whereas the Congressional Budget Office, The Lewin Group, and Coopers & Lybrand analyses make some attempt to account only for costs beyond what is already in place, the Milliman & Robertson analysis does not explicitly do so.

Time Frame for Implementation

Cost estimates are influenced in two ways by the assumed implementation time frame. First, two of the studies make assumptions about where the baseline might be in the future, once federal regulations are finalized and implemented. The baseline of information initiatives is growing rapidly, and what is standard in regard to emergency room utilization, specialist access, and plan offerings is moving into closer conformance with the CBRR, PARCA, and PBRA. As of April 1998, external appeals legislation had been passed in twelve states and more plans are voluntarily offering it as a way to increase enrollee confidence. Eleven states currently require a point-of-service option and others may pass such legislation before any federal action occurs.

Second, phase-in implementation may give organizations the opportunity to develop cheaper means of complying with new regulations. For example, means of disseminating information will continue to become cheaper over time with wider access to the Internet, and a phase-in implementation period for information disclosure would give plans time to incorporate new information into their standard mailings and obviate the need for separate documents. The Lewin Group analysis explicitly builds in assumptions about the time frame for implementation and provides estimates for both a one-year and a three-to-five-year phase-in scenario. Coopers & Lybrand factors in projected market trends across its analyses. The Milliman & Robertson and Congressional Budget Office studies do not make an explicit assumption about the time frame.

Data Sources and Included Costs

Still other factors play into the wide variance between consumer protection cost estimates. Each group used its own databases and its own set of interviews. Assumptions often varied about what costs were included in the analysis. For example, The Lewin Group considers only the administrative costs of external appeals, whereas Coopers & Lybrand adds in the costs for the medical services that plans would be forced to cover upon losing an appeal. The Congressional Budget Office analysis estimates the cost to the federal government in lost taxes due to the substitution of nontaxable employer-paid premiums for taxable wages. As mentioned earlier, the Milliman & Robertson study includes estimates related to "adverse selection against rate increases" and "administrative requirements," which are indirect effects not considered in the other analyses.

The Congressional Budget Office analysis makes assumptions about behavioral changes as a result of patient protections. For example, it calculates the extent to which emergency room visits would increase under a prudent layperson standard (people who are now staying home would be more likely to go to the emergency room), more enrollees would go to nonnetwork hospitals, and hospitals would increase their prices for such care. It also assumes that the external appeals rate per enrollee would go up as a result of federal legislation, even in states that already mandate such appeals processes.

Toward More Precise Language

The studies discussed here present a wide range of estimates of the cost impact of legislated consumer protections. Most of the variation relates to the provisions included in the cost estimates and the interpretation of each provision, because the interpretation affects assumptions about how a particular provision would hamper a plan's ability to manage utilization. The Milliman & Robertson analysis assumes that some of the fundamental aspects of managed care would be prohibited under PARCA, including gatekeepers and capitation.[5] Coopers & Lybrand assumes a more conservative interpretation of the language.

It does not appear to be the intent of lawmakers to go back to pre–managed care days with health care costs again spiraling out of control. Instead, lawmakers seem to want to provide a reasonable set of safeguards to protect consumer interests and restore their growing lack of confidence in the health care system. The language of PARCA, CBRR, and PBRA at the time of these analyses, however, does not always make the legislative intent clear. One response of lawmakers to these cost estimates has been to clarify the language in subsequent drafts of legislation. As the language becomes more precise, we can expect that the cost estimates will begin to converge.

More broadly, the variances described in this chapter argue for legislators to be more critical of cost estimates, to study the underlying assumptions, to compare the assumptions to the actual intent, and then to clarify the language accordingly. As we have seen, it would be dangerous to accept any numbers at face value and use them as a basis for critical decision making.

Notes

1. Milliman & Robertson. "Actuarial Analysis of the Patient Access to Responsible Care Act (PARCA)." Seattle: Author, 1997.
2. Milliman & Robertson, p. 1.
3. Congressional Budget Office. *Cost Estimate: H.R. 3605/S. 1890, Patients' Bill of Rights Act of 1998*. Washington, D.C.: Author, 1998.
4. Milliman & Robertson, p. 1.
5. Milliman & Robertson interpret section 2771(d) of PARCA to "not allow risk sharing arrangements or capitation" (Milliman & Robertson, p. 7).

Index

Appeal rights: in AAHP code of conduct, 247; in Consumer Bill of Rights and Responsibilities, 233–234; under ERISA, 195, 196, 201n.10–11; external, proposed, 183–184, 196–197, 201n.12; for managed care beneficiaries, 181–182; regulation of, 245–246. *See also* Grievance procedures

Appropriateness, in quality of care, 148

Aronson, E., 77

Atkins, G. L., 198

Attachment point, in stop-loss insurance, 192, 200n.5

Audits, of health plans, 103–104

Authorization decisions: and appeal rights, 181–182; as medical decisions, 181–183; wrongful, legal recourse to, 269–272. *See also* Utilization review

Availability of health care services: insurance industry perspective on, 277–278; state regulations on, 43–45

Availability of ombudsman, 128–129

B

Balanced Budget Act, 279

Barents Group cost analysis, 175, 254, 276, 335

Bartlett, American Medical Security Inc. vs., 192

Bass, K., 198

Bast vs. Prudential Insurance, 167

Bator, F. M., 76

Baxley, S. R., 170, 187

Bearden, D. J., 170, 186

Benchmarking, in market-sensitive regulatory system, 260

Benefit packages. *See* Employee benefits

Benson, J. M., 205, 209

Benson, W., 87–88, 117, 124, 133

Berenson, R. A., 179, 187

Berger, M., *xxi*, 2, 53

Bernstein, G., 83

Berwick, D. M., 159

Biles, B., *xxiii*, 88, 135

Blando, P., 239

Blendon, R. J., 205, 209

Blue Cross of Southern California, Wilson vs., 171

Boyd vs. Einstein, 170

Breast reconstructive surgery, hospital length of stay after, 45, 47, 48

Brennan, T. A., 16, 159, 180, 181, 186, 187

Brodie, M., 205, 209

Buchmueller, T. C., 82

Burrage, Pacificare of Oklahoma, Inc. vs., 169

Business of insurance, state regulation of, 40–41, 164, 191, 193, 200–201n.9

Butler, P. A., *xxiii*, 2, 29, 35, 43, 49, 51, 164, 165, 173, 186, 190, 192, 193, 199

Buyers Health Care Action Group, 104

C

California: consumer choice in, 104, 314–315; consumer protection in, government role in, 319–324; experimental procedure requirements in, 44–45; grievance procedures in, 320–322; HMO disclosure standards in, 39; industry self-regulation in, 316–317; insurance contract requirements in, 322–323; market failures in, 317–319; market successes in, 313–315; purchasing cooperatives in, 325–326; quality assurance in, 46, 315, 323–324; regulatory struggle in, 312–329; subsidized health care in, 327

California Insurance Code, 319–320

California Managed Health Care Improvement Task Force, 305; on enabling comparative informa-

Price competition, and erosion of cost shifting, 287

Primary care physicians, access to care by, 136

Princeton Survey Research Associates, 210, 211–214, 225n.4

Princeton University, health plan information at, 105

Principles for Consumer Protection, 304

Private health care regulation: compared to government regulation, 98; examples of, 243–244; and standard setting, 307. *See also* Accreditation; Managed care

Private sector leadership: for access to care, 141–142; for quality improvement, 156, 235; for standard setting, 307

Product quality regulation, 62–66

Providers: and capitation, 83–84; contracting regulations for, 245; due process laws for, 44; network plans sponsored by, 48; shifting risk to, 10

Prudential Insurance, Bast vs., 167

Prudential Insurance Company, Texas Pharmacy Association vs., 200n.3

Public good(s): accountability as, 112–114; subsidizing, 327

Public opinion: on access to care, 217; on consumer choice, 219, 221–222; on cost savings beneficiaries, 219; and evidence for managed care backlash, 211–214; on factors influences health plan decision making, 219, 221–222; on managed care, contradictory findings in, 222–224; on own health plans, 214, 216–217, 218; and public policy decisions, 210, 224–225n.2; on quality of care, 213, 278; on regulation of airlines and banks, 228n.38; on regulation of managed care, 212; on role of government, 77–78, 212

Public opinion polls: error sources in, 225–226n.5; misinterpretation of, 303–304; nonresponse in, 211, 226n.6; research methods, 210–211

Public oversight, under market-oriented managed care system, 33–46

Public-private partnership, for quality improvement, 155–156, 260–262

Purchasers, large, tools of, 314

Purchasing, trends in, 20–21

Purchasing coalition strategy, advantages of, 17

Purchasing cooperatives, state facilitation of, 41, 325–326

Putting Patients First program, 142, 304

Q

Quality: assessment of, 153–154, 248; beliefs about, 99–100; concerns about, 10, 213–214, 229–230, 302; and cost, analysis of relationship between, 236–237; external review of, 46; information on (*See* Quality information); in market-sensitive regulatory system, 258; perceptions of, 64–65; product, regulation of, 62–66. *See also* President's Advisory Commission on Consumer Protection and Quality in the Health Care Industry; Quality assurance; Quality improvement; Quality of care

Quality Assessment and Improvement Model Act, 37

Quality assurance: in California, 46, 315, 323–324; regulation of, 45–46, 151–158, 244; traditional approaches to, 145

Quality improvement: in AAHP code of conduct, 248; AAHP vision for, 257–260; accreditation program for, 151–152, 157–158;